AF709803

RESPONSIBILITY IN HEALTH CARE

PHILOSOPHY AND MEDICINE

Editors:

H. TRISTRAM ENGELHARDT, JR.

Kennedy Institute of Ethics, Georgetown University, Washington, D.C., U.S.A.

STUART F. SPICKER

University of Connecticut Health Center, Farmington, Conn., U.S.A.

VOLUME 12

RESPONSIBILITY IN HEALTH CARE

Edited by

GEORGE J. AGICH

Southern Illinois University School of Medicine, Springfield, Illinois, U.S.A.

D. REIDEL PUBLISHING COMPANY

DORDRECHT : HOLLAND / BOSTON : U.S.A.
LONDON : ENGLAND

Library of Congress Cataloging in Publication Data

Main entry under title:

Responsibility in health care.

(Philosophy and medicine ; v. 12)

Outgrowth of the Eleventh Trans-disciplinary Symposium on Philosophy and Medicine held in Springfield, Ill., on March 16–18, 1981.

Includes bibliographical references and index.

1. Medical ethics–Congresses. 2. Responsibility–Congresses. 3. Medicine–Practice–Congresses. I. Agich, George J., 1947- . II. Trans-disciplinary Symposium on Philosophy and Medicine (11th : 1981 : Springfield, Ill.) III. Series. [DNLM : 1. Ethics, Medical. 2. Physician-patient relations. 3. Interprofessional relations. W1 PH609 v. 12 / W 50 R4346]

R724.R46 1982 174'.2 82-11305

ISBN 90-277-1417-7

Published by D. Reidel Publishing Company,
P.O. Box 17, 3300 AA Dordrecht, Holland.

Sold and distributed in the U.S.A. and Canada
by Kluwer Boston Inc.,
190 Old Derby Street, Hingham, MA 02043, U.S.A.

In all other countries, sold and distributed
by Kluwer Academic Publishers Group,
P.O. Box 322, 3300 AH Dordrecht, Holland.

D. Reidel Publishing Company is a member of the Kluwer Group.

All Rights Reserved
Copyright © 1982 by D. Reidel Publishing Company, Dordrecht, Holland
No part of the material protected by this copyright notice may be reproduced or utilized in any form or by any means, electronic or mechanical, including photocopying, recording or by any informational storage and retrieval system, without written permission from the copyright owner

Printed in The Netherlands

TABLE OF CONTENTS

SECTION IV / LEGAL AND POLITICAL RESPONSIBILITY IN HEALTH CARE MATTERS

ACKNOWLEDGMENTS

The Eleventh Trans-Disciplinary Symposium on Philosophy and Medicine held in Springfield, Illinois on March 16–18, 1981, formed the basis for the present volume. The symposium was the product of many workers, but none deserve greater recognition than Co-director William J. Conroy, M.D. It was a great pleasure to work with him in planning the symposium. He provided an eminently practical perspective which resulted in a superbly staged program.

The symposium was jointly sponsored by St. John's Hospital and Southern Illinois University School of Medicine and generously supported by Illinois Humanities Council Grant RG 5126-0000-0980. (The views expressed in the present volume do not necessarily represent the view of either the Illinois Humanities Council or the National Endowment for the Humanities.)

Particular individuals deserve recognition for their help. Kristina Valaitis of the Illinois Humanities Council provided early encouragement and helpful suggestions in the development of the grant application. Theodore Druhot, St. John's Hospital Executive Vice-President and John Holland, M.D., Chief of Staff, approved the initial financial support which made further progress possible. Patricia Stutler and Barbara Hopgood of the Department of Health Instruction at St. John's competently coordinated the actual meeting. Richard H. Moy, M.D., Dean and Provost of Southern Illinois University School of Medicine, and Glen W. Davidson, Ph.D., Chairman of the Department of Medical Humanities, extended administrative and financial support to the project.

Much appreciation is due Marilyn Flanigan, who saw the project develop largely on her typewriter. The many technical details involved in editing the series of symposium papers for publication were ably handled by Linda Keldermans, without whose assistance this volume would have been longer in coming and shorter in quality.

Finally, a special debt of gratitude must be expressed to H. Tristram Engelhardt, Jr., and Stuart F. Spicker, Editors of the *Philosophy and Medicine Series*, not only for their helpful suggestions and encouragement along the way, but for the trust which their early nomination of the symposium as part of the series of Trans-Disciplinary Symposia on Philosophy and Medicine represented.

November 23, 1981 GEORGE J. AGICH

George J. Agich (ed.), Responsibility in Health Care, vii.
Copyright © 1982 *by D. Reidel Publishing Company, Dordrecht, Holland.*

GEORGE J. AGICH

INTRODUCTION

Medicine is a complex social institution which includes biomedical research, clinical practice, and the administration and organization of health care delivery. As such, it is amenable to analysis from a number of disciplines and directions. The present volume is composed of revised papers on the theme of "Responsibility in Health Care" presented at the Eleventh Trans-Disciplinary Symposium on Philosophy and Medicine, which was held in Springfield, Illinois on March 16–18, 1981. The collective focus of these essays is the clinical practice of medicine and the themes and issues related to questions of responsibility in that setting.

Responsibility has three related dimensions which make it a suitable theme for an inquiry into clinical medicine: (a) an external dimension in legal and political analysis in which the State imposes penalties on individuals and groups and in which officials and governments are held accountable for policies; (b) an internal dimension in moral and ethical analysis in which individuals take into account the consequences of their actions and the criteria which bear upon their choices; and (c) a comprehensive dimension in social and cultural analysis in which values are ordered in the structure of a civilization ([8], p. 5). The title "Responsibility in Health Care" thus signifies a broad inquiry not only into the ethics of individual character and actions, but the moral foundations of the cultural, legal, political, and social context of health care generally.

An alternative title considered for the present volume (and the symposium from which it is drawn) was "Responsibility in the Health Care Team", because much of the inquiry in these essays is undertaken in terms of that complex, multi-level, multi-disciplinary, and interprofessional style of health care which so easily lends itself to description in terms of "teams". However, the impropriety of speaking of *the* health care team (owing to the great number of teams in health care whose composition and functions differ significantly – for example, operating room teams, dialysis teams and primary care teams)[1] and the need to question the status and functions of teams prompted a broader inquiry. In addition, the fact of collective action which appears common to all teams poses questions of the difference between collective and individual responsibility in health care, the responsibility

George J. Agich (ed.), Responsibility in Health Care, ix–xxiii.
Copyright © 1982 *by D. Reidel Publishing Company, Dordrecht, Holland.*

peculiar to formal organizations or bureaucracies which often institutionally support the existence of teams, and the nature of authority, expertise, and power in these complex organizations. These concerns indicated not only the need for a more general title, but helped locate the main inquiry in terms of the history of philosophy.

Although aspects of the problem of responsibility have been prominent in philosophical dicussions since Plato and Aristotle, their philosophical treatment under the concept of responsibility is more recent. Richard McKeon has documented the lineage of the concept of responsibility in political thought during the latter part of the eighteenth century ([8], pp. 6–8). These early treatments of responsibility had their origins in controversies in which the concept or term *responsibility* was not employed. They concerned questions of accountability for one's beliefs and actions and questions regarding the basis of the imputability of moral praise or blame.

Issues regarding accountability and imputation have been central concerns throughout the history of philosophy. On the one hand, human actions have been comprehensively classified as voluntary, involuntary, and nonvoluntary actions. The question of *imputation* involved the question of whether the causality of human actions is essentially the same as the causality of physical motion. As the understanding of causality changed historically, the sense of the question also changed. The problem of *accountability*, on the other hand, involved the interpretation of punishments, penalties, and indemnities imposed by a community to rectify or to prevent injuries arising from crime, misdemeanor, breech of contract, or negligence ([8], p. 11). This set of problems was seen classically as part of the larger problem of justice. Questions of accountability thus brought together political, social, and moral concerns. Whenever justice was the fundamental concept in terms of which accountability was addressed, politics and law naturally assumed importance. Whenever the concept of duty replaced that of justice, however, questions of accountability turned into questions of imputation.[2]

By the end of the seventeenth century the language of natural law and of duties provided a common vocabulary for discussing issues related to responsibility, but not a common philosophical orientation ([8], p. 14). Two alternatives were available for establishing the science of human nature and morality in these circumstances. One could base morality on the assumption that human actions are determined by a causality or necessity similar to that operating in natural science. In this case no special moral cause or imputation is needed. Moral good and evil can be defined by reference to reward and punishment or identified by praise and blame within human society. On the other hand, one could regard the causality of human actions as free – in other words, as distinguished from physical necessity and causation. In this case, law and duty can be based on what uniquely constitutes human action – on will and reason. Any external accountability imposed by power or determined by pragmatic utility or the State must be vindicated morally by reference to an internal law recognized by conscience and reason.

Among others, Hobbes, Locke, and Hume offered versions of the first theme. Common to this approach is the belief that liberty means only the power of acting or not acting according to specific determinations of the will ([7], pp. 315–16). These three philosophers accounted for human actions in terms of an understanding of causality which does not entail a distinction between necessity and imputation. They derived their normative distinctions from external devices of accountability: from the enforcement of civil and criminal law; from the penalties associated with the law of God, the law of political society and the law of fashion or private censure; or from the universal agreement among men discovered in the language of praise or blame ([8], p. 16).

Variations on the second theme focused on imputability. Most notable among these variations is the position of Kant, who based morality on free action. On his view, the possibility of a philosophical account of the practical depends upon being able to distinguish freedom from necessity, persons from things, and being able to provide a satisfactory account of the nature of reason and will – concerns addressed throughout the Kantian corpus. Kant's prime concern, therefore, was with imputation: "Imputation (*imputatio*) in its moral meaning is the judgment by which someone is regarded as the originator (*causa libera* [free cause]) of an action which is then called a 'deed' (*factum*) and stands under laws" ([5], p. 29).

Although the term *responsibility* was not employed in these discussions, its use historically emerged from them in the nineteenth century. The philosophical controversies underlying the introduction of the term *responsibility* into philosophical discourse were naturally translated into issues regarding the concept of responsibility. For example, John Stuart Mill interpreted responsibility in terms of the tradition of accountability – responsibility as punishment generalized beyond the expectation of actual punishment. As Mill expressed it:

> . . . it is well worth consideration, whether the practical expectation of being thus called to account, has not a great deal to do with the internal feeling of being accountable; a feeling assuredly, which is seldom found existing in any strength in the absence of that practical expectation. ([9], p. 289)

In the first philosophical work on responsibility, *L'Idée de Responsabilité*, Lucien Lévy-Bruhl interpreted responsibility in terms of the tradition of imputability. He regarded responsibility as basic to morality and ethical theory, yet argued that the idea had never been studied or analyzed philosophically ([6], p. 5).

These early treatments of the concept of responsibility are important for present purposes because both Mill and Lévy-Bruhl indicated a domain of practical problems which seemingly were unaffected by traditional philosophical differences ([8], p. 22). Mill suggested that the operation of responsibility as punishment uncovers, but does not create, the distinction between right and wrong; Lévy-Bruhl showed that responsibility as a subjective sense of freedom and rationality originated in society and developed with the evolution of society. This congruence has led McKeon to argue:

> If philosophers began with a fact of responsibility in its social context, they might explore and guide its extensions and applications without either deserting basic principles or negating the practical significance of principles by making the choice of principles the center of controversy. ([8], p. 22).

McKeon's recommendation is especially pertinent for medicine and medical ethics. Much attention has been devoted to issues and problems in medical ethics without a corresponding disciplined analysis of the context from which they arise [1].

Since health care is a complex social system with a unique history influenced by political as well as moral factors, the concept of responsibility can function as a regulative idea guiding and unifying otherwise seemingly diverse inquiries – inquiries into the nature of particular social roles, relationships, and institutions. Issues of accountability and imputability naturally come to the fore in these inquiries not as abstract theoretical problems, but as practical problems involving the nature of authority, expertise, and power and their relationship to questions of justice and duty in health care.

In light of these historical considerations, it should be noted that the focus of the essays in the present volume is the health care professional and the institutional and organizational structure of health care. This partially means that questions of responsibility for illness or disease and the relationship of disease and responsibility (for example, criminal liability and insanity) are not directly addressed, though such concerns are implicit in several essays.[3] Whenever an inquiry turns from considerations of justice to the nature of obligation in medicine, concerns about imputation naturally arise. In the present volume expression of these concerns is couched primarily in terms of the clinical practice of medicine viewed as a context in which ethical, political, and social norms and values interplay.

The first section is entitled "Health Care Teams and the Physician-Patient Relationship", and contains essays by historians Theodore M. Brown and Guenter B. Risse. These essays initiate the inquiry into the nature of responsibility in health care by critically examining two ideas vying for prominence in medicine: the health care team and the physician-patient relationship.

Brown's essay, "An Historical View of Health Care Teams", investigates the use of the language of teams and team work in health care during the twentieth century. Brown's main thesis is that much of the language of teams and team care has been employed rhetorically to secure or address change in health care, rather than neutrally to describe actual health care achievements.

In the earliest period which Brown considers (1910–1950), the concept of team work became part of the rhetoric of modernization marshalled against the general practitioner by proponents of scientific and technological medicine. Health care teams were supposed to replace the social component otherwise missing in technologically- and scientifically-based medical practice. Their inclusion in health care would guarantee that the general practitioner was superseded not only in technical competence and organizational efficiency, but in social awareness as well. During the same period, the efforts by nursing to elevate itself to professional status were manifested in advocacy of "group" as opposed to "private duty" nursing within hospitals, an arrangement often labelled "team" nursing. Such arrangements were advocated because they allowed greater solidarity among nurses and an increased sense of their role and mission within hospitals, the repositories of the new medical practice.

The language of the health care team was thus implicated in quests for power, dominance, and professional status by various groups of health care workers. This recognition raises questions regarding the proper definition of the duties and roles of various care-givers in medicine, of authority and its relationship with competence and power in medicine, and of the ethical justification of teams and team language as such – all of which are addressed in subsequent essays.

Risse's essay, "Once on Top, Now on Tap: American Physicians View Their Relationships with Patients, 1920–1970", complements Brown's focus on the development of the team concept in health care. Risse examines the nature of the physician-patient relationship during a period that at least implicitly recognized that the most pronounced shift in the traditional Western therapeutic dyad was "probably a departure from the dyad itself" ([12], p. 31). One consistent concern of physicians involved interpersonal communications with the intent of eliciting confidence and trust from the sick. Implicit in the paternalistic view adopted by most physicians were ideas of laissez-faire entrepreneurship and professional dominance which were never themselves subject to critical discussion.

The rise of group and specialty practice and the growing interest of physicians in objective, scientific data led to decreased personal relationships with patients. Increasingly, physicians blamed scientific and social developments or public attitudes for their ebbing personal contacts with patients. In response to this perception, and the development of compulsory health insurance schemes, and the rise of the patients' rights movement, physicians flirted with questions about the physician-patient relationship but failed to sustain any corollary inquiry regarding the institutional, political, or social context of that relationship. Instead, a new, more public relations-minded approach to patient care emerged in the fifties. Medicine increasingly became what critics had charged – a predominantly economic relationship. This charge was bolstered by physicians' use of business and managerial language and technique in dealing with the primary therapeutic relationship.

The changing ideas and realities of health care analyzed in the first section are reflected on philosophically in the second section, "Authority and Responsibility in the Practice of Medicine". The dramatically changed context of practice – often criticized as dehumanizing for both patients and health professionals – invites questions regarding the nature and relationship of authority, power, responsibility, and rights in medicine today.

In "The Concept of Responsibility in Medicine", George J. Agich argues that medical ethics has tended to focus on paradigmatic cases or problems understood in terms of an ideal physician-patient relationship. Reflecting on the shifting meanings and rhetoric described by Brown and Risse, he argues that philosophers must focus on the actual practice of medicine to uncover the complexity which comprises the proper subject of medical ethics. Responsibility is offered as a heuristically useful concept in that endeavor. Its complex character permits a rich rendering of the ethics of clinical medicine. Arguing for a normative employment of the concept of responsibility which looks toward the future fulfillment of duties and includes a broad understanding of moral offense, Agich stresses the particular duties and values that attach to role responsibility in medicine. Role responsibility on his view cannot be defined without reference to an institutional and social context within which the clinical role develops and operates. In this context of practice, issues of authority and power are confronted especially in terms of competing definitions of responsibility in terms of the performance of tasks.

In "Comments on 'The Concept of Responsibility in Medicine'", Arthur F. Kohrman supports and amplifies the analysis offered by Agich. He argues for the usefulness of the language of responsibility over the language of rights as a basis for reconstructing the role of medicine in society. Reflecting on the demise of the general practitioner and the rise of specialists with their supporting repertories and subsidiary personnel in hospitals, Kohrman questions the possibility of clear definitions of role responsibility in settings in which task responsibility and bureaucratic authority relationships predominate. In these institutional settings responsibilities become unwieldy and often contradictory not only for physicians but also for nurses, who labor under competing senses of responsibility to the hospital administration, patients, and physicians. Kohrman questions whether there is or can be a primary or common role responsibility in medicine and whether the physician-patient relationship can be at once personal and instrumental and managerial.

In "Authority and the Profession of Medicine", Stanley M. Hauerwas approaches the issue of authority as a question of legitimacy. The legitimacy of authority in medicine is often seen as deriving from the coercive nature of illness (which prompts patients to vest authority and power in medical practitioners) rather than from medicine being accorded a legitimate authority independent of its power over disease. Hauerwas argues that this view betrays a dominant political view in which authority is contrasted or opposed to rationality and autonomy (a view which Richard E. Flathman identifies and discusses as the *consensual* model).

Developing his argument on the basis of work by Yves Simon and Alasdair MacIntyre, Hauerwas argues that, when properly understood, authority is required in all human endeavors involving the exercise of judgment. Authority functions as the basis for consensus and involves a shared vision of the goods and values internal to the practice in question. Consensus – and hence, authority – is especially required in a practice in which many different kinds of skill and specialization are necessary to realize a common good. As a result, a conversation or communication between the various specialists and participants – what might be called a tradition – becomes essential. The prerequisite for such a tradition is a succession of authoritative voices. Any understanding of authority, then, requires recognizing that a tradition necessitates a high degree of moral consensus, trust in one's fellow practitioners, a shared vision of the goods internal to the practice, and agreement on the procedures necessary to achieve those goods or values.

For Hauerwas, the common good of medicine is what he terms "the authority of the body" – learning to live with finitude. Professional authority in medicine thus derives not from technical knowledge or skill, but from a shared participation in a practice that embodies particular beliefs and values regarding human finitude. On his view, medicine becomes a sectarian community through a sharing of beliefs and values relating to the fallibility of bodily existence. For these reasons, power and rights are viewed as extrinsic to the practice of medicine.

As with Hauerwas, the notion of a practice comprises the context of analysis of Richard E. Flathman's "Power, Authority, and Rights in the Practice of Medicine". As in his previous work in political philosophy, Flathman defines a practice in terms of two primary concepts: rules and beliefs or values that are not logically part of any set of rules [2]. He discusses two models of medicine on the basis of this vision of a practice. First, in a practice such as medicine, a substantial agreement or consensus regarding beliefs and values is required. Whenever a consensus exists, there appears to be no need for authority or power. This model Flathman terms the *consensual* model, which is consensual to an extent that excludes power and renders authority and rights superfluous if not anomalous. If a consensus regarding values and beliefs is absent, however, consideration of power and rights dominate. This model is termed the *constrained conflict* model.

Because authority is the more complex notion, its place on either model requires attending to certain basic distinctions between *in* authority (authority held in virtue of an office that invests its occupant with authority over some other persons), *an* authority (authority in virtue of knowledge or skill possessed), authorization (the granting of power to act on one's behalf), and the authoritative (that body of knowledge and skills acknowledged as normative by participants in the practice). These senses of authority are employed in an exploration of the connection of authority with the more adversarial concepts of power and rights in medicine.

Flathman trenchantly argues that the concepts of authority, power and rights are inextricably woven into the current practice of medicine, which is best seen in terms of the constrained conflict model. This model is apropos because authority, power, and rights are sustained in it on the basis of an agreement regarding basic objectives or purposes, values, or beliefs. This latter point aligns Flathman's view of medicine with Hauerwas's vision of medicine as a sectarian community which nonetheless excludes power and rights. This point of apparent agreement comprises the starting point for Robert M. Veatch's commentary, "Medical Authority and Professional Medical Authority: The Nature of Authority in Medicine for Decisions by Lay Persons and Professionals".

Veatch argues that both Flathman and Hauerwas fail in their attempts to salvage the concept of authority by not attending to two important distinctions: that between medical authority (the authority for decisions made in the interest of an individual's health care or pursuit of health) and professional authority (the narrower authority based on the historically- and socially-determined expertise of the profession of medicine) and the distinction between technical authority (authority on non-evaluative "facts") and value authority.

Veatch argues that physicians should be recognized for their technical authority as defined by their professional expertise in medicine. This authority, however, relates to non-evaluative facts – not the values and beliefs that we ought to live by. Veatch argues that these kinds of authority are confused by Hauerwas and Flathman, because both seem to assume that disease is best understood in terms of pneumonia or other infectious diseases. In the case of these diseases, there is little dispute regarding beliefs and values: patients simply want to know what drugs will be most effective against the pathogen. However, modern medical dilemmas such as cancer and heart disease are not open to a similar effective technical understanding. Hence, the fundamental questions that arise relate to beliefs and values rather than technical competence.

With only halfway effective interventions, questions of beliefs and values become central and more problematic. A different kind of authority than the authority to treat pneumonia is needed. The relevance of technical authority necessitates that we attend to the more difficult problem of values and beliefs. In such questions the health professional has no legitimate authority. Because the health professional is committed to the special values of preserving the health of the body, Veatch argues, it seems perverse to require that patients also see these professionals as value authorities.

In the third section, entitled "Ethics of Consultation and Interprofessional Relationships", the focus is on critical ethical and conceptual aspects of the social structure of health care. Mark Siegler explores the important but seldom addressed domain of consultation in "Medical Consultations in the Context of the Physician-Patient Relationship". Restricting his exploration to physician consultations, Siegler defines a consultation as a three-way relationship involving the primary physician, patient, and consultant. Much of his effort is descriptive, arguing that prescription must follow description in these matters. He classifies the prominent factors determining the nature and scope of consultations (for example, the decision as to who will select the consultant, the type of specialist consulting, the severity of the illness, and the setting of the consultation) and various reasons or goals for consultations. In the face of these different factors, Siegler argues that the primary responsibility of the consultant is neither to the patient nor the primary physician, but rather to the original physician-patient relationship itself.

Much of Siegler's argument hinges on a view of the physician-patient relationship as "the moral center of medicine". He argues against two alternative positions in which the consultant's primary obligations would center on either the primary physician or the patient. In so arguing, it is clear that his viewpoint is partly empirical, based on the observation that the quality of the care actually provided to patients who enjoy strong primary relationships with physicians is better than those who do not.

The question of the nature and scope of medical consultation and questions concerning the ethics of health care generally have a way of abstracting from the concrete moral agents involved. Especially in hierarchically organized institutions and in team relationships in which power is shared unequally, individual health care workers often experience what they term "ethical crises". In her essay entitled "Integrity in Interprofessional Relationships", Christine Mitchell discusses the moral consequences of neglecting such experiences. Although Mitchell's analysis focuses on the nurse, her observations regarding integrity are intended to apply to others involved in health care.

Mitchell's view of integrity is broad and includes five different senses: truthfulness, fairness, pureness, fittingness, and wholeness. She illustrates how these senses of integrity are compromised in health care situations by discussing two cases in which a nurse is asked and expected to follow different orders regarding the care of two young patients with severe spinal cord injuries. Arguing that each sense of integrity is compromised when the nurse is asked to respond differently to similar patients at the same time, Mitchell synoptically suggests that the question of the individual nurse's integrity involves the broader issue of the integrity of the health care system generally. She sees this problem as arising from a basic tension in health care – between a *mission* model (in which individuals are expected to follow orders to realize a set of goals) and a *sensitivity* model (in which the nurse is expected to identify and respond to multiple and unique needs of patients). These models, she argues, cannot be stably combined in a single personality. Yet in the present health care system, the nurse has a pivotal role in the implementation of each. Hence, the crisis of integrity experienced by the individual nurses represents a systemic crisis for health care.

In "Consulting with Integrity: Some Reflections on Team Health Care and

Professional Responsibility", William B. Bondeson comments on the essays of Siegler and Mitchell. Bondeson first questions Siegler's restriction of his treatment of consultation to physicians and the adequacy of the taxonomy provided. He wonders further about the implications of other consultative relationships in medicine, such as social work or ethics consultations. Bondeson's main criticism is that Siegler does not provide any ethical criteria for deciding when a consultation is appropriate and for judging the actions of consultants in situations of conflict with the primary physician. In fact, he points out that it might be a mistake to locate the ethical conflict between the consultant and the parties in a primary physician-patient relationship because there are overriding obligations to the patient initially and only to the primary physician-patient relationship secondarily (if at all).

In responding to Mitchell's paper, Bondeson points out that her argument can be read in at least two different ways. Her analysis expresses an experience common to nurses and other allied health care workers and also describes the experience in terms of the concept of integrity. Insofar as the expression of the experience can be separated from its description, there is room to disagree with her analysis of the problem in terms of integrity while acknowledging the experiential appeal. Mitchell's analysis could also be interpreted as an account of how the concept of integrity, when properly analyzed, can be employed normatively in health care. Bondeson acknowledges the experiential expression implicit in the descriptive reading of her paper, but wonders about the adequacy of her analysis in terms of the component parts of integrity. In particular, he is concerned about the transition from situations in which an individual's integrity is compromised to institutional considerations. He argues for a more explicit focus on the distinction between different conceptions of responsibility – for example, task, social, and personal – which might be helpful in sorting out the various issues Mitchell synthetically identifies as crises of integrity.

In "Logical Confusions and Moral Dilemmas in Health Care Teams and Team Talk", Edmund L. Erde offers a philosophical analysis of the concept of *team* in medicine. He examines the ethics, ethos, ideology, and rhetoric of teams in health care. Erde regards the language of teams or "team talk" as ethical if it serves genuine moral aims and serves to bind individuals in projects worth pursuing or provide individuals with a sense of belonging to a communal effort. Team talk is unethical for workers if it coerces, misleads, or gives a distorted sense of goals and purposes. Erde views the talk of teams in health care with considerable suspicion because of its propensity to distort legitimate individual and group activities. A central point in his analysis is the way team talk imports democratic rhetoric which often conceals coercive or manipulative maneuvers. In carrying out his analysis, Erde draws on the use of team language in business, the military, and sports to indicate how the employment of such talk in medicine can be coercive or manipulative.

In her commentary, "Responsibility and Health Care Teams: A Health Professional's Perspective", Ruth B. Purtilo is concerned especially with the way that Erde's notions of *teamwork* (activity based on the insightful and shared understanding of the interrelationships of team members) and *team work* (the actual work of the team – patient care) become insidiously confused. In particular, the employment of egalitarian ideals in health care often serves to direct attention and effort away from patient care to improving collegial relationships. This is particularly pernicious when the group in question is not actually constituted as a team having specifically defined goals or purposes or a clearly delineated authority structure, but rather is a loose association of individuals. In these situations team talk can be especially problematic. Patient care decisions can be made anonymously by individuals covered for and protected by appeals to "team" spirit. On her view, other health care workers besides physicians are usually guilty of employing the rhetoric of equality and looking to interpersonal difficulties among caregivers rather than attending explicitly to the question of quality patient care.

The final set of essays deals with "Legal and Political Responsibility in Health Care Matters". In "Legal Responsibility in Health Care: Whose Fault is it Anyway?", Peter C. Williams reflects on the paradoxical difference between legal and moral responsibility. The requirements of morality are sometimes more and sometimes less severe than those of the law. He discusses examples in which the law allows morally culpable individuals to escape punishment for reasons of efficiency in the administration of justice, in terms of a defense such as contributory negligence (where the injured person is barred from collecting damages even from a blatant wrongdoer if the victim was even slightly negligent), or on the basis of the standard of customary practice. Williams also indicates that the law holds individuals accountable even when they are morally blameless, as in cases of liability without fault (for example, vicarious liability and strict liability).

Williams focuses his inquiry on the treatment of what he calls "medical maloccurrences". He argues that the negligence standard or finding of fault so prominent in medical malpractice cases does not adequately serve the four oftentimes competing ends of the liability system – prevention, compensation, retribution, and administrative efficiency. In particular, its ability to compensate victims is restricted. Williams instead proposes an insurance system designed both to compensate medical maloccurrences and to avoid the costs associated with determining that someone was at fault.

The question of legal responsibility is also addressed by Robert F. Rich in "Reaching Closure on Health-Related Controversies". Rich has two related concerns: the nature of closure or final agreement in public controversies regarding science and medicine and the responsibility of physicians, scientists, and public officials in deciding these matters. Rich discusses the debate among political scientists between the technical and political responsibility for public policy. On one view, public officials must involve technical experts in deciding on and in implementing policies which involve technical and scientific components. Scientists engaging in such interactions with government must restrict themselves to technical matters. Another view holds that public officials are responsible for making decisions which protect the public interest. The political system itself provides checks and balances necessary for this decision-making to occur.

Rich argues that in health-related controversies neither of these two pure views of responsibility apply. His main example is the controversy regarding the generic substitution of prescription drugs. Many states have laws which enable generic substitution even though scientific and technical questions involving bio-availability, bio-equivalency, and therapeutic equivalency have not been adequately answered. The question of the proper closure of controversies involving health-related issues is posed by Rich in terms of this example. He suggests that public policies which rely on tenuous or nonexistent scientific evidence do not adequately protect the public interest.

In "Responsibility and Public Policy in Health Care: Commentary on Essays by Williams and Rich", Bruce L. Miller reflects on the complex features of the concept of responsibility. He notes that public policy establishes new patterns of rights and obligations or affords mechanisms for seeking redress of existing rights. Identifying the question of closure as a complicated one, Miller demonstrates how questions of the status of rights and obligations and the responsibility of public officials are interrelated. In critically discussing Rich's essay, Miller argues that the issue of generic substitution is primarily an issue of rights and not of scientific facts, as Rich seems to contend. Miller focuses on the language of rights to dialectically advance political responsibility, whereas Rich implies that technical responsibility should be given primacy. Miller indicates that more argumentation is required to establish how scientific evidence should have implications for public policy on health-related matters than is provided by Rich's analysis.

While he sympathetically supports Williams's preference for a system of strict or no-fault liability over the current system of fault liability for medical maloccurrences, Miller takes issue with some of Williams's arguments. In particular, he argues that Williams eliminates the first two elements of fault liability: reparation or restoration of the injured party to the *status quo ante* (an issue of justice) and cost efficiency considerations. For the most part, compensatory justice and cost efficiency considerations are compatible only when the overriding concern is compensating victims in the least costly way. Miller focuses his analysis on questions of retributive and compensatory justice regarding strict liability. He argues that there are two reasons why it will be difficult to drop the fault component from medical liability law. First, the concept of medical maloccurrence itself contains an element of fault and second, fault and causal factors are interdependent in such a way that their separation in a strict liability system will not be an easy task.

The questions explored in this volume – such as the nature and justification of health care teams, the scope of relationships in health care, and the nature of responsibility and authority in medicine – contribute to an understanding of the ethical basis of health care. This understanding is anchored in an appreciation of medicine as a social practice which is institutionally structured and historically shaped. Taking as their point of origination the concrete practice of medicine, these essays contribute not only to an appreciation of the interdisciplinary relevance of medicine and philosophy, but to a well-articulated philosophical understanding of some of the main problems in health care.

GEORGE J. AGICH

NOTES

[1] Edmund D. Pellegrino and David C. Thomasma make this point in their discussion of teams in health care in a chapter entitled "Social Ethics of Institutions" ([10], p. 256). For an important sociological treatment of teams and their relationship to individual action or performance in the everyday world, see ([3], pp. 77–105).

[2] In this regard, one should consider H. L. A. Hart's notion of the ascription of responsibility. See [4].

[3] For an historical account of the general problem of responsibility in medicine, see [11].

BIBLIOGRAPHY

1. Churchill, L.: 1980, 'Bioethical Reductionism and Our Sense of the Human', *Man and Medicine* 5, 229–242.

2. Flathman, R. E.: 1976, *The Practice of Rights*, Cambridge University Press, New York.
3. Goffman, E.: 1959, *The Presentation of Self in Everyday Life*, Anchor Books, Garden City, New York.
4. Hart, H. L. A.: 1948, 'The Ascription of Responsibility and Rights', *Proceedings of the Aristotelian Society* **49**, 171–194.
5. Kant, I.: 1965, *The Metaphysical Elements of Justice*, John Ladd (tr.), The Bobbs-Merrill Company, Inc., Indianapolis/New York.
6. Lévy-Bruhl, L.: 1884, *L'Idée de Responsabilité*, Hachette, Paris.
7. Locke, J.: 1959, *An Essay Concerning Human Understanding*, Vol. I, Dover Publications, Inc., New York.
8. McKeon, R.: 1957, 'The Development and the Significance of the Concept of Responsibility', in *Revue Internationale de Philosophie* **39**, 3–32.
9. Mill, J. S.: 1884, *An Examination of Sir William Hamilton's Philosophy*, Vol. II, H. Holt and Company, New York.
10. Pellegrino, E. D. and Thomasma, D. C.: 1981, *A Philosophical Basis of Medical Practice*, Oxford University Press, New York and Oxford.
11. Temkin, O.: 1949, 'Medicine and the Problem of Moral Responsibility', *Bulletin of the History of Medicine* **23**, 1–20.
12. Wilson, R. N.: 1970, *The Sociology of Health: An Introduction*, Random House, New York.

SECTION I

HEALTH CARE TEAMS AND THE PHYSICIAN-PATIENT RELATIONSHIP

THEODORE M. BROWN

AN HISTORICAL VIEW OF HEALTH CARE TEAMS*

It should be apparent to anyone who thinks about the issue even for a moment that health care today is no simple matter involving single clinicians and individual patients. Care is provided more often by multiple personnel in complex institutions utilizing several layers of support, consultation, and referral. Yet bioethical discourse still seems focused largely on increasingly fictive one-on-one ideal cases and the somewhat stale concern for individual patient and provider "rights". If bioethical discussion is to remain vital, it must shift its focus away from individual relationships to complex, interactive contemporary realities and the incompletely explored philosophical problems of "authority" and "responsibility" closely related to them. That shift in focus is one major goal of this volume, and for this reason directing attention to the issue of *teams* and *teamwork* in modern medicine becomes important. Teams, or more accurately, the talk of *teams*, has been dominant in health care for at least thirty years. This phenomenon merits both careful historical exploration and serious philosophical attention.

This essay will provide a background and a context for later ethical discussion from an historian's perspective, and will concentrate on the question of why the language of teamwork has been so extensive in recent years.[1] What purpose has the invocation of teams been supposed to serve, and why did their at least ideological popularity begin to crest about three decades ago? Moreover, despite undiminished general enthusiasm for teams these days, why does there seem to be a growing acknowledgement that team language may have become overblown and overextended? As one recent example of current caution, Walter Spitzer and Rosemary Roberts have posed several hard questions about teams in health services ([42], pp. 3–4):

> Does team care provide intrinsically better health service than the sum of the output of its members working separately?
> Is a team the means to an end or the end itself?
> Do patients really prefer health teams?

Since Spitzer and Roberts are not alone in asking these questions it becomes important from an historian's viewpoint to examine what appears to be a dawning awareness that a gap may exist between the rhetoric and the reality

George J. Agich (ed.), Responsibility in Health Care, 3–21.
Copyright © 1982 *by D. Reidel Publishing Company, Dordrecht, Holland.*

of teams ([2], [23], [47]) Why has that awareness emerged in the seventies and early eighties, after the high peak of largely unconditional enthusiasm of the fifties and sixties? This complex question merits an historical answer.

The overriding purpose in this essay, then, will be to raise and answer historical questions about the idea and vocabulary of health care teams. Since teams have meant so many different things at various times to a range of people, historical inquiry could degenerate into hopeless confusion unless precise definitions and clear limitations were specified first. For this reason it seems appropriate to delineate four general categories of team language often encountered in twentieth-century American health care literature: [2]

(1) Team language to describe groups of highly technically competent specialists, sub-specialists, and supporting personnel who join together to execute some dramatic, intense, and usually short-term activity. Examples would be the Mayo Clinic diagnostic "team", the neurosurgery "team", or the ICU "team". (Lewellys Barker's early discussion is an example of this type [3].)

(2) Team language to describe the cooperation of technically-oriented providers (i.e., scientifically specialized physicians) with socially – and/or behaviorally – oriented providers such as social workers. (Numerous examples of this type will be provided in the text.)

(3) Team language used by allied professional groups such as nurses in an attempt to achieve less hierarchic and more egalitarian modes of organization and decision-making in health care settings. (Examples of this type will also be provided in the text.)

(4) Team language introduced manipulatively by physicians or hospital administrators to gain managerial control over allied professionals. Both implicit and explicit in this usage is the notion of the physician as "team leader". (C. E. Lewis's "The Physician as a Care Team Leader" is a classic example of this type [30].)

These four types of team language represent ideal cases among the profuse varieties which can be found in the literature. They neither exhaust all possible categories nor should be taken to suggest that in actual usage team language is precise and specific. Authors often slip from one type of team language to another, and in conversations using the team vocabulary interlocutors sometimes talk past one another (for example, when one person means *team* in sense 3 and the other person simultaneously means *team* in sense 4). It may take the discussants quite some time to realize that a multilevel transaction actually took place during team talk and that neither party fully understood or agreed with the other.

This essay will concentrate exclusively on usages 2 and 3 and will leave the other types and transactional problems aside. This decision has been made for reasons of convenience so as to permit a plausible – even if preliminary and deliberately limited – historical account of the place of teams in twentieth-century American medicine. If the historical account constructed here seems persuasive, then the essay will have provided some justification for pursuing similar directions in greater depth in the more systematic historical investigation of health care teams. Hopefully, this account will have the added benefit of justifying the inclusion of historical perspectives in serious cross-disciplinary discussions of problems in the health care system.

I. TEAMS IN THE RECENT HISTORY OF HEALTH CARE

It seems appropriate to begin with a rough periodization, a periodization that for all its crudeness gives some coherence to the twentieth-century history of health care team talk. The first period covers the years from about 1910 to the Second World War. In this period (which could be termed one of "fitful growth"), conceptions 2 and 3 grew somewhat uncertainly from two different directions. There was initially the recognition by organizational authorities and leading medical spokesmen that conscious efforts should be made to compensate for the increasingly weak social considerations given in medical care as it became more heavily technological and fragmented into narrow specialty subdivisions and more institutionally-centered. There also came the realization by ambitious allied personnel – nurses particularly – that teamwork was a useful alternative to the traditional, physician-dominated, hierarchic organization of health care services.

The second period (which could be termed "high tide") covers the years from the Second World War until the early seventies. In these years, enthusiasm for teams rapidly increased. Most of this accelerated growth was associated first with the dramatic expansion of hospitals and hospital-centered medicine in the post-war period through the fifties and later with efforts to distribute care more equitably in the sixties.

The third period (that of "re-evaluation") began in the seventies and continues today. In this phase it was recognized that more problems may exist in the functioning of teams than have previously been appreciated. A fruitful way of understanding this growing awareness may be to view the third period as the time in which the never-resolved tensions of the first period are re-emerging after the great sweeping wave of the second.

"*Fitful Growth*"

Concern with teams grew between 1910 and 1940 in the two areas already identified. Authorities involved with the new organizational requirements of modern science- and technology-based medicine of the Flexner era felt the appeal of a "replace the missing social component" team notion most eloquently advocated by Michael Davis and Andrew Warner [20]. They were elaborating an idea already introduced by Richard Cabot of the Massachusetts General Hospital, who in 1915 had written about the "teamwork of the doctor, educator, and social worker" while describing a modern hospital out-patient department [14]. Their elaboration of the social component variant of the team idea in the dispensary context allowed them to generalize somewhat more broadly than Cabot had previously.

Davis was director of the Boston Dispensary and a leading advocate of the "efficiency" idea in medicine, which connoted a number of related ideas [28]. First, science-based specialization was a new and welcome development, even though it signaled the demise of the general practitioner. Second, since the new specialists required expensive equipment, they would practice least expensively if they could share resources for diagnosis and treatment. Finally, care would be most rationally organized if it were provided by special facilities – hospitals and dispensaries – rather than by disaggregated and foolishly competitive individual practitioners. Within these special facilities, physicians would cooperate in scientifically-based teamwork. As facilities reached out to patients or sought to supply their social contexts to closeted specialists who would otherwise remain unaware of them, however, a new sort of teamwork had to be developed. This was the give-and-take "social" teamwork between medical social workers and dispensary physicians in which "no plan for a patient should be adopted unless it is based upon the medical opinion and the social facts jointly, as represented by the physician and the social worker together" ([20], pp. 108–109).

The system of scientific physician-medical social worker teamwork was to provide more efficient total care than could the disorganized efforts of solo general practitioners. The G.P. could not hope to equal the specialized physician in technological competence, social awareness, or organizational efficiency. The old-style horse-and-buggy family doctor by this account was a medical neanderthal, and "teamwork" of the social variety was part and parcel of an ideology of modernization marshalled against him. Even at this point teamwork was far from being a politically neutral concept.

Another major expression of the social teamwork notion in the first period occurred in 1932 in the Final Report of the Committee on the Costs of Medical Care (CCMC). The CCMC had been created in 1927 as the organized voice of prominent spokesmen for medicine, public health, and the social sciences [46]. Backed by several major foundations (Carnegie, Milbank, Russell Sage, Rockefeller, and others), the CCMC recommended experiments with prepayment and the "corporate" organization of scientific medicine into multi-specialty group practices closely linked with regionalized hospital centers. Each multi-specialty group, which bore a striking resemblance to Davis's dispensary (Davis was a prominent member of the CCMC), was to deliver both therapeutic and preventive medical services to a defined patient population. To accomplish this purpose most efficiently, groups were to be staffed by specialists, generalists (to assure "the continuing mutual responsibility between patient and physician"), and "subsidiary personnel".[3] These subsidiary personnel would probably have been assigned an even broader role if the CCMC did not try (unsuccessfully) to placate the general practitioners in the AMA with an expanded function for generalist physicians within the groups. In any case, the entire staff of the CCMC's projected groups was supposed to work cooperatively in an optimally efficient manner. Thus, social teamwork contributed by both generalist physicians and subsidiary personnel was woven into this whole-cloth alternative to what was presented as hopelessly out-of-date and prescientific solo practice.

A second area in which notions of teamwork developed during this initial period was that occupied by ambitious allied fields. In this case teamwork was invoked not so much as part of an ideology of modernization but as a device to level hierarchic distinctions and to make for more egalitarian interprofessional relations. Nursing was most significant in this area, but fields such as social work and clinical psychology also played important roles in encouraging talk about teamwork.

The connection between the notion of teamwork and the advance of nursing as a profession in the period prior to World War II is actually rather complex. One insistent reality was the effort by nursing to elevate itself from the status of "technic" to the status of "profession".[4] Nursing leaders knew that if nursing were to achieve this elevation, training had to become relatively independent of the service needs of hospitals. Likewise, training classes were increasingly located in academically respectable schools, and substantially based on the mastery of such disciplines as psychiatry, psychology, and sociology ([16], [37]). In this quest for autonomy and status, nursing leadership recognized the value of public health nurses as role models for the profession as a whole ([9], p. 134). In the same spirit, nursing leadership also pushed for "group" as opposed to "private duty" nursing within hospitals.

Originally because of staff shortages during World War I, patients who had been attended individually by privately-assigned nurses were instead grouped together and looked after cooperatively by a nursing staff [18]. This arrangement (which was quickly labelled "team" or "group" nursing) allowed greater solidarity among nurses and an increased sense of their role and importance in hospitals. In the twenties it was fairly common for nursing advocates to claim that "teamwork" between nurses, physicians, hospital administrators, and patients was essential to make group nursing work [22]. At the same time, the teamwork notion was extended from group nursing to the nurse's general role within the hospital. A series of articles and editorials in the *American Journal of Nursing* in the twenties and thirties both reiterated and elaborated this theme. A sample of the ideas expressed is evident in an article by Dorothy Rogers on "Teamwork Within the Hospital", published in 1932:

> ... it becomes a self-evident fact that the game depends upon no player considering himself the sole performer, or failing to recognize the ability of each member of the team to fill his post with skill and precision, to play the game for the glory of the game itself. What more worthy contest than that of hospital life! What more creditable, or skillful team members are to be found than among the professional personnel of these institutions! ([38], p. 659)

Appeal to the language and imagery of teamwork was intended to raise hospital nurses from their position of subservience.

The same attempted upward thrust via teamwork was also apparent in the twenties and thirties among the social workers, psychologists, and other allied personnel of the "mental hygiene" field. According to an account by John Burnham, psychiatrists during the late teens and twenties encouraged the addition of every imaginable sort of allied professional to the mental health "team" [13]. Whether psychologists, neuropathologists, or social workers, allied workers were welcomed because they might contribute some valuable insight into "the conditions, internal and external, which singly or in combination form the actual somatogenic and psychogenic causal factors" ([13], p. 98). In the thirties, though, presumably in response to economic pressures, psychiatrists increasingly criticized lay members of the team, especially those who had gone into practice on their own" ([13], p. 102). This change in attitude by psychiatrists is significant because it not only indicates the response of specialist physicians to competition in a period of hardship, but also shows indirectly the successful upward thrust certain allied mental health workers were able to make using the team as a steppingstone on their way to fee-for-service autonomy. Invocation of the team notion was perceived correctly by lesser-status psychiatric personnel as a means of liberating themselves from the hierarchic dominance of physicians.

It is obvious that the team notion smacked unmistakably of ideology during the first period in both areas of its development. To those like Michael Davis, who looked to teamwork between physicians and medical social workers to compensate for the progressively excised social side of scientifically modernizing medicine, the idea allowed the possibility of knocking additional nails into the coffin of the general practitioner, who otherwise still showed some vital signs. On the other hand, to nurses and the social workers of the mental hygiene movement, *teamwork* suggested improved status and at least relative liberation from the hierarchic dominance of physicians.

Clearly, *teamwork* meant different things to different people. Growth in the first period was fitful not only because it occurred irregularly and in spurts, but also because it was of a different nature in each area of germination. But these subtleties, tensions, and confusions were rarely noticed for close to three decades – during the second period.

"*High Tide*"

Beginning after the Second World War, the second period extended over a time when the conditions of medical care in this country changed drastically. First of all, the long-term rise of the specialist and decline of the general practitioner rapidly accelerated in this period. In 1940 general practitioners represented 76.5 percent of all physicians in active practice, but by 1949 their percentage had already slipped to 63.8; by 1960 G.P.'s would constitute only 42.7 percent of all physicians in active practice ([43], p. 181). Along with this marked rise of specialists came a phenomenal growth in hospital construction and enlargement of hospital staffs. Between 1940 and 1950 sixty-nine new hospitals were built in the United States and many greatly expanded their facilities. As the best indicator of this extraordinary growth, in those same ten years the number of available residency positions jumped from 4,882 to 18,669, a difference of close to 14,000 new positions ([19], p. 879). Since most of these positions were filled by young men training for specialty careers, America's medical care was quickly on the way to becoming more and more technological and hospital-centered, a development further encouraged by the growth of Blue Cross and commercial hospital insurance ([43], pp. 269–272). The general practitioner was now truly on his way to the grave, despite efforts to mobilize a backlash with the creation in 1947 of the Academy of General Practice and its new journal *GP* ([43], pp. 301–305).

In this post-war environment *teams* were discussed everywhere. They were discussed, for example, in connection with "comprehensive care", one of the great enthusiasms of the fifties and early sixties. As specialty and subspecialty training proliferated at the postgraduate level, comprehensive care experiments were increasingly organized – as if in compensation – at the undergraduate level. They were usually undertaken with substantial foundation support at major medical centers. Commonwealth, Rockefeller, and Kellogg were the leading sponsors; Colorado, Cornell, Harvard, North Carolina, and Temple were among the leading institutional sites. Comprehensive care was offered as a clinical alternative to undergraduate medical students (usually in their fourth year), and it spread with such infectious rapidity that by 1959 there were thirty-two programs in medical schools around the country ([36], p. 393). Although the programs varied, the basic comprehensive care design regularly included the following: reorganization of outpatient services (at least on a pilot basis) into interdisciplinary or "combined" clinics; emphasis on the patient as person rather than as a repository of disease manifestations; consideration of the increasingly dominant pattern of chronic and degenerative disease; and incorporation of psychiatry, preventive medicine, and occasionally, the social sciences.

A special variant of comprehensive care was tried in such innovations as "family care" programs, which were centered on the health needs of family units rather than of individual patients. Robert Haggerty directed a notable program at Harvard in the late fifties that included both medical students and pediatric house officers [24]. With financial support principally from the Commonwealth Fund, Haggerty, a pediatrician, obtained the cooperation of the departments of Medicine, Obstetrics, and Psychiatry and organized a full-time staff consisting of a pediatrician, public health nurse, and a medical social worker. Families were selected after careful screening, and a special clinic area for their integrated comprehensive care was developed.

Obviously, the institutional soil in comprehensive and family care programs within major medical centers was perfect for the growth of the social teamwork conception. All the fundamental conditions that had led Michael Davis to the idea in the teens were now being replicated in the fifties. As a result of these conditions, it would be no surprise to discover the language of teams and teamwork in the literature on comprehensive care. For example, in Haggerty's program at Harvard, basic care was provided by "*teams* consisting of pediatricians, public health nurses, medical social workers, medical students, house officers and various specialist-consultants" ([24], p. 534). Moreover, medical students had to attend conferences and special seminars on topics such as: "discussion of adult health supervision, family planning, the role of health team in medicine today, and community health resources" ([24], pp. 540–541).

The teamwork and comprehensive care notions served major medical centers well. They not only stressed the need to reintegrate specialty-fragmented medicine and to provide missing social components; they also served, ironically, to legitimize the very medical centers that were contributing significantly to those conditions. Since medical students would pass through comprehensive care programs on their way to residency training, medical centers could claim that they were encouraging a broad and socially sensitive view of medicine. Meanwhile, those very medical students or ones much like them would be raised in the same medical centers to the peak of specialty proficiency during postgraduate training. Teamwork, as it had been for Michael Davis, was once again an ideological prop to the advance of technology and science in modern medicine.

Teamwork took on a new flavor in the sixties, which was a turbulently different decade from the fifties. It was the decade in which America "discovered" poverty and racism, felt the full sting of maldistribution and inequity, was torn by the anti-War movement, and underwent an unmistakable revolution in cultural values. These social changes – in their individual expression and their cumulative intensity – had an important impact on medicine and on the place of the teamwork notion within it.

The greatest external impact on medicine came from aggressive new federal initiatives, which were themselves responses to the government's discovery of poverty and its massive associated problems. Federal initiatives took the form of the provision of services which had never been provided before, at least not on the scale and in the manner now attempted. John F. Kennedy's administration provided the watershed. As part of "The New Frontier", Kennedy fulfilled a campaign promise and quickly pushed a hospital insurance program for the aged. Even though this program did not succeed at first, the Kennedy administration continued and then widened its assault in 1963. Neighborhood mental health centers were inaugurated and the Health Professions Education Assistance Act was passed in that year. The former brought organized psychiatric services to the inner city; the latter represented the first direct federal involvement in physician education – after years of retreat in the face of AMA opposition. In 1965, during Lyndon Johnson's campaign for the "Great Society" program, the loan provision of the Manpower Act was amended with a forgiveness provision. Medical students could have up to 50 percent of their loans cancelled if they agreed to practice in a designated "shortage" area. Finally, Medicare was passed in the mid-sixties and was soon followed by Medicaid.

In the midst of these new federal initiatives, neighborhood health centers were established by the Department of Health, Education and Welfare and the newly created Office of Economic Opportunity.[5] The most important feature of neighborhood health centers was that they took the comprehensive care and teamwork ideas from the medical centers of the fifties and injected them into poor and underserved communities, both rural and urban, in the sixties. In that process the already high enthusiasm for teams and the role they were supposed to play in comprehensive medicine expanded further.

Teamwork notions grew primarily because they were linked to new occupational opportunities made possible by health centers. The OEO-funded health centers regularly employed outreach workers recruited from the local population ("neighborhood health workers") at least in part in an effort to absorb safely the political energies recently unleashed in undeserved communities.[6] William P. Brandon has recently summarized the role of these workers with his statement:

> They perform simple medical, social service, and preventive functions in the patients' homes and neighborhoods, insure continuity of care, and facilitate communication between the health center and the patients and communities served. It is primarily the neighborhood health workers who are supposed to mobilize consumers and organize the community ([7], pp. 82–83).

The new health workers joined the physicians and allied professionals already on the health center comprehensive care team. Because the sixties placed such a high premium on participatory decision-making, the health teams which now included neighborhood health workers were expected to function with a spirit of true egalitarianism. Physicians, it was hoped, would not retreat arrogantly into a narrow professionalism, and the "health care delivery team . . . [would] be as democratic as possible" ([7], p. 83).

These ideas clearly had a sixties twist in their broadened social relevance, activist impulse, and pervasive egalitarianism. Yet the fifties lineage of many of these ideas is also clear, as is their more remote ancestry in the social compensation theme of Michael Davis. Teamwork of this style was long supposed to provide the social components increasingly absent in scientific medicine, and teamwork still served that function in the ideology of the Neighborhood Health Center. Because of their target population and historic moment, neighborhood health centers shifted their social concerns into the streets. Nevertheless, non-physician members of the neighborhood health center team still supplied the social components missing from the competence of the technically specialized institutional physician.

As if to confirm this basic continuity, there even seems to have been a transitional model which more specifically connected comprehensive care of the fifties with the neighborhood health centers of the sixties. This was George Silver's Family Health Maintenance Demonstration Project in New York City, sponsored jointly by the Community Service Society, Columbia University College of Physicians and Surgeons, and Montefiore Hospital [40]. Started in 1951, the demonstration project provided total, comprehensive services to 150 families selected at random from the 8,000 families subscribing to the Health Insurance Plan of Greater New York who were members of the Montefiore Medical Group. Silver described the project in the following way:

> Preventive and therapeutic services are provided by a "health team" composed of a physician trained in internal medicine, a psychiatric social worker, and a public health nurse. For children under 13, the evaluation, medical care, and preventive responsibility are lodged in a trained pediatrician. The team operates by dividing responsibility, delineating individual roles, and accepting each other's professional competence. By holding to the democratic team structure, conflict is avoided, and the procedure rendered relatively frictionless. The doctor is responsible for the physical disease. The public health nurse is responsible for collecting information about housing, nutrition, health practices, school and occupational adjustment, and the recreational aspects of family life. The social worker concerns herself with interpersonal relationships and adjustments, the emotional problems of family living ([40], p. 33).

Silver's rationale for the demonstration project follows soon after his description of how the "health team" is supposed to function. Silver described the *team* as a "compound replacement of the family doctor" ([40], p. 34). He expanded this view further with the statement that "scientific advance is inevitably forcing specialization and institutionalizing medical care, and sociological changes which are hopelessly isolating the doctor from the community are making the general practitioner obsolete". He concluded with the observation that "efforts to restore the general practitioner to his preeminent position are doomed to failure" ([40], p. 37). With these comments Silver was foreclosing the possibility of either the primary care movement within Internal Medicine or the creation of a new Board of Family Practice, both of which occurred before the sixties were over.[7]

The term *team* as invoked by social workers and nurses during this second period fared hardly better. Part of the problem was that the language from the first period of "fitful growth" had carried over into the new period of "high tide". A small carryover would not have been troublesome, but in fact there was a great deal more of it. One example was in the publication of a joint committee report of the Association of American Medical Colleges and the American Association of Medical Social Workers. The language of teamwork was very much in evidence:

The management of a patient is no longer a one-man affair, especially in hospital practice. It is now a collaborative effort in which various professionals bring their knowledge and experience to bear on the solution of a medical problem. Doctors, nurses, dieticians, physical and occupational therapists, and medical social workers may all contribute to the care of a patient. It requires a special skill to organize and manage such a team ([26], pp. 13–14).

The changed reality of hospital care is no more evident in this passage than the status-elevating intention of the language used to describe it.

Nursing was also mobilized in 1948, but there were some peculiar twists in the road it traveled to professional elevation during the next two decades. The most notable of these had to do with the altered meaning of teamwork in nursing as a result of changes in hospital staffing patterns caused by World War II.[8] During the war domestic hospitals were affected by massive staff shortages. To keep functioning, hospitals hired large numbers of relatively untrained personnel to provide essential services. This "wide and often strangely assorted variety of personnel" included aides and auxiliaries of various kinds and large numbers of non-graduate, practical nurses ([10], pp. 59–60). When graduate nurses returned to the domestic hospitals after the war, they found an entirely new situation. Personnel hired during the war were either kept on or replaced by others of like kind as hospitals started to expand rapidly. How was the graduate nurse, proud of her recent educational improvements, to respond to these very different circumstances?

One important strategy nurses adopted was to assert the old teamwork notion but to alter its definition to mean graduate nurse leadership of auxiliary hospital personnel. Here is one striking post-war formulation:

. . . we turn to an experiment in total, integrated staffing of a teaching hospital that serves primarily as a diagnostic and surgical center for difficult referred cases. In this institution differentiation according to function has been carried far toward its logical conclusion. The women's wards, for example, utilize the services of ward maids, attendants, trained practical nurses, graduate nurses for specialized aspects of bedside care, sometimes student nurses, and ward secretaries. Each ward is administered by a head nurse who has had advanced preparation for, or considerable satisfactory experience in, ward management . . . . Throughout the hospital emphasis is placed on the role each has to play as a team in the care of patients. Deviation from that role is believed to endanger good nursing care and team relationships, and also the carefully figured budget ([10], pp. 67–68).

Teamwork in this new usage would clearly serve to consolidate graduate nurse leadership in the rapidly evolving post-war hospital and allow the continuation of nursing's quest for professional elevation.

During the fifties and sixties the new meaning of teamwork in nursing achieved considerable popularity. Enthusiastic reports and "how to" manuals appeared with some frequency ([25], [27]). Nursing leadership seemed to like the new language of teamwork, and in 1961 a state-of-the-art review in the *American Journal of Nursing* concluded: "The team method of giving nursing care to patients seems to us to have great advantages as a means of providing this care to patients in the world today and, in the future, so far as we can see" ([8], p. 87). Enthusiasm, the author reported, "has not been dimmed by twelve years of practice".

Nursing also continued its efforts to equalize its footing with physicians. The mid-sixties were notable, in fact, for a series of conferences "For Professional Nurses and Physicians" jointly sponsored by the American Nurses' Association and the American Medical Association. The general aim of these conferences was "to provide an opportunity for representative nurses and physicians to meet informally and away from the pressure of their usual responsibilities to search together for increased understanding and ways to undergird and enhance the quality of patient care" ([35], p. v.). Clearly, this was an effort by nursing to achieve a more egalitarian relationship with physicians. It is also notable, however, that team notions were *not* invoked by nurses in this interprofessional context as they had been before the Second World War.[9] Perhaps the teamwork idea had taken on a special post-war meaning for nursing, and the word would simply have confused matters at conferences between nurses and physicians in the mid-sixties. It is also possible, however, that there was disagreement and ambivalence in nursing about how aggressive it should be in its dealings with physicians. This is certainly suggested in a few public reports ([4], p. 132). In any case, beginning in the late sixties, whenever the more militant wing of the profession wanted to assert nursing's hoped-for increase in status, its representatives resorted to looser and occasionally older uses of the team vocabulary. Henry Silver, Loretta Ford, and Lewis Day, for example, spoke of the "true team relationship" that ought to obtain between physicians and pediatric nurse-practitioners in efforts to provide "increased health care to children in areas with inadequate services and in the offices of private practitioners".[10]

Likewise, Eleanor Brunetto and Peter Birk described the very broad role assumed by the "primary care nurse" working in a neighborhood health center as that of "the generalist in a structured health care team" [12]. Recently, professional leaders have again resorted to the language of "teamwork" in asserting the importance of nursing personnel in inpatient hospital care.[11] What precision of meaning was missing from these aggressive usages was adequately compensated by their vigor of expression.

It becomes apparent that however modified the idea became during the second period, teamwork notions were once again invoked by ambitious allied professionals as they had been in the first period. Social workers in medical-educational and hospital settings, nurses in transformed post-war hospitals, and most recently, assertive nurses in both ambulatory care and hospital settings have all used teamwork ideas in efforts to consolidate their position, enhance their prestige, or vie for power. There was some inconsistency and looseness in all this, which explains why the period appears confusing when scanned in retrospect.

"*Re-evaluation*"

It is easy to see why the last and most recent period, that of "re-evaluation", followed those of "fitful growth" and "high tide". Close scrutiny led rather quickly and naturally to questions about the reality behind the rhetoric of the fifties and sixties. Thus, David Banta and Renée Fox wondered whether "high motivation to work as a member of an interdisciplinary health team in a poverty setting is a necessary, but not a sufficient condition for such a collaborative endeavor" ([2], p. 697). The reality they found behind high-sounding rhetoric was the following:

> ... [teams] did not function as they had been envisioned. The participants were too diverse and too unfamiliar to each other for the teams to function ideally. The peer relationship sought never emerged. Indeed, it was scuttled from the beginning by the practice of assigning a social worker and her supervisor to the same group, and by having experienced, committed physicians and inexperienced, uninterested physicians working together. The nurses reacted to physicians in their traditionally deferential way. And the physicians followed their inclinations and took charge of teams ([2], p. 697).

Re-evaluation here was already far along.

Other voices have also been raised in this period of "re-evaluation". In addition to Spitzer and Roberts (quoted earlier), Barbara Given and Sandra Simmons, for example, concluded that "few interdisciplinary teams now practice in ... [an] ideal way" ([23], p. 166). Moreover, "such teams are hard to form and even more difficult to maintain". Similarly, Saad Z. Nagi noted that studies of teams, where they exist at all, concentrate on the dynamics of team relations rather than on the quality of the care delivered ([33], p. 83). Even Harold Wise, a strong advocate of team-delivered care, reported that at the Martin Luther King Neighborhood Health Center in the Bronx where he worked, "Physicians are more important than other team-members – we do not disagree with them; we wait for them to lead" ([47], p. 541). It has finally occurred to team members themselves that they need to re-examine team relationships in terms of the reality of health care.

II. IMPLICATIONS

What are the wider implications of the history presented here? The answer seems to be rather straightforward and mercifully brief. History has shown that *teamwork* and *team care* as examined in this essay have sometimes been ideologically or rhetorically employed. It can be surmised that teams really have not been tried for as long a time as the language of their use suggests. This inference could lead to the conclusion that interprofessional teams may never have been fully and consciously planned, tried, or studied. This implies, of course, that there is room for further exploration in which philosophy and several other disciplines can play a legitimate role.

The principal pitfall to be avoided is to assume that team care is necessarily a good thing. Since the idea has been used regularly to justify the ascent of the science-based specialist, can it be ascertained that teams definitely do not serve to "dump" functions with which physicians are no longer comfortable? Although the rhetoric might claim that teams compensate for an already missing social component of care, does not historical experience suggest that the opposite tendency could actually be the case – that the invocation of "teamwork" might by used to unburden the physician of onerous tasks? Similarly, while teamwork always evokes a sense of egalitarian cooperation, might it not be the case that in health care some professionals really do know more than others and therefore ought to be in charge of patient care? The ambition of an allied health professional for prestige, while perhaps appropriate in itself, may be irrelevant or, worse, antagonistic to optimal health care. Finally, what happens to patient-provider relationships during power struggles between members of the team? These questions are all suggestive, tentative, and open-ended. History is merely one place to begin to seek thoughtful answers.

University of Rochester

NOTES

* I am grateful to the following colleagues and friends who offered very helpful comments and criticisms on an earlier draft of this essay: William Brandon, Edmund Erde, Stephen Kunitz, Stuart Spicker, and Carolyn Stevens. The faults that remain are of course all my own responsibility. I am also very grateful to Kathleen Parrow, who was a marvelous assistant during the research and writing of this essay.

1 As indicators of and introductions to the vast literature, consider the work of Ducanis and Golin [21], Londey [31], and Tichy [45].

2 It is important to indicate that in my reading I have focused on those discussions which use an *explicit* vocabulary of team functioning and in which the social and institutional context of teamwork is apparent. Even with these restrictions, the four types of usage I have extracted do not, I am sure, by any means exhaust all the ideas about teams that have appeared in the literature, nor do I pretend that these four usages have been mutually exclusive. Historical (and contemporary) reality is often too rich, confusing, and inconsistent to conform to a neat typology. Nonetheless, basic patterns can be discerned with sufficient effort, and their outlines can be conveniently sharpened to make the task of description and analysis more manageable.

3 Among the subsidiary personnel specifically mentioned by the CCMC were visiting nurses who would go out from the group facilities to the patients' homes ([46], p. 114).

4 These were the terms used by physician Esther Loring Richards in an important article on the subject [37].

5 The Office of Economic Opportunity received its official mandate for "neighborhood health centers" in 1966 ([7], p. 81).

6 Stephen J. Kunitz makes this claim with regard to the American Indian community, and he generalizes as follows: ". . . one of the major efforts in the War on Poverty was the creation by OEO of new careers in human services as a means of dealing with both unemployment and community 'disorganization' among the urban and rural poor" ([29], p. 403).

7 See Brown [11]. Some family physicians have even shown themselves partial to the "team" notion, but it would be too large a digression to explore that complication here. Suffice to say that Silver in his remarks was only making explicit what had generally been implicit throughout the fifties and sixties. The concept of teamwork was regularly used, whether consciously or not, to assist the general practitioner into his grave. The sometimes heightened rhetoric about neighborhood health centers accomplished this as surely as did discussion of comprehensive care or Silver's carefully controlled prose.

8 "Accelerated" would probably be a more accurate verb than "caused" in this sentence. Changes in staffing patterns actually began on a small scale before the War ([15], [44]). For example, it was reported: "There is an increase in calls for non-professional workers for hospital service. In 1941 these twenty-four registries had 1,257 calls for hospital service; by 1943 these had risen to 2,089, an increase of 66 percent" ([15], p. 478).

9 However, Dr. Edmund Pellegrino, a leading medical spokesman, freely used the "team" language in his contributions in the period [34]. Also worthy of note is the article by Barbara Bates and M. Sue Kern [5].

10 ([41], p. 302). Also of interest in this regard are the articles by Milvoy Seacat and Louise Schlachter [39] and Ingeborg G. Mauksch and Martha E. Rogers [32].

[11] It is particularly interesting that Bergman's "Typology for Teamwork" ([6], pp. 1618–1620) appeared in the same issue of the *American Journal of Nursing* as Shirley Smoyak's "The Confrontation Process" (pp. 1632–1635). The editors' lead-in quotation in the latter article is the following: "Nurses have been socialized into subservience. A way to regain autonomy is through confrontation. The concept, the process, and the techniques of confrontation are presented." Also very indicative of nursing's current state of mind is the article by Diane Bakdash, "Becoming an Assertive Nurse" [1].

BIBLIOGRAPHY

1. Bakdash, D.: 1978, 'Becoming an Assertive Nurse', *American Journal of Nursing* 78, 1710–1712.
2. Banta, D. and Fox, R.: 1972, 'Role Strains of a Health Care Team in a Poverty Community', *Social Science and Medicine* **6**, 697–722.
3. Barker, L.: 1922, 'Team-Work in Medical Practice', *JAMA* 78, 773–779.
4. Bates, B.: 1970, 'Doctor and Nurse: Changing Roles and Relations', *New England Journal of Medicine* **283**, 129–134.
5. Bates, B. and Kern, M. S.: 1967, 'Doctor-Nurse Teamwork: What Helps? What Hinders?', *American Journal of Nursing* **67**, 2066–2071.
6. Bergman, R.: 1974, 'Typology for Teamwork', *American Journal of Nursing* **74**, 2066–2071.
7. Brandon, W.: 1977, 'Politics, Administration, and Conflict in Neighborhood Health Centers', *Journal of Health Politics, Policy and Law* **2**, 79–99.
8. Brooks, E.: 1961, 'Team Nursing-1961', *American Journal of Nursing* **61**, 87–91.
9. Brown, E.: 1940, *Nursing as a Profession*, 2nd ed., Russell Sage Foundation, New York.
10. Brown, E.: 1948, *Nursing for the Future: A Report Prepared for the National Nursing Council*, Russell Sage Foundation, New York.
11. Brown, T.: 1980, 'The Primary Care Movement in Recent American Medicine', in Stephen J. Kunitz (ed.), *A Study of Four Primary Care Training Programs at the University of Rochester School of Medicine*, An Appendix to the Final Report Submitted to the Robert Wood Johnson Foundation for the Period 1977–1980, Rochester, New York, pp. 1–82.
12. Brunetto, E. and Birk, P.: 1972, 'The Primary Care Nurse – The Generalist in a Structured Health Care Team', *American Journal of Public Health* **62**, 785–794.
13. Burnham, J.: 1974, 'The Struggle Between Physicians and Paramedical Personnel in American Psychiatry, 1917–1941', *Journal of the History of Medicine and Allied Sciences* **29**, 93–106.
14. Cabot, R.: 1915, *Social Service and the Art of Healing*, Moffat, Yard and Company, New York.
15. 'Calls for Nonprofessional Workers Increase', *American Journal of Nursing* **44** (1944), 478.
16. Committee for the Study of Nursing Education: 1923, *Nursing and Nursing Education in the United States*, The MacMillan Company, New York.

17. Committee on the Costs of Medical Care: 1932, *Medical Care for the American People: The Final Report of the Committee on the Costs of Medical Care*, University of Chicago Press, Chicago.
18. Cook, O.: 1922, 'Group Nursing', *American Journal of Nursing* **22**, 253–254.
19. Curran, J.: 1959, 'Internships and Residencies: Historical Backgrounds and Current Trends', *Journal of Medical Education* **34**, 873–884.
20. Davis, M. and Warner, A.: 1918, *Dispensaries: Their Management and Development*, The MacMillan Company, New York.
21. Ducanis, A. and Golin, A.: 1979, *The Interdisciplinary Health Team*, Aspen Systems, London.
22. Geister, T.: 1926, 'Hearsay and Fact in Private Duty', *American Journal of Nursing* **26**, 515–528.
23. Given, B. and Simmons, S.: 1977, 'The Interdisciplinary Health Team: Fact or Fiction?', *Nursing Forum* **16**, 165–184.
24. Haggerty, R.: 1962, 'Family Medicine: A Teaching Program for Medical Students and Pediatric House Officers', *Journal of Medical Education* **37**, 531–580.
25. 'How We Do Team Nursing', *Military Medicine* **116** (1955), 130–135.
26. Joint Committee on The Teaching of Social and Environmental Factors in Medicine: 1948, *Widening Horizons in Medical Education*, A Joint Committee Report of the Association of American Medical Colleges and the American Association of Medical Social Workers, The Commonwealth Fund, New York.
27. Kron, T.: 1961, *Nursing Leadership*, W. B. Saunders Company, Philadelphia.
28. Kunitz, S.: 1981, 'Efficiency and Reform in the Financing and Organization of American Medicine in the Progressive Era', *Bulletin of the History of Medicine* **55**, 497–515.
29. Kunitz, S.: 1977, 'Underdevelopment and Social Services on the Navajo Reservation', *Human Organization* **36**, 398–404.
30. Lewis, C.: 1968, 'The Physician as a Care Team Leader', *Group Practice* **17**, 20–24.
31. Londey, D.: 1978, 'On the Action of Teams', *Inquiry* **21**, 213–218.
32. Mauksch, J. G. and Rogers, M. E.: 1975, 'Nursing Is Coming of Age Through the Practitioner Movement, Pro and Con', *American Journal of Nursing* **75**, 1834–1843.
33. Nagi, S.: 1975, 'Teamwork in Health Care in the United States: A Sociological Perspective', *Milbank Memorial Fund Quarterly* **53**, 75–91.
34. Pellegrino, E.: 1964, 'Nursing and Medicine: Ethical Implications in Changing Practice', *American Journal of Nursing* **64**, 110–112.
35. *Proceedings of the First National Conference for Professional Nurses and Physicians* (Conference Sponsored Jointly by the American Nurses' Association and the American Medical Association), 1964, Williamsburg, Virginia.
36. Reader, G. and Soave, R.: 1976, 'Comprehensive Care Revisited', *Milbank Memorial Fund Quarterly* **37**, 391–414.
37. Richards, E.: 1936, 'Nursing – A Profession or a Technic?', *American Journal of Nursing* **35**, 1165–1173.
38. Rogers, D.: 1932, 'Teamwork Within the Hospital', *American Journal of Nursing* **32**, 657–659.
39. Seacat, M. and Schlachter, L.: 1968, 'Expanded Nursing Role in Prenatal and Infant Care', *American Journal of Nursing* **68**, 822–824.

40. Silver, G.: 1958, 'Beyond General Practice: The Health Team', *Yale Journal of Biology and Medicine* **31**, 29–38.
41. Silver, H., Ford, L., and Day, L.: 1968, 'The Pediatric Nurse-Practitioner Program', *JAMA* **204**, 298–302.
42. Spitzer, W. and Roberts, R.: 1980, 'Twelve Questions About Teams in Health Services', *Journal of Community Health* **6**, 1–5.
43. Stevens, R.: 1971, *American Medicine and the Public Interest*, Yale University Press, New Haven.
44. 'Subsidiary Workers in Nursing Agencies', *American Journal of Nursing* **39** (1939), 759–761.
45. Tichy, M.: 1974, *Health Care Teams: An Annotated Bibliography*, Praeger, New York.
46. Walker, F.: 1979, 'Americanism Versus Sovietism: A Study of the Reaction to the Committee on the Costs of Medical Care', *Bulletin of the History of Medicine* **53**, 489–504.
47. Wise, H., Rubin, I., and Beckard, R.: 1974, 'Making Health Teams Work', *American Journal of Diseases of Children* **127**, 537–542.

GUENTER B. RISSE

ONCE ON TOP, NOW ON TAP: AMERICAN PHYSICIANS VIEW THEIR RELATIONSHIPS WITH PATIENTS, 1920–1970

The most pronounced shift in the traditional Western therapeutic dyad is probably a departure from the dyad itself. Increasingly, the patient is involved not in an isolated two-person social system but in a medical team effort in which the physician is first among equals rather than unique leader ([86], p. 31).

Written in 1970 by sociologist Robert N. Wilson, the above statement on the decay of the physician-patient dyad highlights an almost totally neglected issue in contemporary medical literature on team health care: how can the various healing roles be restructured while still preserving individual relationships deemed essential for patient recovery? Phenomena such as medical malpractice, widespread self-care, discontent with the quality of professional care, and non-compliance with physicians' orders have been blamed on inadequate private rapport between practitioners and their patients ([50], p. 63). How important for healing really is the physician-patient relationship? What are the factors that influence it?[1] How can rhetoric be separated from reality? These questions are central to any understanding of the historical role of medicine and as such need to be examined in detail [30].

If history has a role to play in the ongoing debates about the physician-patient relationship, its value resides in the ability to provide perspectives and facilitate analysis. In spite of numerous pronouncements that the history of relations between healers and sick people is a central topic for research and study,[2] specialized literature on the subject remains elementary and inadequate. Physicians have often been accused in their reconstructions of unnecessarily sentimentalizing the personal relations between physician and patient, thereby contributing to what some perceive as a mystical haze pervading the subject. Indeed, as handmaiden of medical chauvinism or political bias, history often has been employed in the past to defend economic interests and the professional status quo ([56], pp. 62–63).

This brief contribution merely attempts to sketch physicians' published views about relationships with patients for about half a century. The analysis is largely limited to views expressed in the medical literature and designed to uncover leading professional views on the subject. To what an extent they were representative of the American medical profession as a whole remains to be investigated. The evidence shows that practitioners addressing the topic of

George J. Agich (ed.), Responsibility in Health Care, 23–49.
Copyright © 1982 *by D. Reidel Publishing Company, Dordrecht, Holland.*

the physician-patient relationship concentrated on issues related to interpersonal communications designed to elicit confidence and trust from the sick. There seems to have been no significant attention given to the influences arising from profound social and organizational shifts in American society and medicine.

Both external (macrosocial) and personal (microsocial) elements, however, are inextricably linked together, attesting to the complexity and dynamism of the physician-patient encounter. Indeed, past therapeutic interactions reveal a multiplicity of healing roles and relations shaped by socio-economic and cultural factors, epidemiology, medical knowledge, and availability of technology.[3] The only constant in all such relationships has been the universally unsettling phenomenon of illness, causing fear and loss of control in those affected, and therefore demanding reassurance and care to achieve social reintegration.

I. LOSING THE SYMPATHETIC TOUCH

> With regard to the much-talked-of beautiful relationship that exists between doctor and patient – isn't that much overrated and aren't we a bit sentimental about it? ([7], p. 62)

Prior to World War I, physicians expressed rather vague ideas about the nature of their personal involvement with patients.[4] Comments made by James H. Means, a prominent Harvard graduate and professor at M.I.T., aptly express the situation prevailing in the early decades of the twentieth century. "The most vivid thing I remember about the doctor-patient relationship in my early days", asserted Means, "is that I cannot remember having heard much of anything about it . . . . Whatever our doctor-patient relationships were, they were largely unconscious" ([58], p. 727).

Although mostly inarticulated, in the 1920s and 1930s[5] the relationship was seen by physicians as bringing together an independent professional and a usually self-referred sick person in need of help. The practitioner, working in relative isolation from colleagues and considered expert in all general problems of medicine, was expected to provide diagnoses and design effective therapy whenever available. Professional activities were self-regulated, based on codes of ethical behavior. The professional status cast physicians into a service-oriented role collecting fees from patients for their efforts. Their principal obligation was meant to place the welfare of their patients above their own personal interests ([65], p. 450). Constant availability implied long working hours and sacrifices regarding their personal lives and recreations.

Such tasks demanded an intimate association with patients based on mutual trust and obligation. The very fact that they were consulted voluntarily attested to the physicians' availability or reputation. In spite of licensing regulations, workmen's compensation laws, and third party payments from various voluntary insurance schemes, practitioners controlled most of their activities, their independence and authority bolstered by knowledge, skills, and experience. Physicians primarily were accountable to their patients and provided legitimacy to their complaints. As applied scientists, they were expected to display a necessary "affective neutrality" and treat medical problems as objectively as possible. Scientific detachment and accurate judgment precluded excessive intimacy with patients but still allowed for the sympathetic touch.

In this same period patients willingly adopted their hopefully brief sick status on the basis of the presenting disabilities. In turn, they were exempted from normal social responsibilities for the duration while acquiring a new obligation: speedily to seek help from physicians and accept the duties of patienthood. These were obedience and cooperation with doctor's orders, deference to professional judgment in all matters of diagnosis and treatment, including the choice of consultants. As patients themselves admitted, this model conditioned their own approach to the medical profession, creating an "almost instinctive attitude toward the doctor that is of respect and confidence" ([2], p. 710).

The reasons for such a total submission were based on the professional assumption that patients were not competent to help themselves. "The patient has a need for technical services because he doesn't – nor do his lay associates, family members, etc. – know what is the matter or what to do about it, nor does he control the necessary facilities", explained sociologist Talcott Parsons ([65], p. 439). In fact, physicians believed that laypersons had very limited knowledge of medical science, often considerably less than the public presumed to possess. With their rationality clouded by illness and the emotional adjustments demanded by the sick role, physicians thought that patients often exercised notoriously bad judgment.

An important factor derived from Freudian psychology and observed in every physician-patient relationship was transference, an unconscious phenomenon first seen in psychoanalysis whereby patients transferred to their healers attributes taken from parental roles experienced during their childhood. Some practitioners believed that transference could be exploited in somatic medicine for therapeutic purposes. "The physician should be quite willing to assume the role of the omnipotent father", wrote one of them in

1926, "and the patient feels toward the physician much as a little child, looking up to him as a source of great power and helpfulness" ([84], p. 6). Although most nonpsychiatric practitioners at this time repeatedly voiced disapproval of psychoanalytical theory and methodology as inappropriate in medical settings, they nevertheless seemed to subscribe to such a parental dependency model since it symbolically provided them with more leverage: "He (the patient) puts himself in the state of mind of his childhood, and looks to the doctor as a wise, all-seeing parent who will take him under a protecting wing – but who will also be stern with him when necessary" ([41], p. 332). In spite of occasional complaints that they were being manipulated by their patients, physicians felt that they were clearly in charge and on top, prompting sociologists to construct the so-called "paternalistic" model of physician-patient interaction.

However, such a physician-knows-best paradigm was based on traditional, intuitive conventions of "laissez faire" entrepreneurship and customary ideas about professionalism. In the 1920s and especially the 1930s, this model experienced strains as a number of intellectual, social, and institutional transformations in medicine influenced the physician-patient relationship. Some of the innovations and the dilemmas they caused for practitioners emerged as debates between the "science" and "art" of medicine, the latter seemingly eclipsed by the emerging scientific tradition.

Reforms in medical education fueled by the Flexner Report [28] and generous support from private philanthropy increasingly provided society in the 1920s with a new generation of scientifically competent physicians, many of them specialists. These practitioners were seen as being disease- rather than people-oriented, generously exposed to the complexities of pathology and biochemistry but ignorant of the bedside manners attributed to their "horse and buggy" predecessors. "We are losing the sympathetic human touch and this loss is deplorable and the direct consequence of an ever-increasing knowledge of cause", asserted one California practitioner in 1926, adding that "we seek cause with scientific heartlessness. A scientific man is truly a person without a soul".[6]

The charge was perhaps not without foundations. Physicians probably started spending less time with individual patients as they saw more of them and became engulfed in diagnostic laboratory work. They wanted to earn the confidence of the sick through a display of scientific knowledge and dazzling technological skills instead of quaint exchanges of "pleasantries".[7] "Competence is more important than personal relationships", wrote one author in the 1930s, concluding that "today when diagnosis is so much more objective than it was formerly, the personal relationship between physician and patient may be dispensed with entirely" ([81], p. 258).

For some practitioners, playing on the emotions of the sick was actually frowned upon as means usually employed only by sectarians and quacks. Physicians instead were urged to share their diagnostic uncertainties with patients while telling them the unvarnished truth about their condition. The lengthy debates in the medical literature demonstrate that this approach was by no means universal and that it seems to have been resisted by physicians and patients alike. Yet, a degree of impersonality was present especially in surgery and specialty practice: "To have expected any intimate interest on the part of these high-pressure men in my personal problem would have been simply silly", wrote one patient, "I paid my money and received the best attention they were able to provide" ([2], p. 711). Such a statement illustrated the public's somewhat reluctant willingness to forego personalized care for scientifically competent advice if such a choice had to be made.

Group and specialty practice, two increasingly popular forms of medicine, were further macrosocial factors affecting the physician-patient encounter. Critics attempting to preserve their status employed the vision of a steadily decaying relationship to fuel their opposition to the new order. "Specialism tends fundamentally to destroy those intimate relations between physician and patient that constitute the very essence of the healing art", declared one Louisiana practitioner in 1922. His reason for the alleged alienation was "a lack of understanding between the doctor and the patient; the psychological element of sympathy between the two is not likely to prevail" ([27], p. 692). Even the influential spokesman for American medicine, Llewellys Barker of the Johns Hopkins University Medical School, while clearly recognizing the economic and scientific advantages of medical specialization, feared that "the real human costs might actually be enhanced" through the dehumanization of both patients and their physicians ([5], p. 778).

Lack of personal contact between healers and patients was also blamed on the changing setting in which the encounter usually took place. "It is impossible to know people intimately or sympathetically except through some contact with the home", stated one practitioner ([53], p. 322). As it were, medical care was shifting increasingly to physicians' offices and hospitals, thus depriving medical students and practicing physicians of their patients' psychological and cultural contexts so necessary for the development of the much sought-after "human touch" ([40], p. 13).

Moreover, some physicians blamed the remarkable resiliency of sectarians, such as chiropractors and Christian Science healers, and quacks on the depersonalizing aspects of scientific medicine: "I cannot help but wonder whether the modern doctor's mania for admitting uncertainty and for telling the truth is not accomplishing the unexpected result of sending patients to the unscientific irregulars rather than persuading them to the wonders and values of modern medical science," mused Oliver H. P. Pepper, Professor of Medicine at the University of Pennsylvania Medical School ([42], p. 649).

A study carried out during the early 1920s in Los Angeles had already disclosed the rather alarming fact that only 10% of people seeking health care employed regular physicians ([53], p. 322). This survey prompted one practitioner to expound on the lack of grass-roots support for the medical profession. "Always conservative and manifesting an attitude of aloofness, we have never seriously cultivated an interest in the common people and their common needs," he wrote. "Instead we have substituted the laboratory for the bedside and the hospital for the home and left the broad and fertile field of community interests and ailments to be exploited by the ignorant but cunning and mercenary quack."[8]

While most responsibility for the deteriorating physician-patient relationship in the 1920s was placed at medicine's door – especially its impersonal scientific orientation – practitioners also partially blamed the public for the ebbing of friendly contacts. "People nowadays generally have very little faith and very little patience", complained Herbert C. Moffitt, Professor of Medicine at the University of California, San Francisco. "We have been trying the last years to teach them a smattering of medicine and have unfortunately encouraged them to look for quick results in treatment" ([53], p. 324). This author and other physicians especially blamed surgical enthusiasm and a new commercial spirit for encouraging greater expectations and higher costs, thereby fostering inevitable disappointments and unfavorable comments about medical care in general.

In the late 1920s medical leaders began to focus more closely on the issues surrounding the physician-patient relationship.[9] Prominent among those writing and speaking out on the subject was Francis W. Peabody, Professor at the Harvard Medical School. His talk to medical students – entitled "The Care of the Patient" – was published initially in 1927, and to this day remains one of the most quoted articles in the medical literature. Peabody bowed to the inevitable introduction of scientific and business methods into medicine, but sought to reassure his readers that the new schemes would not threaten the personal bonds between healer and patient. "The art of medicine and the science of medicine are not antagonistic but supplementary to each other", he proclaimed, adding that "the significance of the intimate personal relationship between physician and patient cannot be too strongly emphasized, for in an extraordinarily large number of cases both diagnosis and treatment are directly dependent on it and the failure of the young physician to establish this relationship accounts for much of his ineffectiveness in the care of patients" ([66], p. 877).

Peabody especially recognized the depersonalizing aspects of hospital practice but urged his students to reconstruct their patients' social background through a careful assembly of personal facts obtained from the clinical history, information supplied by the social worker, and even visits to the homes of the sick. He also made a foray into psychosomatic disturbances, stressing the therapeutic opportunities that awaited empathetic physicians. For Peabody the greatest reward physicians could hope to achieve was a personal bond with patients, an expression of Aesculapian humanitarianism contained in the now famous phrase "the secret of the care of the patient is in caring for the patient".[10]

In subsequent years, Harvard medical students were exposed periodically to lectures on "the care of the patient" by prominent academics, some of whom further emphasized the need for physicians to understand their patients on a psychological level instead of simply providing "maudlin sympathy" [61]. Yet, while the foreign physicians showed signs of incorporating such psychological insights in medical practice ([33], [49]), American physicians for the most part expressed the opinion that psychology was full of unproven hypotheses and fads. Physicians thought that they knew plenty about human nature by virtue of their practices. Their true instincts and subsequent experiences molded the communicative skills necessary for success.[11] A prominent medical writer, Walter Alvarez, listed a supplemental series of pragmatic recommendations designed to achieve a "state of personal rapport": a thorough history and physical examination coupled with prompt diagnosis and treatment [1]. If the suggestions were followed, the patient invariably developed confidence in the practitioner ([77], [68]). Moreover, physicians in the 1930s were enjoined to recognize the potentially destructive role of fear in patients – "a fear ignored is a fear confirmed" – and ordered to ameliorate it by a judicious display of confidence and fragmentary truthtelling, not by the rather harmful "let-it-all-hang-out" stance favored by certain practitioners [67].

Lawrence J. Henderson, a prominent biochemist with broad interests in the philosophy of science and medical sociology, pursued the subject a step further. In a speech delivered at a Harvard Medical School colloquium in December of 1934, Henderson first reassured his audience that the personal relations between the physician and patient remained "nearly what they have always been", presumably referring to the traditional paternalistic model ([40], p. 819). He then went on to lament, like others before him, that the new scientific facts and expanding technology had powerfully engaged the minds of his medical colleagues to the detriment of their personal relations with the sick. While admitting that any previous knowledge about the relationship was intuitive and empirical, Henderson attempted to place it on a more respectable intellectual level by applying the prevailing systems theory of the biological sciences. "A physician and a patient make up a social system", he proclaimed, and therefore the sentimental interaction of healer-patient was "hardly less important than gravitational attraction in the solar system" ([40], p. 820).

In addition to providing the relationship with scientific respectability and sociological foundations, Henderson also envisioned it as a mechanical model of reciprocal emotional exchanges that could be fruitfully exploited for therapeutic reasons. Interviewing practices borrowed from industry and avoidance of unnecessary moralizing were recommended to practitioners for enhancing personal contacts. Once established, physicians should "endeavor to act upon the patient's sentiments according to a well-considered plan" and promote important attitudinal changes [39]. The final goal of Henderson's emotional manipulation was the restoration of patients to their healthy equilibrium.

Henderson also suggested that healers, while manipulating their patients' feelings within the framework of a close personal relationship, remain emotionally aloof, since expression of their sentiments could be potentially harmful in certain surgical practices and drug administrations. "The physician should avoid, so far as possible, the action of the patient's sentiments upon his own and above all upon his own speech and behavior", he wrote ([39], p. 16). His prescription was copied by other authors who also argued that the restrained and distant physician was merely behaving in the best interests of patients. "The doctor who is oversympathetic, i.e. in the derivational sense of the word 'suffering with' his patient, may be lacking in intellectual or unemotional qualities that are prerequisite of good judgment," wrote one physician ([42], p. 13). In fact, to be effective in both diagnosis and treatment, critical reasoning demanded a "detachment of objectivity" unobstructed by emotions [55].

As organized medicine escalated its campaign for "laissez faire" practice before World War II by opposing several health insurance and prepayment schemes, the physician-patient relationship quickly became embroiled in political and economic debates, emerging, in the words of one writer, as the "chief bulwark against socialization" ([45], p. 1416; [73]). In the late 1930s and early 1940s the tone and content of the debate in medical journals shifted away from concerns regarding the scientific impersonality of physicians and concentrated instead on the threats of compulsory health insurance and patients' need of free choice in the selection of practitioners and payment for care.[12] Even some of the recent hardnosed proponents of scientific medicine, "men who had previously looked askance on discussions of human relationship as the vaporings of undisciplined thought" [45], now eagerly flocked to a new rallying point. Numerous publications insisted that third party medical payments only sowed distrust and destroyed confidentiality between healers and their patients ([60], p. 881; [37]).

The Second World War apparently placed a brief moratorium on further discussions. The relative shortage of physicians stateside seemingly squelched many complaints: "The public is willing to put up with treatment minus the art of medicine," announced one physician, who feared that the military experience would only accentuate the cold and efficient regimentation of scientific medical care ([49], pp. 724–25). Indeed, "it is idle to look back for a return to 'normal' in the sense that prewar medical practice was normal", concluded another practitioner a few years later. "Medical science has received its own dose of jet propulsion during the past six or seven years and it promises to keep all of us moving faster in the discharge of our duties" ([21], p. 860).

After World War II the Truman administration supported new legislative efforts to enact a national compulsory health insurance. Strong resistance by organized medicine was reflected also in the medical literature on the physician-patient relationship. Some writers argued rather strenuously that the mutual trust and confidence deemed essential for a successful transaction between the two parties could occur only in an atmosphere of economic freedom. The argument was expressed forcefully by Alphonse M. Schwitalla, Dean of St. Louis University School of Medicine: "When the benefits of the physician's services are received by the patient and the payment is made by some other agency extraneous to the two parties between whom the real contract exists, we are endangering the sanctity and the exclusiveness of the patient-physician relationship and we are exposing that relationship to the desecration of commercialism" ([76], p. 1466). Physicians' service orientation and personal dedication to the sick were jeopardized. "We are bartering for coin the devotion and loyalty and confidential intimacy of the physician, together with the confidence and trust and the need for sympathy of the patient", concluded Schwitalla ([76], p. 1466).

Some members of the medical profession and the public expressed skepticism about the true motives behind this call for freedom of choice. For them the "slogan-mongering" seemed more like a smokescreen concealing professional resistance to changes in the economic relationships of medicine ([45], p. 1416). The new payment plans posed a direct threat to the power and financial autonomy of practitioners, but how could they affect the already declining sympathy dispensed to patients? In effect, for many patients financial constraints precluded seeing doctors in the first place. "If one can't pay for it [the personal relationship between physician and patient], he isn't going to get it", concluded one medical critic ([7], p. 96). In addition, how could patients even come close to surgeons when many of them insisted on being paid in advance? ([81], p. 258).

Reflecting on the recurring image of a selfish and often greedy American practitioner [19], such a sudden concern for close personal relations impressed many people as being hypocritical: "Medicine's ace in the hole, or Sunday punch, is the sacred relationship between doctor and patient. Besides being an ace in the hole and a Sunday punch, the sacred relationship is a bag of bones. Common kindness is sacred, but it isn't medical. ... The doctor's only sacred relationship ... is to his profession" ([57], p. 31). Moreover, patients who indeed could afford to consult physicians often found their relationship noticeably impersonal and cold. "That 'subtle and intimate relationship' so essential to the successful practice of medicine had no more existence in that office than it would have had in a socialized Soviet clinic or a German public health station" grumbled one anonymous patient after returning from a visit to a New York specialist ([2], p. 711).

By the early 1950s an era in the physician-patient relationship was ending. Armed with a $2,250,000 war chest, organized medicine temporarily had defeated the forces fighting for compulsory health insurance. A massive public relations effort stressed that a national scheme was superfluous given the excellent health of the American people [62]. Yet greater demands for individual medical attention followed new breakthroughs in surgery and antibiotic therapy. The highly publicized political battles between the government and the AMA and the idealized accounts of medicine's new miracles made the public more inquisitive and interested in health matters. Provided with greater knowledge as well as skepticism, many patients found the traditional paternalistic relationship with their healers outmoded and even insulting. Perceptive physicians quickly responded by recommending a "new look" for medicine, its centerpiece a better appreciation of the patient. "In days gone by when public curiosity was less keen and the physician's word represented unquestioned authority, the doctor's grunt was somewhat more passable if no less ill-mannered. Today, however, it connotes just one thing: a public-be-damned independence which insults the patient's dignity" ([21], p. 859).

II. UNSTUFFING THE MEDICAL SHIRT

> A revolution has been taking place quietly in the healing arts. The patient has found his voice .... Today's layman, quick in his reaction to professional doubletalk and gobbledygook, avoids the physicians who will not meet him on an equal conversational plane. He demands a partnership with the physician ([42], p. 145).

Physicians quickly realized that unfavorable views about the aims and functions of American medicine strongly influenced the attitudes patients brought to their relationships with physicians. Thus, the early 1950s witnessed supplementary efforts aimed at improving the tarnished image of the medical profession. Reflecting a growing sophistication of psychological studies and consumer surveys, medical organizations hired consultants to research public and professional opinions concerning the practice of medicine.

The expressed goal was a restoration of the physician-patient relationship to former levels of intimacy. "Such a renaissance could prove to be medicine's strongest bulwark against all those schemes for the distribution of medical care which impersonalize the services", declared Ernest Dichter, a psychologist hired in 1951 by the California Medical Association.[13] Dichter based his observations on a study of physicians then practicing in Alameda County, California. His final report concluded that medicine had lost its historical heritage of community orientation and leadership because professional views concerning the physician-patient relationship had remained static in the face of rapid social change. Confronted with rising malpractice suits, complaints about excessive fees, and incompetent practitioners, Dichter diagnosed the presence of a "psychological lag" between physicians and their patients ([26], p. 222).

Among the principal factors uncovered by Dichter's survey and considered responsible for the perceived crisis were the demise of the "ideal doctor" of yesteryear, the gradual intrusion of economical factors in professional activities, and the changing role of patients. For the passing of the general practitioner, Dichter recommended a replacement: a general manager or family doctor "who can guide the patient through the confusing maze of modern medicine in his search for an economically fair and consistently good medical product" ([82], p. 96). Like his counterpart in industry, this manager had to possess enough skills and wisdom to integrate and correlate pertinent medical information. Dichter recommended the term "personal physician" for this kind of a practitioner as a public relations device to suggest intimacy. Wide use of the term, he thought, would dramatize patients' needs and desire for such a physician-patient relationship. The slogan "a personal physician for every person" was urged in conjunction with efforts by organized medicine to publicize the virtues of entrepreneurial practice.

For the festering problems of expensive medical services and fee collecting, Dichter gave physicians "moral permission" to charge their fees, a felicitous phrase describing their right to set a price on humanitarian services. To generate a feeling of "rightness" on both sides of the relationship, the following justification was offered to patients: "Your personal physician is your modern medical general manager; your investment in his fee is always a wise investment in good management of your total medical problem" ([82], pp. 99–100).

Finally, the Dichter Report grappled with the changing role of patients. A fair amount of public misunderstanding and antagonism was laid at the door of an autocratic medical profession unwilling to share its knowledge. As one practitioner had argued, "medicine must learn about this new status of the layman. The day of the elevated eyebrow is long gone when doctors could be dryly amused at the misinformation of the layman, gently spiked with unconscious humor" ([43], p. 145). In effect the term *layman*, emphasizing the priesthood of medicine, carried similarly a pejorative connotation, placing patients in "an intellectually and socially inferior position" ([43], pp. 104–107; [34]). To make patients feel as participants in treatment even further, Dichter recommended the use of charts, popular booklets, and slides to educate them. Others suggested cosmetic changes in physician's offices. Their waiting rooms were to be showcases for a new attitude that regarded patients as guests, welcomed by friendly receptionists who acted more like hostesses. The hopefully brief waiting periods could be made more palatable with comfortable chairs, piped-in music, and interesting reading material, a veritable home away from home for the distressed ([43], p. 108; [72]).

In all, the report concluded on an optimistic note and a renewed call for action to formulate images favorable to the medical profession. In Dichter's eyes the trouble was that medicine had witnessed miraculous scientific progress without corresponding advances in human relations: "It is as if the scientifically modern physician's gleaming new hundred-horsepower medical engine were anachronously hitched to the old family doctor's one-horse human relations buggy. Both doctor and patient are getting a rough, unpleasant, and dangerous ride. A modern human relations engineering job is indicated" ([82], p. 108).

As president of the Institute of Research in Mass Motivation, Dichter made another series of recommendations to practitioners at a meeting of the New York Medical Society in 1953. Recognizing through his surveys that the physician-patient relationship was deteriorating, Dichter hammered away at the deleterious effects of practitioners' authoritarianism, rugged individualism, and aloofness. "The modern citizen, and thus the modern patient has been invited to become a participant rather than a passive recipient", he warned. "He insists on his right to ask questions. He wants to be loved, not in a condescending, paternalistic fashion but as an equal partner in the fight against the difficulties of modern life"([26], p. 226).

The full impact of Dichter's recommendations still needs to be studied. In California the report prompted the State Medical Association to establish a research division for the study of issues related to the physician-patient relationship. Headed by Richard H. Blum, another psychologist, a staff of more than twenty experts conducted interviews, administered questionnaires, and designed tests between 1956 and 1960. The results and conclusions appeared in a series of publications covering hospital practice and malpractice suits, culminating with the release in 1960 of a book fittingly entitled *The Management of the Doctor-Patient Relationship.*[14]

While Dichter's report suggested practical ways for physicians to improve their image, it also challenged them to improve their own vague understanding of illness, psychology, and interpersonal dynamics occurring between healers and their patients ([6], [64]). A statement by Avery B. Weisman, a prominent Harvard psychiatrist, epitomized the new and earnest quest spearheaded by psychiatry and supported by the budding behavioral sciences (sociology, anthropology, and clinical psychology): "The doctor-patient relationship becomes more and more important as increasing attention is paid to the psychic factors of illness. It is furthermore in treatment that the relationship becomes more important, often meaning the difference between success and failure" ([83], p. 1144).

Weisman sought to articulate many of the factors operating in the relationship. With the help of case histories, he described the complexities inherent in specific healer-patient encounters, pointing out the rich variety of preconceived and frequently contradictory notions, attitudes, and expectations existing on both sides. Their intricacy and manner of interaction failed to always guarantee satisfaction and effective relations. Physicians especially needed to understand the importance of language and manners, the impact of topics discussed during interviews, and the type of treatment recommended ([83], pp. 1149–50). Equally important, practitioners needed to assess their own personalities and emotional needs. Self-knowledge, wrote another psychiatrist, was a primary obligation since physicians' personal qualities decisively influenced the kind of rapport they could establish with patients [78].

Not surprisingly, a majority of medical students displayed personality traits inimical to a systematic study of psychology. Preference for the "hard" facts of science and concrete phenomena predominated. The students were uncomfortable with areas of knowledge lacking definite limits and precision, identifying sympathy, kindness, and generosity with weakness [63]. Yet medical educators insisted on the importance of cultural determinants in health behavior, the importance of emotions in health and disease, and the necessity for acquiring good communication skills [24].

Thus, the 1950s witnessed a dramatic growth in educational programs designed to introduce the sciences of human behavior to medical students. Most of the courses initially were sponsored at the preclinical level by departments of psychiatry and often were titled "human ecology" or "growth and development" ([20], [32]). Gradually, a number of psychologists and sociologists were appointed to selected medical school faculties and charged with the responsibility of teaching the social sciences to medical students. In turn the Russell Sage Foundation began publishing a series of books on the subject written in part by these early teachers. The goal was an understanding of the whole patient, not just his disease. Concluded the 1952 Report of the Commonwealth Fund, a private philanthropy interested in medical education: "Scientific medicine has hitherto been weakest in relation to the patient's affective life and social environment. The behavioral sciences are already helping the doctor to rely less on intuition and more on systematized knowledge as he approaches these facets of the patient" ([8], p. 21).

The new "comprehensive" approach required novel schemes of medical care, notably the establishment of teams. Many of these teams included social workers and clinical psychologists ready to deal with the social and psychological components of illness. However, such a shift from the traditional healing dyad was perceived by many practitioners as another external threat to the already fragile physician-patient relationship. A typical example of the new tensions between team and solo management was furnished by the proceedings of a 1954 conference organized by Molly Harrower, a prominent New York psychologist. Organized under the auspices of the Macy Foundation, the meeting addressed the issue of an expanding incidence of chronic diseases. Physicians, nurses, clinical psychologists, and other health personnel were encouraged to assemble in interdisciplinary teams and cooperate in treatment [34]. As expected, several papers presented at the conference dealt with the physician-patient relationship. Fears were expressed that role conflicts within teams would destroy such relationships unless physicians remained firmly in charge. "The great danger is to overlook the importance of the broadly-trained, psychologically oriented internist as the key figure in the management of chronic diseases" claimed one rheumatologist, although he was aware that specialists with such training were scarce ([36], p. 14).

Psychiatry in the 1950s not only spearheaded educational reforms designed to include training in behavioral sciences, but also contributed to an understanding of medical practice through the formulation of three basic models of physician-patient interaction. Two psychiatrists, Thomas S. Szasz and Marc H. Hollender, sought in 1956 to identify specific types of relationships based on prevailing clinical conditions [79].

The first model of *activity-passivity* generally occurred in very serious medical emergencies such as diabetic coma, in which the patient was unconscious. In sharp contrast with the physician's active intervention, the patient – akin to an infant – was passively subjected to life-saving procedures. These clearly contrasted roles were followed by a second model of *guidance-cooperation*, employed in acute infections and postoperative situations based on powerful healers who know best and cooperative patients who obey orders ([79], p. 586). Finally, the authors postulated a third paradigm of *mutual participation* based on situations of near equality between physician and patient. Their adult "partnership" could be equally forged during psychoanalytical sessions or the management of chronic illnesses. In fact, the physician's role became more one of a helper, assisting patients in helping themselves. Szasz and Hollender noted that this model had until now been rare in medicine, but changes in epidemiology and awareness of the social aspects in chronic disease demanded that physicians enlist the cooperation of patients in long term management of incurable disabilities ([79], p. 587). They concluded that "the steady drift in social relations – in America as well as in most parts of the world toward increasing acceptance of and often insistence on 'democratic' patterns of behavior – exerts pressure on medical relations to conform to a similar pattern" ([80], p. 527).

Szasz and Hollender also stressed that "each of the three types of therapeutic relationship is entirely appropriate under certain circumstances and each is inappropriate under others" ([79], p. 591). Their formulations were extremely useful in showing the dynamic nature of the relationship and its partial dependence on clinical characteristics. As the numbers of the elderly expanded and long-term management of degenerative diseases increased, the partnership model began to predominate. The authors explained that the mutual participation model required a more complex psychological and social organization from both sides of the partnership, and therefore concluded that "the greater the intellectual, educational, and general experiential similarity between physician and patient the more appropriate and necessary this model of therapy becomes" ([79], p. 587).

The early 1960s witnessed efforts by the medical profession to learn to actually "manage" the physician-patient relationship. "Both the doctor and his patient may cling to images of each other that are rooted in the past, but the pressure for change is relentless" affirmed Lester J. Evans, Executive Director of the New York State Committee on Medical Education ([9], p. 8). His words appeared in the preface of a new book, *The Doctor and His Patient*, written by the sociologist Samuel W. Bloom, a pioneer in the introduction of the social sciences into medical education [10]. Bloom's work summarized five years of teaching at Baylor University School of Medicine. His aim was to subject the hitherto inarticulated "art" of medicine to a disciplined and systematic analysis with the help of the social sciences: "The basic assumption is that a body of knowledge is available sufficient to guide human beings toward more rational and effective relationships with each other" ([9], p. 33).

With the aid of several diagrams, Bloom constructed a much more complex transactional social system than the previous models elaborated by Henderson and Parsons. It distinguished a general socio-cultural matrix, a contemporary body of biomedical knowledge providing the necessary information, and the two protagonists to the dyad: healer and patient, each guided in behavior by special societal groups: the medical profession and the family. Based on insight obtained from small group dynamics, Bloom also distinguished two levels of interaction: specific tasks (instrumental) and an emotional process of communication (expressive) ([9], p. 247). In all, this model stressed the importance of culture in shaping the attitudes and actions of both physicians and patients.

Other medical publications followed suit, stressing the systematic management of the physician-patient relationship because of its potential therapeutical value ([31], [38]). In one of his books, Richard Blum reiterated what many physicians saw as the most pressing contemporary need: "Without information about patient psychology, even the most skilled and dedicated doctor may find himself frustrated, upset or, upon occasion, sued by the troublesome patient" ([13], p. ix).

Blum's book was a practical manual primarily written for practitioners. Its premise was that society's image of medicine was the result of individual physician-patient interactions; therefore, improving these associations would ameliorate widespread criticisms and decrease malpractice suits. He contended: "Good public relations for the profession facilitates the management of individual physician-patient relationships; good doctor-patient relations improve medical public relations" ([13], p. 298). A psychological profile of suit-prone patients and physicians was presented together with an analysis of factors responsible for suit-prone hospitals ([13], pp. 216–217, 286–287; [18]).

To understand their patients further, practitioners were informed about the cultural and psychological factors influencing patients' definitions, attitudes, and reactions to illness. Chapters on office and hospital care followed separate and detailed descriptions of the unreasonable, uncooperative, and ignorant patient. A psychological test – the Patient Attitude Test devised by Blum's staff – provided early warnings about individuals with "unreasonable" expectations of medical science, fees, or the physician's competence. Not surprisingly, most so-called "unreasonable" patients were from lower socio-economic backgrounds and included more women than men ([13], pp. 110–118). Lack of cooperation was defined as not following physicians' instructions and was observed mainly in patients from those minorities only recently acquainted with Western scientific medicine. Another test – the Patient Uncooperativeness Test – was constructed especially to anticipate immature and untrustworthy patients.

An extensive discussion focused on patients' ignorance regarding health-related matters. Blum was emphatic about the dangers posed to the physician-patient relationship by this lack of knowledge. Not only were practitioners enjoined to teach health, hygiene, medical terminology, and the limitations of science, but their patients should also receive information on medical economics, health insurance, and conventions of medical practice, all with the help of pamphlets and books. Roadblocks along the path of patient enlightenment were identified as communication gaps based on the physicians' propensity to use medical jargon and provide insufficient information: "Words are part of the communication process, and good communication is necessary to achieve the broader goal of a satisfactory doctor-patient relationship" ([12], p. 127).

Blum's manual only made passing references to external factors such as the cultural bases for illness definition, and generally concentrated on the interpersonal dynamics between physician and patient – assuming that the former was engaged in a customary individual and fee-for-service practice. Yet the rather turbulent decade of the 1960s witnessed major challenges to traditional organizations and payment schemes of health care that had profound consequences for physician-patient interactions. Implementation of the "Great Society" programs (including the "war" on poverty and disease) meant assistance financed through Medicare and Medicaid to hitherto neglected sectors of the population, notably the elderly and poor.

Central to government-sponsored schemes were primary health care teams providing what was termed "comprehensive" services. Predictably, many of the recipients lived in inner-city ghettos and had until now been separated from most health professionals by barriers of class, education, economics, and values. A growing influx of foreign medical graduates, many of them from Asia, created further linguistic and cultural obstacles. Clearly, two distinct worlds – one representing the patient and another the physician – were intersecting, but not always with harmonious results. In fact, Eliot Freidson, a sociologist who had closely studied the Montefiore Hospital in the Bronx, prominently articulated the new experiences for medicine. He noted that "the separate worlds of experience and reference of the layman and the professional worker are always in potential conflict with each other" ([75], p. 209).

Sources for differences were the diverging definitions of what constituted a health problem and judgments regarding the relevance of the means employed to control it. Perhaps unsurprisingly, it was discovered that patients actually went through rather precise steps in handling their own illnesses, frequently consulting family members and other lay-persons before seeking professional help. Such lay referral systems were strongly shaped by cultural values and socio-economic status. Thus, the separate realms of experience offered a continuous source for possible disagreement and strife. But as Freidson and others were quick to point out, clashes between healers and patients based on diverging viewpoints and values were not a new experience suddenly thrust on the scene by changes in urban America. "Struggle between patient and doctor seems to have gone on throughout recorded history", he asserted, providing examples from the Hippocratic writings to prove the point ([75], p. 207–208).

The prominence of the patient in the 1960s, however, was novel. Buttressed by the contemporary trends in consumerism and individual rights, patients possessed an unprecedented amount of scientific health information. Once again, far-reaching social and organizational shifts in society decisively influenced the role and attitudes of physicians and patients. "Intimate physieian-patient contact is a vestige of a more highly individualistically oriented society," wrote one physician in 1967, adding that the differences in role behavior expectancy currently held by many physicians and patients had unleashed a wave of anti-medical sentiment in the general public and defensive hostility in practitioners, some of whom actually went on strike for higher salaries ([54], p. 168–169). With solo medical practice declining in favor of group and team health care, chances for close physician-patient relationships seemed to diminish. These changes were noted frequently in the medical literature ([44], [25]). "The doctor", observed Freidson, "instead of being a consultant, is becoming more or less a servitor, someone that the patient calls when he thinks he needs it" ([29], p. 42). Now physicians, like other professionals, viewed themselves truly just "on tap" ([22], p. 287).

III. SUMMARY

The complexity of this survey precludes sweeping generalizations or final conclusions. The importance of a personal physician-patient relationship for curing is hardly a settled question. From anthropological field work on healing roles to biochemistry of the placebo effect, researchers are attempting to uncover the foundations of a phenomenon said to have been a "spontaneous, unplanned development of social structure" ([65], p. 460). This phenomenon is still the subject of much speculation. In their writings before and after World War II, physicians expressed a belief in the utility and intrinsic therapeutical value of the physician-patient relationship, while at the same time assuming a rigorously scientific and emotionally detached stance. Noting the possible consequences of that attitude, one author wryly commented that "the milk of human kindness has been curdled by molecular biology" ([11], p. 449). To this day, the inherent tensions between a universal and impersonal "science" and a particular and intimate "art" of medicine continue to fill the pages of medical journals here and abroad.

While political and economic developments in American society continually influenced the medical marketplace, shaping and disturbing the physician-patient relationship, authors in part tended to ignore these connections in print or, having no apparent control over societal events, pragmatically set out to restore or improve physician-patient rapport by issuing a series of prescriptions. Physicians assumed that society's image of medicine was merely a composite view of single relationships. Their tendency was to propose correcting problems involving health care organization and economics by conducting individual public relations campaigns and "managing" their personal contacts with patients as if they were medical problems.

Improving communications and learning the psychology of patients was the aim. In the two decades after World War II these efforts gradually became more formal and systematic, reflecting the dramatic growth of the behavioral sciences. Since patients' personalities played a fundamental role in the production of illness and since somatic ailments could severely affect the mind of those suffering from them, the emotional dynamics between physician and patient became a legitimate field of medical endeavor. By the mid-1960s, a list of specific issues was being discussed in the medical literature, all of which demanded psychological knowledge and interpersonal skills. This list ranged from the psychic effects of stillbirth to the mental preparation for death. From caring for cancerous or dying children to dealing with alcoholics, from developing therapeutic alliances with adolescents to managing widowhood, practitioners were instructed in psychological management, patient compliance, iatrogenicity, and the psychodynamics of medication. Physicians also were asked to define their own emotional boundaries and gain insight into the value systems and resultant biases that guided their own dealings with their patients. Even non-verbal communications were seen to play an important role in the new psychosomatic orientation of medicine. Although the thoughtless grunts and raised eyebrows of yesteryear hopefully were fading, a practitioner's voice, facial expression, and body posture were seen as important elements in the promotion of good contact with patients [16].

Above all, in their writings physicians sincerely felt that control of the physician-patient relationship was an essential component of their practices; they reacted strongly to any external factors which threatened to interfere or diminish this management. The earlier model of paternalistic benevolence allowed physicians enough mastery over their work so that they in fact defined and then dispensed what they believed to be compassionate care ([3], p. 939). Some critics, however, charge that this focus on the uniqueness of interpersonal relations was evidence of an attitude designed to preserve control or dominance and insure a steady flow of patients. Thus, physicians were prevented from recognizing that patient-physician encounters shared many similarities with other organized systems of social behavior, a connection that implied the interchangeability of practitioners ([69], p. 200). Moreover, as the public became increasingly frustrated and actually critical of entrepreneurial medicine in the 1950s, physicians reactively promoted the image of a necessary and close personal relationship with their patients as an ideology designed to protect professional status and authority.[15]

Finally, questions remain about the gradual shift to a more egalitarian model of physician-patient interaction, either in the traditional dyad or involving team care. As Szasz and Hollender demonstrated, the clinical variability of ailments significantly shapes and changes the relationship. In their introduction to a recent work titled *Psychological Basis of Medical Practice*, both authors recognize the prominent role played in such permutations by the so-called diseases of civilization: "The role of the physician has changed over the past fifty years from one of concern with acute, lifethreatening infections and traumatic disorders to concern with chronic diseases involving multiple, interactional causative factors. This change necessitates having an approach which recognizes and makes use of the broad interrelationships that affect health" ([17], p. viii).

The public has steadily increased its sophistication regarding health-related knowledge to such an extent that physicians, as well as other professionals, no longer occupy positions of privilege in society. Thus, changes toward new relations based on equality and cooperation are a reflection of the erosion of Aesculapian power and authority. Among informed individuals "doctor shopping" has become rampant [48]. In fact, "treatment has become a question of controlling, maintaining and rehabilitating processes in which patients themselves play the major role" [87]. To be successful, these relationships require a good deal of openness, communication, and negotiation between the parties. Even compassion can be seen as the result of mutually agreed-on attitudes ([3], p. 943).

Unfortunately, the rhetoric of negotiated and collegial models of physician-patient interaction[16] ignores the existence of considerable communication gaps arising from rapidly accumulating scientific knowledge and technological complexity. Also, certain types of clinical decision-making require speedy and decisive action and so are not amenable to protracted bargaining. At the same time, social class and educational difference among the members of the therapeutic dyad still pose inordinate difficulties. If varying degrees of dependence, helplessness, anxiety, and even irrationality are universal characteristics of patienthood, they invariably will place limitations on the power of the sick. For the same reason, physicians will continue to draw power from the technical competence which they possess and continue to project charismatic characteristics inherent in the healing role.

The University of Wisconsin at Madison

NOTES

[1] For an excellent summary that explains the nature of healing and need for personal relations between healer and patient, consult Eric J. Cassell [23].

[2] In an essay read before the California Academy of Medicine in San Francisco, March 11, 1940, the prominent medical historian Henry E. Sigerist declared that "in every medical action there are always two parties involved, the physician and the patient, or, in a broader sense, the medical corps and society. Medicine is nothing else than the manifold relations between these two groups. The history of medicine, therefore, cannot limit itself to the history of the science, institutions, and character of medicine, but must include the history of the patient in society, that of the physician and the relations between the physician and patient" ([46], p. 26).

[3] T. S. Szasz *et al.* ([80], p. 528) make the point: "Awareness of the cultural relativity of the doctor-patient relationship should make us skeptical of the assumption that our current practices are 'good' or the 'best possible'." See also G. B. Risse, "Patients and Their Healers: Historical Studies in Health Care" [71]. The paper sketches five historical patient-healer relationships including prehistory, ancient Greece, Medieval Europe, eighteenth-century England, and late nineteenth-century Germany.

[4] W. J. Jones made the rather cryptic comment: "In the practice of medicine there is as much use for sympathy as for the hypodermic syringe or the judicious application of mustard and hot water" ([47], p. 640). For some views prior to 1920, consult B. Sicherman's essay in Chapter 5 of *Nourishing the Humanistic in Medicine* ([74], pp. 95–124).

[5] For one of the early analyses of medical roles and the physician-patient relationship as carried out in the 1940s in Boston, see Talcott Parson's essay on social structure and dynamic process ([65], pp. 428–479).

[6] The statement was made by T. C. Edwards, a practitioner from Salinas, California. See H. D. Lawhead ([53], p. 323).

[7] Wrote Frank Smithies, Professor of Medicine at the University of Illinois School of Medicine in Chicago: "While we may have neglected human psychology, one must not forget that the various maneuvers of laboratory diagnosis exert a psychology probably as satisfactory as what you term bedside psychology." See Lawhead ([53], p. 234).

[8] ([53], p. 322). The issue of "cultist" medicine benefiting from impersonal scientific exchanges with patients was also expressed in a somewhat later Harvard lecture by D. Guthrie, entitled "The Care of the Patient" [35].

[9] Beginning in 1925 with volume 10 of the *Quarterly Cumulative Index to Current Medical Literature*, edited by the AMA library staff in Chicago, appears the rubric: "Physician-relations to patient." For the first years there were usually only one or two entries per year, but after 1929 the section expanded rapidly.

[10] For more information on Peabody, see T. F. Williams ([85], pp. 462–481).

[11] L. J. Henderson says that "the little scientific knowledge that we now have of the relations between persons is the professional concern of the psychologists and the sociologists, but in general, we have little to learn from them for they are often unaware of the application to everyday life and to practice of what they know" ([39], p. 10). Another article espousing this position is by W. R. Miles [59].

[12] H. J. Hartman makes the comment: "That type of medical practice which preserves the personal relationship between the physician and the patient, that maintains the

practice of medicine as a profession and not a business and that has withstood the test of centuries must be preserved for the interests of both the public and the medical profession" ([37], p. 442).

13 The so-called "Dichter Report" first appeared in a summary prepared by R. Waterson and W. Tibbits and approved by the California Medical Association [82].

14 The series of publications by Richard Blum include: *Physician-Patient Relationships, Survey and Action* [14]; *The Psychology of Malpractice Suits* [15]; *Malpractice Suits: Why and How They Happen*, [12]; and *The Management of the Doctor-Patient Relationship* [13]. It is interesting to note that at least one author claimed that since 1974 malpractice suits had increased 250–350% ([70], p. 256).

15 Even one of the presidential candidates espoused this view; see excerpts of General Eisenhower's campaign speech, delivered in September 14, 1953, and quoted by J. H. Means ([58], p. 725).

16 For a full description of these models, see A. Lazare *et al.*, "Studies on a Negotiated Approach to Patienthood" ([30], pp. 119–139); and T. Parsons, "Epilogue" ([30], pp. 445–455).

BIBLIOGRAPHY

1. Alvarez, W. C.: 1931, 'The Art of Medicine', *Minnesota Medicine* **14**, 227–232.
2. Anonymous: 1930, 'A Patient Looks at Doctors', *Harper's Magazine* **161**, 710–719.
3. Barber, B.: 1976, 'Compassion in Medicine: Towards New Definitions and New Institutions', *New England Journal of Medicine* **294**, 939–943.
4. Barber, B. (ed.): 1970, *L. J. Henderson on the Social System, Selected Writings*, University of Chicago Press, Chicago.
5. Barker, L. F.: 1922, 'The Specialist and the General Practitioner in Relation to Team Work in Medical Practice', *JAMA* 78, 773–779.
6. Bartemeier, L. H.: 1951, 'The Attitude of the Physician', *JAMA* **145**, 1122–1125.
7. Bernheim, B. M.: 1939, *Medicine at the Crossroads*, W. Morrow Company, New York.
8. Berry, G. P.: 1953, 'Medical Education in Transition', *Journal of Medical Education* **28**, 17–42.
9. Bloom, S. W.: 1963, *The Doctor and His Patient: A Sociological Interpretation*, Russel Sage Foundation, New York.
10. Bloom, S. W.: 1959, 'The Role of the Sociologist in Medical Education', *Journal of Medical Education* **34**, 667–673.
11. Blumgart, H. L.: 1964, 'Caring for the Patient', *New England Journal of Medicine* **270**, 449–456.
12. Blum, R. H.: 1958, *Malpractice Suits: Why and How They Happen*, California Medical Association, San Francisco.
13. Blum, R. H.: 1960, *The Management of the Doctor-Patient Relationship*, McGraw-Hill, New York.
14. Blum, R. H.: 1956, *Physician-Patient Relationships, Survey and Action*, California Medical Association, San Francisco.

15. Blum, R. H.: 1957, *The Psychology of Malpractice Suits*, California Medical Association, San Francisco.
16. Bogdonoff, M. D.: 1965, 'The Doctor-Patient Relationship: A Suggested Practical and Purposeful Approach', *JAMA* **192**, 45–48.
17. Bowden, C. and Burnstein, A. G.: 1979, *Psychosocial Basis of Medical Practice: An Introduction to Human Behavior*, 2nd ed., Williams and Wilkins, Baltimore.
18. 'Breakdown in Doctor-Patient Relationship Is Shown by Malpractice Suits, Say Psychologists in C.M.A. Study', *Bulletin of American College of Surgeons* **44**, (1959), 137–140.
19. Burnham, J. C.: 'The Golden Age of American Medicine: Changes in Criticisms of the Profession, 1900–1960' (unpublished manuscript).
20. Cameron, N.: 1952, 'Human Ecology and Personality in the Training of Physicians', Report of the Conference on Psychiatric Education, *Psychiatry and Medical Education*, American Psychiatric Association, Washington, D. C.
21. Cardle, A. E.: 1948, 'New Look in Medicine', *Minnesota Medicine* **31**, 857–861.
22. Carr-Saunders, A. M.: 1955, 'Metropolitan Conditions and Traditional Professional Relationships', in R. M. Fisher (ed.), *The Metropolis in Modern Life*, Russell and Russell, New York.
23. Cassell, E. K.: 1976, *The Healer's Art: A New Approach to the Doctor-Patient Relationship*, J. B. Lippincott Company, Philadelphia.
24. Chesler, J.: 1959, 'The Medical Student and Human Relations', *Journal of Medical Education* **34**, 1101–1105.
25. Cruikshank, N. H.: 1967, 'The Public's Expectations in Changing Health-Care Programs', *Journal of Medical Education* **42**, 713–717.
26. Dichter, E.: 1954, 'Do Your Patients Really Like You?', *New York State Journal of Medicine* **54**, 222–226.
27. Dowling, O.: 1923, 'Public Confidence and the Medical Profession', *Southern Medical Journal* **16**, 691–696.
28. Flexner, A.: 1910, *Medical Education in the United States and Canada*, A Report to the Carnegie Foundation for the Advancement of Teaching, Carnegie Foundation, New York.
29. Freidson, E.: 1975, *Doctoring Together: A Study of Professional Social Control*, Elsevier, New York.
30. Gallagher, E. B. (ed.): 1978, *The Doctor-Patient Relationship in the Changing Health Scene*, Department of Health, Education and Welfare, Washington, D. C.
31. Gee, H. H.: 1960, 'Learning the Physician-Patient Relationship', *JAMA* **173**, 1301–1304.
32. Group for the Advancement of Psychiatry: 1962, *The Preclinical Teaching of Psychiatry*, Report No. 54, New York.
33. Grund, G.: 1929, 'Psychologische Grundlagen der Anamnese', *Muenchener medizinische Wochenschrift* **76**, 49–51.
34. Guess, J. D.: 1952, 'Medicine's Tragic Failure', *Journal of South Carolina Medical Association* **48**, 151–153.
35. Guthrie, D.: 1939, 'The Care of the Patient', *New England Journal of Medicine* **221**, 679–682.
36. Harrower, M.: 1955, *Medical and Psychological Teamwork in the Care of the Chronically Ill*, Charles Thomas, Springfield, Illinois.

37. Hartman, H. J.: 1935, 'The Patient-Physician Relationship Should be Maintained', *Journal of Iowa Medical Society* **25**, 440–442.

38. Hastings, G. E.: 1968, 'Teaching Psychiatry *in vivo*', *Journal of Medical Education* **43**, 741–744.

39. Henderson, L. J.: 1936, 'The Practice of Medicine as Applied Sociology', *Transactions of the Association of American Physicians* **51**, 8–22.

40. Henderson, L. J.: 1935, 'Physician and Patient as a Social System', *New England Journal of Medicine* **212**, 819–823.

41. Henry, B.: 1940, 'Faith and the Doctor', *Journal of the Association of American Medical Colleges* **15**, 330–335.

42. Herrick, J. B.: 1936, 'The Successful Doctor and the Human Side of Practice', *New England Journal of Medicine* **214**, 9–15.

43. Hodges, F. T.: 1955, 'Layman's Stake in Medicine', *General Practitioner* **12**, 145–149.

44. Hodgins, E.: 1969, 'Whatever Became of the Healing Art?', *Annals of the New York Academy of Science* **164**, 838–846.

45. Houston, W. R.: 1938, 'The Doctor Himself as Therapeutic Agent', *Annals of Internal Medicine* **11**, 1416–1425.

46. Ibañez, F. M., ed.: 1960, *Henry E. Sigerist on the History of Medicine*, M. D. Publications, New York.

47. Jones, W. J.: 1923, 'The Physician's Sympathy is a Psychological Remedy of Great Value in the Treatment of Disease', *Virginia Medical Monthly* **50**, 639–640.

48. Kasteler, J. *et al.*: 1976, 'Issues Underlying Prevalence of "Doctor-Shopping" Behavior', *Journal of Health and Social Behavior* **17**, 328–339.

49. Kattwinkel, E. E.: 1945, 'Medical Care of the Patient', *New England Journal of Medicine* **232**, 724–725.

50. Kleinman, A.: 1978, 'The Failure of Modern Medicine', *Human Nature* **1**, 63–68.

51. Krehl, L.: 1928, 'Krankheitsform und Persoenlichkeit,' *Deutsche medizinische Wochenschrift* **54**, 1745–1750.

52. Korsch, B. M., Gozzi, E. K., and Francis, V.: 1968, 'Gaps in Doctor-Patient Communication: Doctor-Patient Interaction and Patient Satisfaction', *Pediatrics* **42**, 855–871.

53. Lawhead, H. D.: 1926, 'The Relation Between Physician and Patient', *California and Western Medicine* **25**, 321–325.

54. Lesse, S.: 1967, 'The Changing Faces of Medicine, Physicians, and Patients', *American Journal of Psychotherapy* **21**, 168–169.

55. Lunt, L. K.: 1938, 'Attitudes in Relation to Illness', *New England Journal of Medicine* **219**, 557–559.

56. Magraw, R. M.: 1966, 'The Doctor-Patient Relationship: Professional Shibboleth, Political Slogan, or Psychological Reality?', in *Ferment in Medicine*, W. B. Saunders Co., Philadelphia, pp. 62–83.

57. Mayer, M.: 1949, 'The Dogged Retreat of the Doctors', *Harper's Magazine* **199**, 25–37.

58. Means, J. H.: 1953, 'Evolution of the Doctor-Patient Relationship', *Bulletin of the New York Academy of Medicine* **29**, 725–732.

59. Miles, W. R.: 1934, 'Psychology in Relation to Medicine', *Yale Journal of Biological Medicine* **6**, 603–608.

60. 'Mutual Trust Between Physician and Patient in Medicine', *JAMA* **107** (1936), 881.
61. 'Notices', 1930, *New England Journal of Medicine* **203**, 1270.
62. Numbers, R. L.: 'The Specter of Socialized Medicine: American Physicians and Compulsory Health Insurance', (unpublished manuscript).
63. Parker, S.: 1958, 'Personality Factors Among Medical Students as Related to their Predisposition to View the Patient as a Whole Man', *Journal of Medical Education* **34**, 736–744.
64. Parkinson, J.: 1951, 'The Patient and Physician', *Annals of Internal Medicine* **35**, 307–314.
65. Parsons, T. (ed.): 1951, *The Social System*, Free Press, New York.
66. Peabody, F. W.: 1927, 'The Care of the Patient', *JAMA* **88**, 877–882.
67. Pepper, O. H. P.: 1935, 'The Handicap of the Patient's Fears', *Journal of Nervous and Mental Disorders* **82**, 639–651.
68. Pepper, O.H.P.: 1937, 'The Importance of Detail in the Art and Care of the Patient', *New England Journal of Medicine* **216**, 773–779.
69. Pratt, L. V.: 1976, 'Reshaping the Consumer's Posture in Health Care', in E. B. Gallagher (ed.), *The Doctor-Patient Relationship in the Changing Scene*, Department of Health, Education and Welfare, Washington, D. C., pp. 197–214.
70. Regan, L. J.: 1955, 'Physician and Patient', *JAMA* **158**, 256.
71. Risse, G. B.: 'Patients and Their Healers: Historical Studies in Health Care', in W. K. Bell (ed.), *Who Decides? Conflict of Rights in Health Care*, Humana Press, Clifton, New Jersey (in press).
72. Roberts, C. L.: 1952, 'Blueprint for Improved Patient Relations', *JAMA* **149**, 1194–1196.
73. Robinson, G. C.: 1939, *The Patient as a Person. A Study of the Social Aspects of Illness*, Commonwealth Fund, New York.
74. Rogers, W. R. and Barnard, D.: 1979, *Nourishing the Humanistic in Medicine*, University of Pittsburgh Press, Pittsburgh.
75. Rose, A. (ed.): 1962, *Human Behavior and Social Class*, Houghton-Mifflin, Boston.
76. Schwitalla, A. M.: 1946, 'The Physician in the Patient-Physician Relationship', *New York State Journal of Medicine* **46**, 1463–1467.
77. Smith, T. A.: 1933, 'What Do Patients Expect from Physicians?', *Journal of the Medical Society of New Jersey* **30**, 641–648.
78. Stockes, A. B.: 1952, 'Psychological Effects of Patient and Doctor', *Medical Clinics of North America* **36**, 585–592.
79. Szasz, T. S. and Hollender, M. H.: 1956, 'A Contribution to the Philosophy of Medicine: The Basic Models of the Doctor-Patient Relationship', *American Medical Association Archives of Internal Medicine* **97**, 585–592.
80. Szasz, T. S., Knoff, W. F., and Hollender, M. H.: 1958, 'The Doctor-Patient Relationship and Its Historical Context', *American Journal of Psychiatry* **115**, 522–528.
81. Tannenbaum, S. A. and Branden, Paul M.: 1935, *The Patient's Dilemma: A Public Trial of the Medical Profession*, Coward-McCann, New York.
82. Waterson, R. and Tibbits, W.: 1951, 'The Doctor-Patient Relationship – A Psychological Study', *General Practitioner* **4**, 93–109.
83. Weisman, A. D.: 1950, 'The Doctor-Patient Relationship: Its Role in Therapy', *American Practitioner* **1**, 1144–1151.

84. White, W. A.: 1926, 'Dynamics of the Relation of Physician and Patient', *Mental Hygiene* **10**, 1–11.
85. Williams, T. F.: 1950, 'Cabot, Peabody, and Care of the Patient', *Bulletin of the History of Medicine* **24**, 462–481.
86. Wilson, R. N.: 1970, *The Sociology of Health: An Introduction*, Random House, New York.
87. Zola, I. K.: 1963, 'Problems of Communication, Diagnosis and Patient Care: The Interplay of Patient, Physician and Clinic Organization', *Journal of Medical Education* **38**, 829–838.

SECTION II

AUTHORITY AND RESPONSIBILITY IN THE PRACTICE OF MEDICINE

GEORGE J. AGICH

THE CONCEPT OF RESPONSIBILITY IN MEDICINE

Achieving agreement in medical ethics is particularly difficult in light of the confusion surrounding the identification of what constitutes medical ethics.[1] Alasdair MacIntyre contends that this difficulty is but a characteristic of our broader culture, which has no systematic way of using such words as "ethical" and "moral" that does not already embody a particular and contentious morality ([20], p. 3). As a consequence, the conflict over how morality is to be defined is itself a moral conflict. Different and rival definitions cannot be defended apart from defending different and rival sets of moral principles.

Nevertheless, MacIntyre argues that what can be rescued from this situation can be determined partly by considering the historical sources of the dilemma. To do so, however, means that philosophers cannot restrict themselves to the task of analysis because their cultural inheritance is limited to a variety of fragments, some of which are mutually inconsistent and unusable by those committed to rational discourse. Rather, they are obliged to engage in what he terms "a conceptual reconstruction", which must be "morally partisan" since a morally neutral foundation cannot be secured ([20], p. 40).

If contention and disagreement are characteristic of the present situation – and I agree with MacIntyre that they are – then theories and concepts applied to medicine *ab extra*, no matter how carefully formulated, will not prevent ethical objection. The usual approach in medical ethics, however, has been to take a problem- or issue-based approach. Larry Churchill explains:

> This model seems particularly well-suited for biomedicine *if* one conceives of that field as one populated by exotic, save-or-let-die options. It seems, indeed, to have captured the imagination of bioethicists, and dominates our notion of what it means for human beings to act as moral agents. On the terms of this model, moral aspects of biomedicine are couched as problems and stated in cases which then issue into options suitable for a decision. Recent anthologies in bioethics reflect precisely this mode of thought ([5], pp. 230–31).

Churchill criticizes this approach because its proponents seem to forget that ethical problems are rooted in an ethos: " 'Ethics' derives from 'ethos,' and the notions we hold of what is good and right have their roots, not only in some explicit belief system, but also in the moral ambience of customs, communities, professions, and institutions" ([5], p. 235). An important

George J. Agich (ed.), Responsibility in Health Care, 53–73.
Copyright © 1982 *by D. Reidel Publishing Company, Dordrecht, Holland.*

question for the reconstruction of medical ethics thus becomes: How can the practice of medicine be opened to reflection and the main features of its ethos defined?[2]

Implicit in the problem- or issue-based focus of medical ethics is the belief that the physician-patient relationship is the proper social structure in terms of which to discuss the ethics of medicine. Certain facts, however, belie the importance which philosophical reflection has accorded this relationship. Contemporary medical care is unthinkable without the involvement of many kinds of health care providers besides physicians. This point is often obscured by the assumption that conflicts in values and perceptions associated with new scientific and technical developments are at the core of most ethical problems in medicine ([15], p. 4). Because of the dominance of physicians in health care, these developments naturally are interpreted in terms of their impact on the physician-patient relationship.

The growing philosophical interest in the ethics of nursing and other health care providers as evidenced by recent publications, however, indicates the need for greater sensitivity in discussing the social and institutional context of health care [4]. It is not surprising that many health care professionals are starting to challenge the view that medical ethics is basically physician-ethics extended throughout the health care system. Nonetheless, the predominant view seems to be that the bureaucratic organization and impersonal style characteristic of medicine is attributable to advances in science and technology which cannot be readily assimilated into what is basically a humane and caring enterprise modeled on the physician-patient relationship. On the basis of Guenter Risse's essay, "Once on Top, Now on Tap: American Physicians View Their Relationships With Patients, 1920–1970," it seems appropriate to question these assumptions regarding the physician-patient relationship by suggesting that the organization of medical care according to industrial and managerial ideals perhaps contributes more than science and technology to the complex character of ethical problems in the practice of medicine today. That these ideals are hardly politically neutral becomes evident with the recognition that the concept of the physician-patient relationship has been employed rhetorically and that the ideal of team care – often offered as a corrective to organizational impersonality – similarly has been manipulated, as Theodore Brown demonstrates in "An Historical View of Health Care Teams." The alternative, then, is to seek the sources of the present problematic situation from within the subject matter itself – namely, the practice of medicine – and to view this practice in its social and political context.[3]

I. THE CONCEPT OF RESPONSIBILITY

The concept of responsibility brings to the forefront elements which are significant in properly defining medical ethics. Responsibility serves this function partly because it is such a richly ambiguous and complex concept ([34], pp. 330–332). Its complexity, though problematic in other contexts, allows a full incorporation of the main elements contributing to ethical conflict in medicine. It does so by raising to prominence not only the social and organizational structure of health care, but also the manifold senses in which individual moral agents and groups are accountable for their actions. As a consequence, it raises the question of what *accountability* means in practical terms. For example, the kinds and distribution of authority, expertise, and power in relationships between physicians, nurses, other health care workers, and patients influence the provision of care in ways basic to medical ethics. Until now, these have been viewed as interesting sociological or political facts peripheral to ethics.[4] It is noteworthy, however, that these "facts" are important determinants of what historically has been regarded as comprising the subject matter of medical ethics [35]. The concept of responsibility brings these elements into question by identifying the clinical practice of medicine as the primary concern of medical ethics – over, for instance, biomedical research, public health, and health care administration.[5] In so doing, a morally partisan position is taken which views the clinical practice of medicine as the benchmark for undertaking the philosophical project of conceptual reconstruction.[6] In making this assumption, it is necessary first to examine the main features of the concept of responsibility: accountability, liability, rationality, and absence of negligence ([12], [17], [18], [34]).

Senses of Responsibility

The requirement of *accountability* is basic to all uses of "responsibility" in ethics. A responsible agent must be able to give an account or reasons for his actions. This presupposes what H. L. A. Hart has termed "capacity responsibility" ([12], pp. 227–30) and involves what Sumner Twiss has termed "capacity requirements" ([34], p. 334). This means that to identify an agent as responsible in the sense of being accountable, certain conditions must be met, such as the ability to understand what conduct is required in specific situations, to be able to deliberate and reach decisions regarding courses of action, and to be able to say what the agent is doing and why he is doing it.

In the absence of these conditions, it is awkward to speak of an individual as ethically responsible.

Second, a responsible agent is liable for the consequences of his actions. *Liability* involves reference to an agent's knowledge and intention, as well as the causal connection between the action and its consequences. It is important to note that not all judgments of liability have the same meaning. They are employed in at least three distinguishable ways – in assessments of (moral) blame, (legal) punishment, and compensation. In each of these employments, "liability determination" has a different meaning and involves different issues depending on the kind of liability in question ([8], pp. 25–37). This point is often forgotten or ignored in discussions of fault in medicine.

Implicit in the notions of accountability and liability is the assumption that a responsible agent will "take his responsibility seriously" [13]. This assumption implies two further features: *rationality* and *absence of negligence*. A responsible agent is one who exhibits rational deliberation regarding his actions. He considers his actions and their consequences before acting. Similarly, a responsible agent does not act negligently, but takes due care in the performance of his actions. The interdependence of these features permits convenient pairing: accountability/liability and rationality/absence of negligence. The latter requirements generally indicate the importance of character and disposition for responsibility. They also point to the institutional and ambient social environment in which character is formed and so raise the question of the proper interpretation of this environment. Nevertheless, the pairing of these elements indicates that in any application of the concept of responsibility, each pair (and element within a pair) will influence the other ([25], pp. 13–14). Although one pair (or element within a pair) may occupy the thematic focus, the other will be present in the background. The complexity of the literature on responsibility is due partially to the way one or another of these features assumes prominence.

Collective and Individual Responsibility

Twiss has noted correctly that the literature on responsibility tends to focus either on the moral implications of the free will/determinism controversy or the legal implications of theories of human causation and action ([34], p. 332). In addition to moral and legal treatments of responsibility which employ the features discussed here, the question of whether (and in what sense) responsibility can be predicated of groups also has been treated ([8], pp. 222–51; [9]; [26]).

In medicine the question of group or collective responsibility is raised both for the profession as a whole and in the context of health care teams ([21], [22]; [23], pp. 244–65). The distinction between individual and collective responsibility is particularly important in connection with team care, especially in light of the way the concept of team care has been employed. Most philosophical discussions approach the individual/collective responsibility distinction in terms of either of two questions: Can collectives be said to perform actions or exercise power such that liability and causality can be assigned to them? Or, can collectives be regarded as persons such that they can be said to exhibit rational decision-making? These questions are important in that they bear on the definition of accountability and liability within groups such as health care teams and within complex institutions such as hospitals. Insofar as these questions are framed on a level removed from medical practice, the concrete norms and values which guide individuals and groups in medical practice are often ignored. As a consequence, even if one could answer affirmatively the question of whether a group can be regarded as a person (in the sense that it can be said to exhibit rational decision-making), it is not clear that the question of the responsibility of individual members of a health care team is thereby decided. Similarly, if groups are uniquely liable insofar as they can be said to perform actions or exhibit causality, it does not follow that individual members are free of liability or moral accountability or unable to act on their own. The very fact, however, that these are issues open for philosophical discussion indicates the heuristic richness of responsibility for framing ethical questions in the highly organized, technically sophisticated centers of clinical practice so prevalent today. When employed as a methodological guide, the concept of responsibility thus lends a richness and breadth to the analysis of health care.

II. RESPONSIBILITY AND MEDICAL ETHICS

To reiterate, the main attraction of the concept of responsibility involves a judgment of what is wrong with medical ethics. One view of the current state of medical ethics that accords with MacIntyre's general assessment is presented by John Ladd in a paper entitled "Legalism and Medical Ethics" [18]. By loosely following Ladd's argument and supplementing it at key points, it becomes possible to outline the main significance of the concept of responsibility for the reconstruction of medical ethics and thereby indicate the sense in which this reconstruction is "morally partisan". Ladd's article is important because it argues for a view of responsibility which seems to minimize the importance of institutional and organizational arrangements in health care. For this reason, his advocacy of the concept of responsibility in medical ethics needs to be considered critically.

Rights vs Responsibility

Ladd's aim is to develop a criticism of the concept of moral rights – moral rights that share the logical properties of legal rights – and to propose the language of responsibility as a firmer foundation for medical ethics. While this project is appealing initially, the approach tends to turn primarily methodological concerns into a substantive preference for a particular view of responsibility insofar as his positive concept of responsibility is constructed on the basis of a criticism of the legal view of *rights* functioning in medicine.

The three logical properties of legal rights which Ladd considers important are: the peremptory nature of rights, the impersonal and adversarial relationship presupposed by rights, and the distinction between possessing and exercising a right. First, rights claims are unique moral claims in that they are peremptory: "In general, when a person's rights are involved, many sorts of actions are authorized that would otherwise be impermissible" ([18], p. 16). Second, because rights are appealed to when "the person against whom it is asserted threatens, neglects, or otherwise appears unwilling to accede to one's requests, needs, or demands," they imply a particularly adversarial relationship between the parties involved ([18], p. 17). Finally, it is important to note that an individual possesses a right if he can choose not to exercise it. In this sense, rights are a reflection of the concept of a person as free and capable, in the sense of competence, to make decisions regarding rights.

On Ladd's view, these properties make the language of rights inappropriate for medical ethics. As an alternative he proposes an ethics based on the concept of responsibility. First, the kinds of considerations relevant to moral decisions based on responsibility involve judgment. That is to say, deliberation, reflection, consultation, and discussion are essential components of responsibility, whereas rights normally do not require or even permit consideration of facts other than those directly related to the status of the right itself and an individual's ability to do what the right requires. Second, attitudes are an essential ingredient in an ethics of responsibility; however, they are pertinent in the context of rights only if attitudes legitimately can be claimed as a right. Third, in a relationship of responsibility there is a certain antecedent inequality between the parties as far as their needs and abilities are concerned. By definition rights presuppose a basic equality much like that assumed to exist between parties entering into a contractual agreement. Finally, responsibility relations are dynamic – they change and develop through time as the needs and abilities of persons develop and their conditions change. Rights, however, pre-exist and are determined before the decision-making process even starts.

From this characterization it is easy to see why the language of rights is seen by Ladd to be inadequate for medical ethics. Rights presume a lack of trust and a situation characterized by conflict and lack of concern. Just the opposite supposedly is necessary for health care. By recognizing the inequalities of parties to health care and the importance of attitudes, the concept of responsibility allows judgment a greater function in the dynamic relationships characteristic of health care. So while the juxtaposition of rights and responsibility is helpful as a methodological objection – namely, that the language of rights encourages the view that medicine is dominated by problems, issues, or life and death decisions, whereas responsibility permits a fuller analysis of the ethos of medicine – it does not logically require that the substantive and positive function which the language of rights serves in medicine be denied. Although this point is acknowledged by Ladd in passing, it is only inadequately provided for in his account and he neglects entirely the broader and potentially more troublesome use of the language of rights in health care as a way of promoting or sustaining discord among health care providers.

Rights are valuable because they protect individuals from the impersonal decision-making of institutions and from other individuals who hold a disproportionate share of power. A claim to rights thus is often a strong moral counterweight to an argument that rests on, for example, what the rules of a hospital require, what is customary in the profession, or what the practitioner usually does in such cases. The language of rights, though, also encourages argument not only regarding the rights of patients, but also regarding the rights of physicians, nurses, and other health care workers. So, while the moral protection provided by rights is attractive, the language of rights fosters a Punch-and-Judy version of ethical discourse, of assertion and counter-assertion. In this sense, it is symptomatic and not diagnostic of problems facing the reconstruction of medical ethics. The language of rights consequently leads to the unfortunate view that the main philosophical task is that of clarifying and evaluating various claims to rights in health care without clearly requiring an examination of the context or practice from which such rights emerge and without even requiring that the rights in dispute be vindicated ([18], pp. 31–33). Similarly, since many ethical problems in medicine simply bypass questions about rights because none of the parties involved find it necessary to appeal to or to exercise their rights, the language of rights restricts the scope of ethical inquiry in medicine.

It therefore seems important that medical ethics be guided by an alternative concept. It is also important, however, that this alternative approach retain the positive functions of rights in medicine by allowing the institutional and organizational aspects of medicine (which seem to encourage the language of rights in the first place) to come to the fore. Ladd's approach unfortunately makes this difficult if not impossible.

Descriptive and Normative Responsibility

To understand why responsibility should include the institutional and organizational aspects of medicine, it will be helpful to differentiate two approaches to responsibility termed by Ladd the *descriptive* and the *normative* approach.[7] Descriptively, responsibility is used to refer to an *actual* relationship between an actor and a state of affairs (usually a past state of affairs). Normatively, it refers to a relationship which *ought* to exist between them (usually a future state of affairs). This distinction is important because the prospect of an ethics of responsibility in medicine depends upon being able to reconstruct a rationally defensible, future-oriented, or normative sense of responsibility rather than in developing an acceptable "after-the-fact" or descriptive sense – the main concern of most legal treatments of responsibility.

Descriptive responsibility almost always involves judgments regarding undesirable states of affairs, that is, judgments involving blame or assessment of liability. The states of affairs referred to in descriptive assessments of responsibility (such as causes) usually are specific and determinate. By determining the causal agent involved, descriptive responsibility usually is closed and exclusionary; that is to say, descriptive responsibility usually is fixed on an object or person to the *exclusion* of others. (For example, "If John is responsible for the mess, then no one else could have caused it.") These features make descriptive responsibility ill-suited for the task of conceptual reconstruction. Taken alone, descriptive responsibility can trivialize ethics by attempting to resolve such conflict in terms of causality alone.

Normative responsibility, on the other hand, need not be restricted to determination of causality because responsibility in this sense pertains mainly to the fulfillment of duties in the future. It includes a broader understanding of moral offense than descriptive responsibility by extending beyond the transgression of rules or principles to include the question of the fulfillment or loss of moral values ([29], p. 210). In other words, most individuals have responsibilities over and above those that arise out of their past actions and omissions. Normative responsibility therefore is used prospectively to point to an individual's accountability and future liability for performing actions. In general terms, this sense of responsibility is open and inclusionary. That is to say, because a particular agent has a duty, it does not follow that no one else has this duty. Others are also usually covered by the duty. It should be noted that the inclusionary character of normative responsibility is graded; thus, it is possible and sensible to speak of one individual as being more or less responsible than another in a normative sense. The responsible person is expected, by means of rational deliberation, to decide to what extent he is duty-bound to act in a certain way or to follow a certain course of action. Similarly, he is expected to act with care and to avoid untoward consequences. Descriptive and normative responsibility consequently must be distinguished on logical grounds even though they are importantly interrelated.

Normative responsibility can arise from descriptive responsibility. For example, "Because John caused the mess" (descriptive responsibility), "he must clean it up" (normative responsibility). This connection is predicated on the interrelationship of the four general features of responsibility discussed earlier – accountability, liability, rationality, and absence of negligence. Twiss explains this interconnection in the following way:

> For example, if agent A is held responsible (liable) for the harmful outcome of his action, then A is assumed to have had the reason and foresight to avoid that outcome (if he had exercised his judgment or not been negligent); or, from the other side, if A is deemed to be responsible in the rational sense, then A is assumed to be aware of his accountability and liability for his actions and their consequences ([34], pp. 333–34).

The inference is that John, though perhaps not only John, is accountable and liable in a future and normative sense for rectifying the wrong done, namely for cleaning up the mess he caused.

Although this inference seems natural, it is often forgotten that it is supported by institutional and social frameworks. These frameworks represent the ambient values and particular norms in terms of which judgments of responsibility – and the specifics of such judgments in terms of accountability and liability, for example – are made. In other words, without a shared framework of norms and values, normative judgments of responsibility would be impossible. One important consequence of employing the concept of responsibility methodologically is that it opens social and institutional values and norms for reflection. By being employed normatively, however, the concept of responsibility morally commits the inquirer to a reconstruction which involves a particular set of values and norms. It at least implicitly projects a vision of medicine and health care. In Ladd's case, the vision of medicine seems particularly restrictive and out of touch with contemporary realities.

Responsibility as a Personal Relationship

Ladd's approach to responsibility, as well as that of other advocates of the concept of responsibility in medicine, is clearly normative ([3], [21], [22]). His approach, however, is unique in that it focuses on the responsibility relationship itself. This restriction tends to isolate the responsibility relationship from the institutional context which supports it. In so doing, it prevents Ladd from developing the possibilities inherent in the normative approach to responsibility and provides instead a restrictive vision of the ethics of medicine.

Ladd argues that responsibility relationships cannot be casual or transient relationships such as those existing among strangers, but rather are like personal relationships of a more permanent nature ([18], p. 22). It is the *personal* character of the responsibility relationship which is central in his account ([14], p. 40). As Ladd expresses it: "The relationship of giving and receiving set forth here is therefore *personal* in the sense that it binds particular persons to other persons, rather than persons to persons generally" ([18], p. 25).

Several implications follow from this characterization. The first is that personal relationships should not be confused with social roles which are defined by the set of rules determining rights and duties that attach to roles.[8] Social roles are viewed as impersonal in that they require action without regard to the specific individuals involved in the relationships, whereas responsibility requires actions which grow out of the immediate interpersonal relationship itself. Not only are responsibility relationships not to be confused with social role relationships on this view, but responsibility relationships are supposed to involve a relatively high degree of intimacy and familiarity which cannot be found in relationships with strangers. These implications already point to the inadequacy of Ladd's characterization of responsibility for conceptualizing the ethics of medical practice.

To say that responsibility in medicine involves a personal relationship is problematic, particularly when personal relationships are to be distinguished from social or role-defined relationships. There are crucial differences between the physician-patient relationship (and other health care provider-receiver relationships) and more intimate relationships such as husband-wife and parent-child. It must not be forgotten that being a physician, nurse, or other health care worker is above all an occupation – and perhaps a profession. In defining responsibility as a personal relationship, a serious problem of interpretation must be faced. What can "personal" mean when applied to relationships defining responsibility in medicine if "personal" relationships are to be contrasted with role-defined relationships?

Even in the cases of parent-child, husband-wife, or friend relationships, there are differing degrees of intimacy and distance involved. So, when responsibility is seen as involving a personal relationship, with friendship and parent-child relations serving as the paradigm, no specific emotional quality or proximity is automatically conveyed. It thus is logically possible to admit a variety of attitudes and emotional responses in any of the abovementioned relationships without destroying the meaning of the relationship. Acceptability of any particular attitude or emotion in the relationship will depend partly on an assessment of the values and aims of the individuals involved, the circumstances of their interaction, and partly on the particular relationship itself. There is no general rule that will adequately cover all cases, however.[9] The moral considerations are actually quite complex.

In seeing responsibility as a personal relationship, Ladd might have in mind what has been termed "face-to-face" encounters. Such encounters are seen as essential to personal relationships but absent from social or role-defined relationships. Phenomenological and sociological evidence suggests, however, that this view is simplistic ([27], [28]). In many respects the presentation of self in everyday encounters, even with close associates and friends, significantly involves social role-playing and behavior or putting on public "faces" ([10], [11]). This behavior is even more in evidence in institutional contexts. For these reasons, the sense in which personal relationships are to be distinguished from social relationships, especially those involving strangers, is unclear. In fact, R. S. Downie argues that "while 'person' or 'human being' cannot be regarded as an assemblage of roles, 'person' is itself a role-concept . . . . But to say all this is not to say that 'person' simply names yet another role" ([6], pp. 131–32).

Downie says there are two ways in which a person's responsibility cannot be analyzed completely in terms of the rights and duties of his role. First, the morality of an individual's voluntary acceptance of his role is not necessarily reducible to that of the role which is accepted.[10] Second, the qualities an individual brings to his role are not necessarily analyzable in terms of the role itself. Rather, it is necessary to refer to the sense of "person" beyond the role and to the freedom which underlies all action – the basic presupposition of morality itself [16]. This reference to freedom as the foundation of morality, however, does not help in understanding why personal relationships are distinguished so strikingly from social or role relationships in Ladd's account. The direction of his thought becomes obvious, though, in light of his peculiar criticism of rights.

The language of rights is apropos for contexts in which moral relationships have broken down, in which moral relationships cannot be assumed to exist, or in which genuine moral conflict exists. In each case, the appeal to rights represents an effort on the part of the rights claimant to establish his autonomy or freedom of action and decision and to give concrete expression to his decisions. It is important to note that the language of rights functions very differently in each of these situations. For example, when moral relationships break down – such as in a case of marital discord – the appeal to rights can serve to protect the individual's sense of self or the need for privacy or peace to deal with stress without necessarily implying that the break in the relationship is irremedial and adversarial. In contexts wherein moral relationships cannot be assumed to exist – such as between strangers potentially in conflict – rights can serve to sustain a minimal relationship in which the mistrust attributable to unfamiliarity may be overcome. In contexts wherein genuine moral conflict exists – such as in paradigmatic "cases" in medical ethics – rights peremptorily serve to sustain the individual's autonomy and freedom of decision. Ladd, though, seems to assume that rights language is apropos only for cases in which moral relationships are absent or where they cannot be assumed to exist. (Here the example of strangers comes to the fore.) He fails to consider situations of genuine moral disagreement (either between strangers or intimates) or the possibility of strangers not having to appeal to rights because social role relationships themselves prevent the erosion of trust, which actually undermines the possibility of moral relationships between strangers.

Ladd's restrictive definition of responsibility as a personal relationship as opposed to a social role relationship arises in part from these oversights. The discerning reader thus is forced to conclude that he has presented an extremely abstract and inadequate view of responsibility in medicine. This point can be validated by contrasting what Ladd calls task or official responsibility – a peculiar version of responsibility within institutions – with the richer notion of role responsibility. The confusion of task responsibility with role responsibility seems to underlie Ladd's restriction of responsibility to personal relationships.[11]

Role vs Task Responsibility

Role responsibility is attached to social roles and role relationships which usually serve a significant social purpose (for example, parent-child, lawyer-client, physician-patient). These relationships can be contrasted with more casual and socially less significant or *ad hoc* relationships based on agreements or contracts ([34], p. 338). The contrast is predicated not on the duration of the relationship, but on its social significance and bearing. Social roles therefore are paradigmatically understood in terms of parent-child, husband-wife, or physician-patient relationships, because these relationships serve *basic* social functions and values.

In medicine the clinical role, whether in the form of a physician-patient relationship or nurse-patient relationship, exists to achieve certain aims or ends relative to the welfare of patients. These aims range from the most *immediate aims*, which include the specific tasks having to do with ministering to the patient's medical or other health care needs, to broader *institutional aims*, which guide how immediate aims are achieved – how tasks are identified, divided up, and performed within the particular patient care context – to *background socio-moral norms*, which justify and constrain task and institutional aims regarding the specific clinical role ([34], p. 341). Role responsibility is therefore a fairly complex concept which encourages analysis at several levels. For medical ethics, however, institutional aims are the most important insofar as they define the unique features of the clinical role.

The style and structure of the institutional context within which the clinical role develops and operates has important implications for responsibility arrangements. These arrangements have to do with the type and distribution of authority and power within the institution and among the various role-players. For this reason, they help determine how individuals are called to account for their actions and what accountability means in practical terms. Within highly organized, bureaucratically structured institutions it is obvious that not all individuals can be equally free agents; some require supervision. Joel Feinberg points out that authorization can take two very different forms, depending on the kinds and degree of discretation granted to the agent ([8], pp. 226–27). On one hand, there is the agent who is authorized to act only within strict limits. Such an agent is the mere tool of his principal – he is a "mere agent" or a "bound agent" as opposed to a "free agent". On the other hand, an agent may be hired because of professional expertise and be expected to exercise professional judgment on behalf of and in the name of his principal. He may be given complete independence to act as he deems best within the confines of his expertise. These distinctions are particularly important in the practice of medicine, where high degrees of role specialization encourage a plethora of different kinds of health care workers. The institutional and organizational needs of clinical medicine thus introduce what Ladd has called a task-definition of responsibility alongside, and sometimes in competition with, role responsibility. It develops naturally as a version of the "bound agent" who is seen as a mere worker or employee.

The contrast between task and role responsibility therefore seems especially pertinent in that task responsibility seems to be what Ladd has in mind when he excludes social roles from responsibility relationships. He says that official or task responsibility

> ... is institutional; it is the kind of responsibility that goes with offices, jobs, and functions .... A characteristic logical feature of this kind of responsibility is that it is divided up and limited like the jobs that it is associated with. "This is my responsibility, not yours." "That is your responsibility, not mine." "That is their responsibility, not ours." and so on ([19], p. 181).

Rather than focusing on the welfare of others, task responsibility is oriented toward the tasks or jobs required by an individual's position within an organization such as a hospital. This definition of responsibility seems particularly problematic when the jobs or tasks in question involve patient care, because in such cases the interactions are not practically reducible to technical performance, but instead are interpersonal, involving judgment and negotiation of the definition of health care needs.

To apply the earlier discussion of different approaches to questions of responsibility, task responsibility can be said to resemble descriptive responsibility in being exclusionary and to resemble normative responsibility in generating prescriptions for conduct ([17], pp. 116–18). Unlike role responsibility, task responsibility is oriented primarily to the objective action to be performed rather than to the recipient of the action. In fact, task responsibility receives its basic justification from the fact that bureaucratic organizations are structured hierarchically along lines of authority. This structure of authority promotes an external accountability regarding actions rather than a subjective accountability in terms of rationality and judgment.

In institutional settings such as hospitals, authority is delegated to subordinates by superiors who in turn are responsible to their superiors. In this sense responsibility means *answerability* to one's superior. For this reason it has to be exclusionary in that it is associated with the kind of authority and tasks that are delegated to a subordinate by a superior. ("It is John's job, not Mary's, and he alone will have to answer for it.") Task responsibility differs from both descriptive and normative responsibility in that the "duties associated with offices are alienable" ([17], p. 117). In other words, task responsibility can be delegated, transferred, created, and extinguished, whereas neither descriptive nor normative responsibility can be so alienated. ("John ordered Mary to do it, so she is now responsible.") Patient care consequently can take on some of the worst qualities of an interaction between strangers.

It has been argued that this concept of task or official responsibility does not adequately characterize the responsibility typical of social roles, particularly the role of physician, nurse, or other health care providers ([34], pp. 337–38). Because task or official responsibility is defined in terms of authority and tasks delegated by a superior, this concept seems inadequate to account for the responsibility which defines the social roles of health care providers. For one thing, the duties associated with these roles are not alienable in the same sense that a bureaucrat might pass on assigned tasks. There are senses of fundamental need and basic aspects of caring which cannot be delegated or abrogated without at the same time violating the normative features of the clinical role itself. For this reason, the concept of task responsibility is important in medicine since for many health care workers there is an all-too-vague definition of the normative features of their particular roles. This seems to encourage appeals to task-defined responsibility: "It's not *my* job" or "It's not *your* job" with corresponding consequences on patient care.

This clarification brings up a final difference between task and role responsibility. Task responsibilities are usually determinate and specific. Performing them requires only limited rational deliberation and judgment. An individual is expected merely to exercise due care and avoid negligence, but not to reflect and critically assess patient needs. Role responsibility, on the other hand, is generally like normative responsibility in that it is diffuse and indeterminate. Hence, judgment or rational deliberation is necessary. While these distinctions are logical in that they involve the concepts of role and task responsibility, they gain practical import insofar as they help explain the basis of many disputes in health care regarding professional status (since professional status is supposed to assure an independent domain of judgment for the professional) [3]. More importantly, however, these distinctions indicate the need for epistemological investigation of the division of labor in medicine and of the definition of various health care specialties in terms of how knowledge (construed broadly, of course, to include cognitive knowledge and practical skills) can be critically related to particular role responsibilites.

Role responsibility thus stresses the duties which are inherent in a relationship directed toward the needs of the role recipient and which sustain the integrity of the relationship itself ([34], pp. 342–43). Accountability accordingly is directed primarily toward the role recipient.[12] Task responsibility, on the other hand, restricts accountability to answerability to one's superior. It poses the problem of moral action within institutional frameworks possibly insensitive to ethical values and raises the question: How can institutions exercise oversight and supervision of individual health care workers without encouraging task definitions of responsibility? To answer this question necessitates facing a more fundamental issue, one raised by Richard Zaner:

> What, after all, can it mean "to care", in those commonly accepted terms, "health-care"? Stripped of rituals, guises and disguises, what is called "health-care" most often goes on among strangers, in settings which seem structured more to encourage than to ameliorate strangeness: the large, highly bureaucratized, technologized and impersonal urban health-centers [36].

Ladd's stress on the personal character of responsibility relationships is on track, but is like an engine going in the wrong direction. It still shares an assumption with the language of rights, namely, that morality is fundamentally individual and that morality is to be understood exclusively in terms of relations between autonomous individuals who come together. It ignores altogether the institutional and communal context of morality and health care and so fails to develop a view of responsibility adequate to these situations ([14], p. 42).

III. SUMMARY

The concept of responsibility affords a significant access to the clinical practice of medicine. By its very complexity and openness to the organizational and institutional aspects of medicine, responsibility draws attention to the ethical issues involving the definition and distribution of authority, power, and expertise in health care. Responsibility thus is central to the project of reconstructing medical ethics. It permits a wide range of analysis and conceptualization of medical ethics, but is uniquely sensitive to the communal aspects of medical ethics in which care-giving roles are defined.

Working with examples involving kidney disease and dialysis, Zaner has argued that the responsibility relationship in medicine must be understood as

> . . . a fundamentally *communal, consociate* or *interindividual* phenomenon: it is neither autonomous nor heteronomous in Kant's sense. The person afflicted with ESRD [End Stage Renal Disease], as afflicted, is the presence to other, non-afflicted persons of a moral entreaty which is compelling to others precisely *by* its having been unasked-for, *by* its having been neither chosen nor deserved [36].

This intersubjectively experienced sense of need or affliction marks the core and foundational phenomenon of responsibility in medicine.[13] Illness or affliction compels response. The response solicited is not abstract or general but particular, and involves the interaction of individuals – an interaction which is sustained by a social and institutional context or practice.

One implication of this reflection on responsibility, then, has to do with what should comprise a theory of needs and what constitutes the relationship of needs and desires in health care. The concept of responsibility heuristically indicates that such a theory must focus on the intersubjective meaningfulness of expressions of need, particularly in cases of affliction and illness insofar as these expressions ground the institutionally determined patterns of response in medicine. Here, the epistemological task has been mapped out by H. Tristram Engelhardt, Jr., who argues that disease language is derivative of the language of illness, and that the world of the pathologist is secondary to that of the clinician [7]. Disease language thus is not only value-laden, but derives its basic sense within the practice of medicine from patient complaints, even though the interaction between complaint of illness and diagnosis in terms of disease language is exceedingly complex and involves sociological and historical considerations beyond philosophical analysis.

What remains largely unexplored, however, is how particular care-giving roles are related to underlying expressions of affliction and need. In other words, what is required is an analysis and definition not only of disease language and its relation to needs and desires, but of the ways in which this language institutionalizes certain kinds of response to affliction in terms of specific clinical roles. This kind of analysis is essential, as Stephen Toulmin has argued, for understanding the very meaning of professionalism and professional ethics in medicine [32]. The concept of responsibility is basic to this endeavor insofar as it encourages questioning what are the roles of physician, nurse, and other health care providers from a conceptual rather than empirical, sociological viewpoint. It should be obvious that this is not a single question, but a series of questions which must be posed for each of the various kinds of care-givers in medicine.[14]

If the language of rights serves so well as a peremptory appeal in an adversarial context, then an alternative language of responsibility in medicine seems essential for conceiving the ethics of clinical medicine. But because medicine is such a highly structured and complex social institutuion, the analysis of action and responsibility in specific roles is a *sine qua non* for this endeavor. In this sense, the concept of responsibility allows inquiry in medical ethics to embrace epistemological inquiry in the philosophy of medicine and so greatly enhances the prospects of the philosophical understanding of medicine.

One final point remains to be made. The language of responsibility encourages reflection on the social and institutional structure of medical practice in ways that reveal the sources of ethical conflict. The reconstruction of medical ethics in these terms is "morally partisan" because it forces the articulation of a particular vision of relationships between individuals and groups within health care, a vision predicated on relating the definition of needs with the social practice of medicine. To do so requires the assumption of a moral stance regarding the recognition of needs as well as the definition of medicine's various roles in meeting those needs.

Southern Illinois University
School of Medicine

NOTES

[1] For a discussion of various problems in defining medical ethics, see [1], [2], [18], [21], [22], [23], [30], [31], [36].

[2] In like manner, Churchill proposes a broadly "phenomenological" methodology emphasizing "the lived world of moral actors" ([5], p. 239). I am advocating a similar orientation for medical ethics, but one which particularly would utilize an accepted ethical concept – that of responsibility – and would focus on the social and institutional structure of health care.

Although I will speak of the methodological employment of responsibility, methodological issues as such will not be treated. My claim regarding the use of the concept of responsibility in medicine is rather modest. Responsibility simply offers important heuristic advantages. My treatment thus hardly addresses (much less resolves) serious questions of methodology raised by Churchill's appeal to phenomenology.

[3] To move to a social and political view of the practice of medicine does not represent an abandonment of ethics, but rather a recognition that ethics itself naturally gives rise to social and political concerns.

[4] It is useful to distinguish jurisdictional disputes and arguments regarding professional status in health care from arguments regarding the ethics of care. To be sure, how power, authority, and expertise are distributed among health care workers not only has important ramifications for patient care, but involves questions of justice for health care

workers as well. The struggle to gain status and power in health care, however, can compromise the basic aims and values undergirding the entire enterprise of patient care, a point often missed in the rhetoric advocating the professionalization of health care. I have dealt with some of these concerns elsewhere [3].

[5] For a discussion of the relationship of responsibility in biomedical research, public health, health care administration, and the relation of these to clinical practice, see Twiss [34].

[6] I take medical centers, hospitals, or at least highly organized clinic settings to be paradigmatic for the clinical practice of medicine and hence for medical ethics, not only because such centers are so visible in medicine today, but because they exhibit the main issues involved in medical ethics in such stark terms.

[7] I am not entirely satisfied with terming these approaches *descriptive* and *normative* since both have normative elements. A more accurate – though more cumbersome – terminology is *before-the-fact* and *after-the-fact* responsibility. The descriptive approach focuses primarily on normative features, albeit features observed or reflectively noted after-the-fact. Similarly, the normative approach includes factual elements, such as the agent's abilities and causal intentions, in projecting duties into the future. However, for the sake of consistency, I will continue to speak of descriptive and normative responsibility.

[8] Apparently insofar as rules can be said to define social roles, Ladd views social roles as excluding personal relationships. Why? For one thing, Ladd seems to think that rule-defined action is inconsistent with personal relationships on the grounds that the latter are spontaneous and derive from freedom, whereas rules can only be overridden by other rules ([18], p. 13). Surely though, a Kantian would be quick to point out that overriding a heteronomous rule is itself an action which must in principle be capable of being understood in terms of freedom. Nothing about rules logically precludes such an understanding. Nothing about rules as such precludes an agent's freely willing the action they prescribe as his own, either.

[9] It is ironic that Ladd, who argues against rules, should implicitly seem to appeal to a rule of conduct in defining personal relationships.

[10] Here it would be useful to compare Pellegrino's notion of the "act of profession" ([24], pp. 46–7).

[11] Twiss similarly attends to the distinction between task and role responsibility. He argues, however, that Ladd's notion of official or task responsibility is wrong, for the responsibility that typically attaches to social roles is not a correlate of authority and tasks delegated by a superior ([34], p. 337). Although he is right as far as he goes, task responsibility *is* important heuristically for posing the question of the meaning of accountability and authority in medicine. For this reason, I prefer to distinguish task-defined (Ladd) responsibility from role-defined responsibility (Twiss) in order to elicit some of the main problems for constructing an ethics of clinical medicine.

[12] Because accountability in the responsibility relationship is directed toward or has its source in the patient or role recipient, the language of rights becomes crucially important when factors intervene to break down accountability. In this sense, rights remind us that there must be accountability within a caring relationship. Like the concept of liability, rights logically function as a corrective when faulty action occurs or threatens to occur.

[13] Pellegrino indicates the same point by the phrase "the fact of illness" [28]. The actual absence of rational explanation in the experience of illness or affliction is partly

at the basis of the view that the sick person should be exempted from responsibility or liability for his condition.

[14] In other words, I am proposing that the epistemological inquiry which Toulmin has initiated for the physician-patient relationship be deepened and broadened to consider the multiple roles defining the clinical practice of medicine today [33].

BIBLIOGRAPHY

1. Ackerman, T.: 1980, 'What Bioethics Should Be', *Journal of Medicine and Philosophy* 5, 260–75.
2. Agich, G. J.: 1981, 'The Foundation of Medical Ethics', *Metamedicine* 2, 31–34.
3. Agich, G. J.: 1981, 'Professionalism and Ethics in Health Care', *Journal of Medicine and Philosophy* 5, 186–99.
4. Benjamin, M. and Curtis, J.: 1981, *Ethics in Nursing*, Oxford University Press, Oxford and New York.
5. Churchill, L.: 1980, 'Bioethical Reductionism and Our Sense of the Human', *Man and Medicine* 5, 229–242.
6. Downie, R. S.: 1971, *Roles and Values: An Introduction to Social Ethics*, Methuen, London.
7. Engelhardt, H. T., Jr.: 1980, 'Doctoring the Disease, Treating the Complaint, Helping the Patient, Some of the Works of Hygeia and Panacea', in H. T. Engelhardt, Jr., and D. Callahan (eds.), *Knowing and Valuing: The Search for Common Roots*, Institute of Society, Ethics and the Life Sciences, Hastings-on-Hudson, pp. 225–49.
8. Feinberg, J.: 1970, *Doing and Deserving: Essays in the Theory of Responsibility*, Princeton University Press, Princeton.
9. French, P.: 1979, 'The Corporation as a Moral Agent', *American Philosophical Quarterly* **16**, 207–15.
10. Goffman, E.: 1967, *Interaction Ritual: Essays on Face-to-Face Behavior*, Anchor Books, Garden City, New York.
11. Goffman, E.: 1959, *The Presentation of Self in Everyday Life*, Anchor Books, Garden City, New York.
12. Hart, H. L. A.: 1973, *Punishment and Responsibility: Essays in the Philosophy of Law*, Clarendon Press, Oxford.
13. Haydon, G.: 1978, 'On Being Responsible', *Philosophical Quarterly* 28, 46–57.
14. Hoffmaster, B.: 1978, 'Comments on "Legalism and Medical Ethics"', in J. W. Davis, *et al.* (eds.), *Contemporary Issues in Biomedical Ethics*, Humana Press, Clifton, New Jersey, pp. 37–42.
15. Hunt, R. and J. Arras: 1977, 'Ethical Theory in the Medical Context', in R. Hunt and J. Arras (eds.), *Ethical Issues in Modern Medicine*, Mayfield Publishing Company, Palo Alto, California, pp. 1–48.
16. Kant, I.: 1913, *Kritik der praktischen Vernunft*, Paul Natorp (ed.), Königliche preussische Akademie der Wissenschaften, Berlin.
17. Ladd, J.: 1975, 'The Ethics of Participation', in J. R. Pennock and J. Chapman (eds.), *Participation in Politics, Nomos* XVI, Lieber-Athernton, New York, pp. 98–125.

18. Ladd, J.: 1978, 'Legalism and Medical Ethics', in J. W. Davis, *et al.* (eds.), *Contemporary Issues in Biomedical Ethics*, Humana Press, Clifton, New Jersey, pp. 1–35.
19. Ladd, J.: 1975, 'Policy Studies and Ethics', in S. Nagel (ed.), *Policy Studies and the Social Sciences*, Lexington Books, Lexington, Kentucky, pp. 177–84.
20. MacIntyre, A.: 1978, 'How to Identify Ethical Principles', *The Belmont Report* Appendix, Volume I, National Commission for the Protection of Human Subjects of Biomedical and Behavioral Research, DHEW Publication No. (OS) 78–0013.
21. Newton, L.: 1979, 'A Framework for Responsible Medicine', *Journal of Medicine and Philosophy* **4**, 57–69.
22. Newton, L.: 1978, 'Hippocrates Lost, A Professional Ethics Regained: Reflections of the Death of the Hippocratic Tradition', in J. W. Davis, *et al.* (eds.), *Contemporary Issues in Biomedical Ethics*, Humana Press, Clifton, New Jersey, pp. 140–60.
23. Pellegrino, E. D. and Thomasma, D. C.: 1981, *A Philosophical Basis of Medical Practice*, Oxford University Press, New York and Oxford.
24. Pellegrino, E. D.: 1979, 'Towards a Reconstruction of Medical Morality: The Primacy of the Act of Profession and the Fact of Illness', *Journal of Medicine and Philosophy* **4**, 32–56.
25. Pennock, J. R.: 1960, 'The Problem of Responsibility', in C. J. Friedrich (ed.), *Responsibility, Nomos* III, Liberal Arts Press, New York, pp. 3–27.
26. Risser, D. T.: 1978, 'Power and Collective Responsibility', *Kinesis* **9**, 23–33.
27. Schutz, A.: 1971, 'Making Music Together', in A. Brodersen (ed.), *Collected Papers II: Studies in Social Theory*, Martinus Nijhoff, The Hague, pp. 159–78.
28. Schutz, A.: 1971, 'The Stranger', in A. Brodersen (ed.), *Collected Papers II: Studies in Social Theory*, Martinus Nijhoff, The Hague, pp. 91–105.
29. Silber, J.: 1967, 'Being and Doing: A Study of Status Responsibility and Voluntary Responsibility', in J. M. Edie (ed.), *Phenomenology in America: Studies in the Philosophy of Experience*, Quadrangle Books, Chicago, pp. 197–254.
30. Spicker, S. F. and H. T. Engelhardt, Jr. (eds.): 1977, *Philosophical Medical Ethics: Its Nature and Significance*, D. Reidel Publishing Company, Dordrecht, Holland, Boston, U.S.A.
31. Thomasma, D. C. and Pellegrino, E. D.: 1981, 'Philosophy of Medicine as the Source of Medical Ethics', *Metamedicine* **2**, 5–11.
32. Toulmin, S.: 1977, 'The Meaning of Professionalism: Doctors' Ethics and Biomedical Science', in H. T. Engelhardt, Jr. and D. Callahan (eds.), *Knowledge, Value and Belief*, Institute of Society, Ethics and the Life Sciences, Hastings-on-Hudson, pp. 254–278.
33. Toulmin, S.: 1976, 'On the Nature of the Physician's Understanding', *Journal of Medicine and Philosophy* **1**, 32–50.
34. Twiss, S. B.: 1977, 'The Problem of Moral Responsibility in Medicine', *Journal of Medicine and Philosophy* **2**, 330–75.
35. Waddington, I.: 1975, 'The Development of Medical Ethics – A Sociological Analysis', *Medical History* **19**, 36–51.
36. Zaner, R. M.: 'Chance and Morality: The Dialysis Phenomenon', in Victor Kestenbaum (ed.), *The Phenomenology of Physical Illness,* University of Tennessee Press, Knoxville (in press).

ARTHUR F. KOHRMAN

COMMENTS ON "THE CONCEPT OF RESPONSIBILITY IN MEDICINE"

As a physician and medical educator, I am stimulated by George Agich's essay, "The Concept of Responsibility in Medicine," in that it represents an effort to look at common activities in a new light. His is a rich analysis, from which I can pick only a few points of departure. First, I agree with the perspective of *responsibilities*, rather than *rights*, as a basis for discourse and as a framework upon which to begin reconstruction of the presently uncertain role of medicine in our society. The appeal to rights of patients, physicians, and institutions in times of change is an admission of the failure to communicate and to enlighten through dialectical means.

As Agich suggests, the language of rights is the language of adversaries. It further polarizes and fragments a discourse which should be seeking to bring the various actors closer, to reassert the common purpose of medicine – the care of persons with illnesses. The choice of "illnesses" rather than "diseases" is deliberate. Many contentious issues, which are reduced to issues of "rights" between the care-takers and those taken care of, arise from differing perceptions of illness, with consequent differences in the desired actions to be taken [4]. I have refrained from speaking of "health" because the medical profession is trained and organized to manage illness, whether initially perceived by the patient or discovered by the physician [5].

With this brief endorsement of Agich's approach, I will move quickly to a discussion growing out of his distinction between *role* and *task* responsibilities. In the late 1930s and early 1940s, my father was a rural general practitioner in northeastern Ohio. I have recovered his daybooks, the terse yet revealing notes of his patient encounters which also served as account records (although payment was as often in kind as in cash). They reveal the simple expectations of both physician and patient. The physician was expected to be caring, available, and capable of making reasonable estimates of prognosis (competence was presumed, if untested). On the other hand, the patient was expected to be trusting and supported by family and neighbors (and if possible, to make some payment). It is clear from reading those daybooks that the core of the physician-patient relationship was caring and trusting. Issues of "compliance" never arose; the physician's counsel was assumed to reflect the state of the medical art. He was responsible and

George J. Agich (ed.), Responsibility in Health Care, 75–81.
Copyright © 1982 *by D. Reidel Publishing Company, Dordrecht, Holland.*

accountable for that portion of the patient's destiny in which medicine had some commonly understood role. Cure was of course desired. The physician was viewed, at best, as the agent of cure (if it occurred), whether the source was medical science, the deity, or chance. Because patients and the public generally considered their physicians to be in control of only a minor part of all the intervening forces, however, they could not be held ultimately liable for the outcome.

If it became necessary for my father to send a patient to the local hospital, he continued to be clearly responsible and accountable. The hospital in a sense was one of the instruments with which he carried out his role responsibility. There he performed or at least assisted in all surgery on his patients and knew all the nurses, technicians, and functionaries. In fact, many of them were also his patients. Few patients died in the hospital. If the outlook was grim, patients went home to die, among familiars, attended still by their physician. Thus, the perceived role responsibility of physicians such as my father in the institutional setting was virtually the same as that in the office or in the patient's home – a logical and controllable extension of the primary physician-patient relationship. To be sure, the fiduciary role responsibility (presumably focused on the welfare of the patient) was perceived and negotiated in various ways; however, the relationship usually involved only patient and physician or at most, additionally, immediate members of the patient's family.

What has happened to the physician's role since those simpler times? Within the doctor's office (rarely now in the home), the one-on-one relationship of trust is still maintained, although strains are sometimes evident. Outside the office, though, the situation has changed dramatically. An explosion of skills, knowledge, and technology has led to the creation of subgroups of specialists needed for and occupied in their use. Although some of these physician-specialists carry into their encounters a number of the same expectations my father had, their roles often are reduced to elaborate task responsibilities when they function as consultants for a specific organ, system, or disease.

Do these specialists, as they go about their more or less technical tasks, have the same view of their role as my father had? Often their primary clients are consulting physicians rather than patients. It is unlikely that all the physicians – much less the non-physician technical personnel – who participate in the care of the contemporary patient have the same fiduciary role responsibility.

To the practice of medicine have also been added many other layers of interested parties – hospital administrators, medical school faculty and administrators, third party insurers, and local, state, and federal agencies. Their visions, as expressed in their jobs and through their decisions, hardly correspond to my father's understanding of his role as a physician. Thus, there now have emerged many groups of actors, each with private and differing senses of responsibility. Most of them see their function in terms of task accomplishment, of accountability to one or another hierarchy, system, or tradition. These physicians most often are responsible only to their patients for a certain level of technical competence in performance of their special tasks. Yet, the unspoken (and untested) assumption is that the aggregate of the professional and technical task responsibilities somehow results in a continuation of the role responsibility embodied in the uncluttered, traditional, single physician-single patient relationship.

At the same time, there has been a steadily increasing "medicalization" of life, with growing recourse to medicine and its institutions for solutions to life problems and dilemmas, a situation which has generated increased demand for the services of medical professionals. This new dependency – and the predictable disappointments which so often occur in dependency situations – arises from several sources. Among them are: the disappearance or fragmentation of other traditional support structures; the great American love affair with expertise and experts; and increasing inequality of knowledge (and thus of power) between patients and experts.

Consequently, there has evolved an enlarging gap between patients and their physicians at the same time that the classic fiduciary role responsibilities are more necessary than ever. Nowhere is this tension better exposed than in the dominant institutional setting of medicine, the hospital. It is useful to look at hospitals not only as the most common of the institutions of medicine, but also as exemplary of how *all* the institutional settings beyond the individual office encounter conspire to confound the physician's sense of responsibility to the patient.

First, it must be acknowledged that hospitals are *not* rational extensions of the role responsibilities of the physician from the office to an institutional setting. Rather, hospitals are multi-functional accidents of history, geography, and convenience. As an institution, the hospital increasingly has become the repository – the most convenient "parking place" for services and technologies – for functions not otherwise served in society. Those functions have wide range: from that of a "garage" for the efficient mechanical application of technology to patients, to an arena in which social rituals such as dying are played out, to a refuge of last recourse, such as the use of hospitals for protective detention of abused children.

In institutions with so complex a mission, there is an overriding need for order – for management, for conservation of resources, and thus, for authority and power structures. In addition, within each of the professional or technical specialities sustained by this institutional setting, there are variously well-developed forces of professionalization and guild behaviors which in turn are focused upon concerns of relative position in the institutional hierarchy and the power, both authoritarian and economic, which derives from that position.

What, then, is the role responsibility of the physician in *this* setting, wherein tasks and authority relationships dominate? How can the sense of responsibility established in the original physician-patient relationship be maintained? How is the fiduciary character of that relationship to be preserved? What can the physician do to insure the effective discharge of the initial and fundamental role responsibility of his relationship to the patient?

In the hospital setting, the primary care physician finds himself confronted by various forms of responsibility to the patient. He is the guarantor of competence of all those specialists and technicians who perform their tasks upon and in behalf of the patient. Thus, the physician is assumed to be liable for the aggregate actions (or failure to act) of the members of the "health care team". Such a guarantee is hard to uphold in many cases for two major reasons: it requires that each of the accountability structures (hierarchies, guilds, and bureaucracies) of the specialists is a consequence of the impossibility of any single physician having all of the requisite contemporary knowledge and skills. To some degree, therefore, the primary physician – like the patient – is dependent upon assumptions of competence, hearsay, and faith in evaluating the competence of each of the partial care-takers and the commitment of each to fiduciary role responsibilities similar to that on which the original physician-patient relationship is based. It is not surprising, given the multiplicity of responsibilities and roles which the hospital setting demands of both primary physicians, specialists and technicians, that motives, intentions, and goals are often misunderstood. As a consequence, there is a very real risk that medical care will become "an interaction among strangers".

Nurses sit at a crucial point in this complex arrangement. They are with patients and families continuously. The other actors – even the primary physicians – are episodic participants who have usually not communicated directly with each other but only (if even then) by means of *post facto* chart notes. Nurses must try to put all these disparate pieces into a rational care plan, interpret and deliver this plan to their patients, and maintain, integrate (and often referee) the many orders of each of the specialists. Nurses themselves are at the center of yet another set of competing senses of responsibility: to the hospital administration (in this case, are nurses merely employees and subject to task responsibility alone, or are they professionals and thus subject to role responsibility?); to patients (do nurses have a separate and different role responsibility from physicians?); to physicians (are nurses physician-surrogates, physician-extenders, or simply instrumental agents of physicians' wishes, with no autonomy?). It is quintessentially in the analysis of the nurse's role that the "free agent-bound agent" dilemma discussed by Agich becomes most apparent.

It is no wonder, then, that there is continuing uneasiness between physicians, nurses, and administrators. Similar tensions exist between other professional and technical groups in the hospital. Unless and until there is a deliberate confrontation concerning the vague and multiple concepts of responsibility held by the various professionals in the complex settings of modern medical practice, this uneasiness and confusion and tension will persist and increase.

A great deal of the current negative reaction of physicians to oversight, peer review, and regulation appears to be an expression – at times inchoate or even misguided – of the frustration felt by those who find that the proper discharge of their role responsibility is thwarted by the very institutions of medicine presumably designed to help them and their patients. Most important for this argument is the belief that hospitals generally are assumed to represent and insure the natural extension of physicians' individual values and role responsibilities toward patients. The argument that all the professionals and technicians in the hospital setting operate under the same imperatives and values as do physicians in the performance of their tasks further complicates the situation.

There is a paradox here, if not a contradiction. The assumption that medicine's institutions, its specialities, subspecialties, supporting professions, and occupations, are animated by the same *primary* sense of responsibility (that is, a common role responsibility in Agich's terms) is either false or at least not apparent to most observers. The traditional role responsibility of the physician in the hospital has fallen victim to other imperatives as a consequence of institutional development and organization. As Agich states, the classic social role of the physician and the duties (*not* the tasks) associated with that role "cannot be delegated or abrogated without violating the normative features of the clinical role itself". When those duties are translated into a series of tasks performed by multiple individuals, each with a unique and different "epistemological view of the division of labor in medicine", something is lost.

What, then, is needed to understand this situation, to permit restructuring of institutions and practices in order to adapt better to changing demands and roles? Initially, an analysis of the assumptions underlying our thinking about medicine is in order. Particular emphasis should be paid to the ways in which the division and redivision of tasks in medicine has affected the continuity and effectiveness of the role responsibility of the individual physicians and of the profession itself. As Agich suggests, there must also be a move toward a new epistemology of illness and disease, medical care, and the division of labor in medicine, one which will place medical care-seekers and the multiple groups of medical care-givers under the same semantic umbrella.

An important related inquiry is a re-examination of the ways in which the physician-patient relationship is personal and particularistic (including the necessary consequences of and boundaries to that relationship) and the ways in which it is instrumental and managerial. With these new tools, we may then begin a reconstruction of educational programs and of medical institutions – a reconstruction which will reflect new insights and generate a direction toward better service to both patients and professionals. It is essential, however, first to agree that attempts to understand contemporary complex medical institutions based solely on perpetuation of the belief in a collective and institutional role responsibility identical to and extended from the traditional physician-patient encounters, are inadequate.

It must be acknowledged, finally, that rational explication of responsibility will occur only after serious effort to discover the diverse elements which comprise the present roles. Toward that end, I propose an intensive ethnography of medicine – an anthropological field study of the highest order. The beginnings of such an ethnography have already appeared and taught us much about ourselves ([1], [2], [3]). After all, medicine satisfies all the criteria of a distinctive, exotic culture (with its own language, rituals, dress, and hierarchies) and thus ought to be as fit a subject for study as any remote South American tribe. Out of such an ethnography, an intense study of how patients, physicians, and others in medical institutions *in fact* behave, a new epistemology can begin, in which more satisfactory and useful definitions of role and task responsibility can emerge.

La Rabida's Children's Hospital and Research Center, University of Chicago

BIBLIOGRAPHY

1. Bosk, C. L.: 1979, *Forgive and Remember: Managing Medical Failure*, University of Chicago Press, Chicago.
2. Fox, R. and Swazey, J.: 1974, *The Courage to Fail*, University of Chicago Press, Chicago.
3. Fox, R.: 1980, 'The Evolution of Medical Uncertainty', *Milbank Memorial Fund Quarterly* **58**, 1–49.
4. Kleinman, A., Eisenberg, L., and Good, B.: 1978, 'Culture, Stress, and Care', *Annals of Internal Medicine* **88**, 251–258.
5. Pellegrino, E. D.: 1979, 'Toward a Reconstruction of Medical Morality: The Primacy of the Act of Profession and the Fact of Illness', *Journal of Medicine and Philosophy* **4**, 32–56.

STANLEY M. HAUERWAS

AUTHORITY AND THE PROFESSION OF MEDICINE

I. AUTHORITY AND MEDICINE: SOME GENERAL CONSIDERATIONS

To broach the subject of authority and medicine is for many an invitation to launch an attack against what they consider the paternalism and arrogance endemic to current medical practice. Patients are encouraged to reclaim their autonomy against the usurped authority of doctors and other health professionals. Though some of these claims may be valid, it is not the purpose of this paper to provide yet another variation on that theme. Instead, a constructive account of authority and medicine will be presented in such a way as to demonstrate why finding a balance between autonomy and paternalism is an inadequate moral goal. I trust the reader will realize that such a balance reveals a misunderstanding of the concept of authority with regard to medicine as a moral practice.

The lack of an adequate philosophical account of authority certainly contributes to the confusion of so complex a topic. Although sociologists like to refer to Max Weber's famous distinction between charismatic, traditional, and legal-rational authority [20], this typology fails to clarify what it means to acknowledge an authority as legitimate.[1] Authority is fundamentally a political-moral concept; therefore, its meaning must be correlative to understanding the nature of human community and the moral good. In this regard, Alasdair MacIntyre argues that the lack of consensus concerning the latter makes it impossible to formulate an intelligible concept or practice of authority [12]. If MacIntyre's contention is correct, it is easy to understand how frustrating it can be to address the subject of authority in the practice of medicine.[2]

In spite of confusion regarding the general question of authority in our society, medicine actually may be able to provide some insight into the concept of authority. For medicine does seem to be one of the few areas of modern life where some sense of authority remains viable. It is important to recognize, for example, that MacIntyre's argument turns not on the inherent character of medicine, but on society's lack of any common consensus and tradition through which the variety of goods can be ordered in a coherent manner. The problem of authority in medicine, therefore, is not peculiar to

George J. Agich (ed.), Responsibility in Health Care, 83–104.
Copyright © 1982 *by D. Reidel Publishing Company, Dordrecht, Holland.*

medicine, but rather is another indication of the general problem of authority today.[3]

There can be no doubt that physicians individually and as members of an elite profession continue to command *de facto* authority. For example, part of my duties is to teach seminarians who have no experience and little conception of the past power and authority of the priesthood. Most assume they are entering a devalued profession in which any authority they may attain depends largely on their personal characteristics. To help them at least understand the authority of the priesthood as role and office, I call their attention to how they regard their physicians. By revealing their willingness to accept direction from their physicians even when they often know little about the basis for such advice, I try to give them a sense about how people once looked to priests for direction. By its very nature, then, authority seems to involve people's willingness to accept judgments of another as superior to their own on the basis of that person's office and assumed skills ([12], p. 200).

A number of people might argue with the choice of such a parallel, especially if they infer incorrectly that priests should behave like physicians. From their perspective there could be no poorer paradigm than medicine for providing a resource for rethinking the nature of authority. This contention is based on the charge that reliance on physicians is justified neither morally nor medically. When patients give such power to physicians, poor medical care results because they are robbed of their own resources to maintain health. Attributing such authority to physicians encourages a medical authoritarianism and cultivates an almost uncontrollable resentment against the medical profession in general.

Although physicians may still be able to command *de facto* authority, this authority is by no means always legitimate. Why, then, have physicians individually and as a group been able to continue to command such authority in spite of what seems to be a widespread dissatisfaction with them? It is a singularly interesting question. Richard Blum notes that the "average citizen places the medical profession and its members at the top rung of social prestige".[4] While prestige is not the same as authority, it does suggest the level of respect that contributes to the authority of the profession of medicine. Physicians (unlike priests) are perceived by the majority to possess a particular moral commitment and special expertise by which they perform an irreplaceable service – to make people well when they become ill. Herein lies the contrast with the loss of authority in the priesthood – people are rather unsure whether they need saving, but they are certain that they want to get well when they are ill.

The critic of the authority and power of medicine may well respond that this contrast is exactly the point. For the authority of the physician is morally suspect *because* it derives from and exploits fears of illness and mankind's hopeless attempts to avoid death. Authority attributed to medicine (an attribution made all the more compelling by medicine's often exaggerated claims of being a science) is based on false and self-deceiving presuppositions of the power of medicine to cure. Though patients are the ones who confer such power on medicine, physicians are morally culpable for reinforcing, if not positively encouraging, such mistaken attitudes. The very illnesses that drive people to seek aid in the first place are used unfairly by physicians to reinforce their unjustified power over patients' lives. Rather than offering a defensible paradigm of authority, medicine remains one of the last institutions thwarting the individual's claim to rightful autonomy against all illegitimate authorities of the past.

Yet the authority of physicians shows no signs of crumbling. If those who approach these issues from a sociology of knowledge perspective are even close to being right, physicians are in an impregnable position. In fact, if physicians ever run short of diseases or illness it seems they are capable of helping to discover new ones. Medicine has the ability to make people sick as well as healthy. In this way, the necessity of physician services is assured, as well as the necessity of remaining under their authority.[5] Moreover, the moral commitments that physicians use to underwrite the autonomy of their profession turn out to be yet another way they are able to increase what is essentially their illegitimate power.[6]

It is important to note, however, that a number of these attacks on medicine draw on a political philosophy which presupposes that the autonomy of the individual renders all relations that are less than fully "voluntary" morally problematic.[7] Hence, all claims of authority are suspect. Insofar as illness is perceived to be a coercive condition, the power of physicians cannot help but be seen as illegitimate and a source of continued resentment. It seems, therefore, that the task must be to make the physician-patient relationship conform as nearly as possible to a contract between two voluntary agents.[8]

Such an ideal, however, not only distorts the kind of relationship that often does and should evolve between physician and patient, but it also assumes a false political and ethical ideal for all human relations. In contrast, the claim in this essay is that medicine does offer an alternative conception and practice of authority that can help in an appreciation of how other forms of authority should function in morally healthy societies. To be sure, physicians often misunderstand and abuse their authority, but this is not a sufficient reason for denying all authority to physicians. Instead, it is more desirable to try to understand the sense in which the authority exercised by physicians is valid.

Part of the difficulty of trying to develop a constructive account of medical authority is that the dominant moral and political conceptions of authority make it hard to acknowledge the different kinds of authority that still function in some social institutions. Richard Sennett has observed that the current dilemma of authority is that people feel attracted to strong figures not considered to be illegitimate; therefore, they try to protect themselves by denying authority to these figures or, even more self-deceptively, by claiming that no one (not even these strong figures) has power over them ([16], p. 26). Those forms of authority which people do find in their lives, moreover, inextricably appear destructive because they appear to lack the nurturance which authentic forms of authority provide. Simply to provide an alternative conception of authority, then, is insufficient. It is more important to try to elicit a sense of how authority can function legitimately.

II. AUTHORITY IN A LIBERAL SOCIETY: MACINTYRE'S CHALLENGE

An account of authority that may prove helpful in understanding the authority in and of medicine is that presented in MacIntyre's "Patients as Agents" [12]. MacIntyre's essay may seem to be an odd choice since the thrust of his argument is that maintaining an intelligible account of the practice of medical authority is no longer possible. He concludes that patients must become "agents" – autonomous, as nearly as possible, since they have no other alternative. What is particularly interesting about MacIntyre's argument is that his recommendation is not based on a view of autonomy as a moral good, but as a last resort in a society that lacks any means of determining how goods such as life, health, and freedom are related to one another ([12], p. 210).

Contrary to many philosophical accounts of authority, MacIntyre's does not contrast authority with rationality and/or autonomy. Indeed, he argues that authority and tradition are the necessary conditions for rationality ([12], p. 201). In support of this claim he appeals to recent arguments in the philosophy of science which indicate that any progress of natural science depends on the willingness of the scientific community to move into areas where agreement within the community cannot yet be secured.[9] That such is the case should not be surprising, according to MacIntyre –

authority is required in all human endeavors that involve the exercise of judgment.[10]

The nature of this authority is very much like that of a judge in the common law tradition. MacIntyre draws this parallel, stating that "in each case there is a rule-governed form of practice in which judgments as to how best to understand particular cases or in some cases how best to reformulate the rules in the light of particular cases are entrusted to certain individuals in virtue of recognition of their having a certain kind of experience and a consequent capacity for judgment".[11] Such judgment is not a mechanical procedure since it often has to go beyond existing precedents and current generalizations if it is to work out the anomalies in the tradition or meet demands of a new day. The prerequisite for the carrying on and growth of a tradition is a succession of authoritative voices. Thus, science has been able to grow because it has refused to adopt as adequate any specific methodology and instead has relied on the judgment of those skilled in the practices that constitute the scientific tradition.

According to MacIntyre, the flourishing of such a tradition and a correlative understanding of authority requires a high degree of moral consensus – trust in one's fellow practitioners as well as a shared vision of the goods internal to that practice and the procedures necessary to achieve those goods. Such a consensus is also required by the very nature of specialization required of those pursuing the particular goods within a community. While not everyone can master the same skills, specialization is encouraged because the limits of each specialist are underwritten and balanced by other community goods. Also required for the proper functioning of authority is an allocation of roles and rights within the practice and a shared acceptance of the constraints necessary to keep the practice from being distracted by external goods such as power, money, and fame ([12], pp. 201–202). (Needless to say, this is easier said than done.)

MacIntyre contends, therefore, that an authority which is internal to a practice is quite different from one required by organizational necessity. The latter presupposes inequality of power – authority becomes but a name for the power that some are given to insure compliance by others. This form of authority is necessary because an organization, in contrast to a practice, exists entirely to serve extrinsic purposes.[12] MacIntyre does not deny that often the role of authority in a practice may become so obscure that authority as an organizational necessity is required. It is part of the pathos of modern society that almost all forms of authority must become organizational to varying degrees.

To pursue further MacIntyre's distinction between a practice and an organization is unnecessary in the context of this paper.[13] More appropriate are some of MacIntyre's substantive, but insufficiently explicit, assumptions about community with respect to authority. The heart of his case involves an attempt to defend an account of authority that does not make the necessity of authority a correlative of human weakness. Authority is required not because human beings lack something or are innately evil. Rather, it derives from common participation in worthy endeavors. In this respect MacIntyre's basic intuitions are very similar to those of Yves Simon's account of authority [17].

Simon contends that authority originates in plenitude of human purposes rather than in the deficiency of human nature.[14] In contrast to political theorists such as Robert Dahl, who assume that the problem of authority is how "to reconcile personal choice with my nature as a social being",[15] Simon contends human nature is social exactly because community provides the means whereby the many goods people rightly desire can be actualized. Consequently, there should be a plurality of means in the pursuit of a community's common good. Indeed, the pursuit, or the conversation necessary for that pursuit, is in many ways the common good. For any conversation to occur a plurality is required, as well as a sufficient method of steadily procuring unity of action. Authority, therefore, is exactly that power which allows unified common action for the achievement of the common good ([17], pp. 47–48).

Authority is needed, according to Simon, because "it is desirable that particular goods should be taken care of by particular agencies" ([17], p. 72). (The diversity of skills and activities necessary for communities to flourish is a case in point.) It is because those goods are not known by necessity, but rather must be discovered through concrete judgments that authority is essential for the pursuit of the common good. In other words, if moral and political truth were necessary or universal, there would be no need for authority. Since truth involves judgment, however, people cannot seek it unaided. Put differently, all moral goods can be known through a political process.

MacIntyre's case for authority seems to presuppose something very much like this understanding of the nature of human community. His view becomes particularly important in light of his discussion of the exercise and legitimacy of traditional medical authority. The background and practice required to make intelligible the willingness of patients to let physicians take responsibility for them – responsibility not simply in terms of advice, but responsibility that *tells* patients what they must do – involves a cultural setting in which there is a clearly established view of the human good and in which there is a rational consensus on the order of human goods. The variety of human practices can be normatively ordered in terms of the goods internal to them. For each practice there is a profession which specifically pursues that good and cultivates those virtues necessary to achieve it. For example, the goods related to rational inquiry and the virtues of intellectual honesty, self-criticism and theoretical thinking are entrusted to the learned professions. The good of health is given to the medical profession with its concomitant virtues. There is accordingly a moral division of labor in society which requires that each part of society has to trust the other. The distribution of powers in this way is justified by the relationship of professions, goods, and virtues ([12], p. 206).

MacIntyre, like Simon, presupposes that the common good is served by "particular goods being taken care of by particular agencies". He does not assume that any society has perfectly institutionalized this pattern, but he argues that something approaching this pattern has provided the basis for professions in the past, particularly medicine.[16] It is only against this background that the current situation can be assessed: in the absence of any shared moral consensus about the goods necessary for individual and community flourishing, traditional medical authority cannot be vindicated or sustained. Thus MacIntyre argues that a profession today is something anomalous:

> ... not quite a craftsman's guild, not quite a trade union of skilled workers, not quite anything. Its various characteristics have lost their connection with the principles which made of their variety a relatively unified whole. This is what has happened in our culture, so I am suggesting, to such professions as schoolteaching and medicine, and it at once makes their peculiar claims to authority implausible and unintelligible. The recognition of authority and the concept of profession are inseparably linked.[17]

MacIntyre's account of authority aids in understanding why medicine's authority does not derive directly from the scientific or technical skill of the physician or surgeon. The authority of the doctor is not that of the "expert", at least not in the sense in which that term is currently used.[18] Rather, a physician's authority derives from physicians' and patients' common moral benefits and shared participation in a practice that embodies those beliefs. The physician's authority thus is based upon mastery of the moral and practical skills involved in that physician's commitment to care for and never abandon the ill and the dying. Obviously, this view involves a particular understanding of medicine.

III. WHAT MEDICINE PROFESSES: THE AUTHORITY OF THE BODY

To sustain the argument about the nature of authority necessitates nothing less than a philosophy of medicine that at least makes credible the claim that medicine is a practice of the kind suggested above. Edmund Pellegrino and David Thomasma have provided some insight as to what an adequate philosophy of medicine entails [15]. They reiterate that medicine is a complex activity and as such is difficult to characterize philosophically. For example, they argue that medicine is neither art nor science, but a *tertium quid* involving both but distinct from each. Medicine is the "cognitive art of applying science and persuasion through a complex human interaction in which a mutually satisfactory state of well-being is sought, and in which the uniqueness of values and disease, and the kind of institution in which care is delivered, determine the nature of the judgments made" ([15], p. 69). Or medicine is "a relation of mutual consent to effect individualized well-being by working in, with, and through the body" ([15], p. 80).

One aspect of Pellegrino and Thomasma's account which is crucial to any understanding of the kind of authority medicine does or at least should have is the insistence that whatever else medicine may involve, the overriding commitment of physicians is to care for individuals who come to them with complaints of illness. They conclude that "medicine *as* medicine is a process aimed at an action taken in the interest of a specific patient. Its chief aim is not discovery of laws of nature. The end of medicine, its justifying principle, is, in the final analysis a moral one: the good of a person seeking help" ([15], p. 147).

Pellegrino and Thomasma thus make the interesting suggestion that medicine is not only science and art, but also a virtue. They argue that what constitutes medicine is the accumulated wisdom of well-reasoned and concrete judgments about the "capacity to act with regard to the things that are good or bad for man" ([15], p. 148). The practice of medicine is thus "a habit of the mind" that embodies the good inherent in the process of healing. Since health is a good, it follows that medicine must be a virtue, because a virtue "must make right choices about the ends and purposes for which the decisions and actions are produced. Medicine must not only perform well but also act well. It must choose what should be done to heal a particular whose good is the true end of the whole activity" ([15], p. 148).

Surely the claim that medicine is a virtue is an odd one, because a virtue is a disposition of a particular agent. Pellegrino and Thomasma, on the other hand, interpret medicine to be a relation. Of course, it is true that Aristotle called justice and friendship virtues, though each is clearly a quality of a relation rather than a good inherent to the self.[19] That a relation may be subject to virtuous formation is but a reminder that all virtues require formation through the practical judgments shaped by the wisdom of a community's translations. Medicine, therefore, is a virtue insofar as it is the name for a tradition of wisdom concerning good care of the body. As such it is not a "means" to health, but rather is part of the activity of health – an activity that involves as much the participation of the patient as the physician.

Pellegrino and Thomasma's case for medicine as a moral profession goes well beyond the notion that health is a normative category.[20] The issue is not simply that medicine involves values in decisions concerning the care of particular patients, but that medicine is an activity which requires as well as enhances a virtuous life.[21] In this context, the physician is not the sole participant in the activity; rather, medicine becomes a relation that inextricably involves patient and physician. This does not mean that patients need to possess the skills of their physicians; it is sufficient that patients have moral reasons to trust physicians to support their patients' life projects insofar as those projects involve a well-functioning body.

The very willingness of patients to permit physicians to be present as well as to lay hands on them in times of crisis is a telling indication of physician dependence on patients. In this respect, perhaps the best way of thinking about the medical relation is to see it as fundamentally an educational process both for doctor and patient, in which each is both teacher and learner [13]. It is from patients that physicians learn the wisdom of the body. Both physicians and patients must learn that each of them is subject to a prior authority – the authority of the body. The form and practice of medicine may change throughout history and differ from one cultural setting to another, but these differences in the end are merely reflections of different attitudes toward the body and are regulated finally by the body. Medicine thus represents a trans-cultural practice of learning to live with finitude.[22]

Pellegrino and Thomasma, however, properly insist that "the body" is by no means a straightforward category ([15], pp. 73–74). Each person is not simply a physical body, but a "lived body" which organizes a whole field of perceptions in addition to being the subject of a history of experiences.[23] The body sets the norm for medicine because it is the "artist of its own healing" ([15], p. 79). The task of medicine is to aid that process so that individuals may better learn to live in and through their bodies, since they cannot successfully live beyond or without their bodies. Medicine is therefore a tradition of inherited wisdom and practices through which physicians acquire the responsibility to remember, learn, and pass on the skills of learning to live with a body.

As mentioned before, there is little evidence to support the claim that the health of a population is a result of the practice of medicine. Except for the contentions of those persons who try to justify the special privileges of medicine in this light, the claim should not be viewed as a judgment against medicine. Those who justify privileges are responsible in part for the eventual perversion of medicine, since medical authority cannot long be sustained by promising more and more cures through technological advances.[24]

Wise physicians, on the other hand, have learned their craft better. As Eric Cassell notes, the primary task of physicians is to remove the world of illness from the unknown to the known world where it can become subject to human care ([6], p. 131). Their task, however, is not limited to those who become ill. By steadfastly identifying with the ill, physicians become teachers also for the healthy. Part of the physician's vocation, therefore, is to serve as a bridge between the world of the sick and the world of the healthy.

The sick constitute a threat to us by making us aware of the frailty of our own connectedness, the thinness of our shield of reason and the limit of our control over the world. By segregating the sick in hospitals having special rules of behavior, the threat for us and the sick is somewhat mitigated, if not entirely eliminated. It is not surprising that we do not often discuss or even secretly recognize the essential characteristics of sickness, because it would be too frightening to do so. This carries over into medicine itself. Cassell points out: "Ostensibly, the physician deals only with disease elements of the illness. His manifest function is the cure of disease, but his latent function, healing, which involves restoring the sick to the world of the healthy, is a secret even to himself" ([6], p. 46). Because physicians have this task, they stand as a constant reminder that the worlds of the sick and the healthy are actually one world joined by common destiny.

In his book *The Healer's Art*, Cassell provides impetus for the contention that medicine is primarily an educational process by showing how physicians act as arbitrators between patients and their bodies ([6], p. 47). Yet as important as Cassell's explicit thesis is the way in which he uses examples to make his case. These examples nicely reveal how he was in fact educated by his patients to understand what medicine is about.[25] The wisdom manifest in Cassell's book is therefore a witness to the wisdom of the body that teaches "what life is really about underneath the social conventions."[26]

This point is exemplified in Cassell's observation that it is possible, and even a duty, for a physician to teach patients how to die – "to give his patients in this final stage of life the same kind of control that can be taught in earlier stages of living" ([6], p. 203). This is not to say that teaching patients how to die is the first priority. Cassell admits that the primary duty of a physician is to aid in patients' recovery. He is not suggesting that the physician can give the patient control for which the patient does not already have the resources. Patients cannot and should not be made to die better than they have lived.[27] Likewise, medicine should refrain from substituting technology for a patient's lack of moral resources. Physicians, however, can help their dying patients to acquire the "innate ability to command the body, and then enlist the aid of those who surround him – family, friends, and physician. It is dependent on what humans have within themselves; to that extent it is a lonely thing, as is death itself. But the dying are also dependent on others and relationship is based on trust. Both inner resources and trust in others are required because the enemy of control is fear" ([6], p. 204).

It is ironic, though, that what people fear is loss of control. That fear is so all-consuming an indication of the common misunderstanding of what control of the body entails. To control the body does not mean to "manage" or even, as Cassell suggests, to "soar" over the body ([6], p. 146), but rather to appreciate how the body's limitations are also the source of the most creative and interesting possibilities available to us.[28] Cassell concludes:

> I think that those who die well and in control have something to teach the living about the body and about living. They show us that it is possible to come to peace with the body, both to be controlled by its limitations and to control it to a far greater extent than unlearned existence would suggest. They teach us that control is not denial or repression. That which we deny or repress about ourselves or within ourselves controls us by the very fact of our constant need to deny rather than to come to terms. Control implies acceptance of limitations plus an awareness that the limitations provide room for the continued exercise of self, even into death. The beauty and potential of growth lie not only in intellectual transcendence and the formation of transcendent emotional bonds, but also in the possibility of dynamic unity with the body. In that state the fear of death, an essentially backward look, becomes unimportant ([6], p. 228).

Medicine is therefore a learned profession because it literally learns from patients the skills necessary for acceptance of the possibilities and limits of the body. It is a tradition comprised of the skills of caring for, and sometimes even curing, those who are ill. Medicine is a profession because it has learned how to teach and initiate new agents into that tradition and how to govern the practice of their skills. That even neophyte physicians have authority indicates that medicine as a practice does not begin *ex nihilo* with each new generation. On the other hand, young physicians acquire their skills in a manner that makes them their own. Learning is thus fundamentally a moral training because the skills are of the sort that can be mastered only by watching a master perform them. Such learning is necessary not only in order to pass on tradition, but also because it is the source of critique and innovation of tradition.

In summary, medicine constitutes a community formed by an authority not too unlike MacIntyre's understanding of authority. People are participants in a community based on common bodily existence that has the potential to sustain the authority of medicine as an educational practice. Specialization, or, preferably, the calling of some members of the community to become physicians, is justified by the community's need to have some of its members committed to practicing the wisdom of the body. That such a calling is required and justified indicates the kind of knowledge which can be gained through learning from the body, as well as the kind of skills necessary to care for individuals who are ill. This knowledge and these skills are not universal truths that can be known by just anyone. Rather, they are matters of learned judgments and wisdom which can only be sustained by those willing to place themselves under the guidance of an acknowledged master.

IV. THE COMMUNITY OF AND REQUIRED BY MEDICINE

Even if this account of medicine is persuasive (and there obviously are powerful challenges to the arguments raised here), it remains unclear whether these arguments successfully respond to MacIntyre's challenge. MacIntyre might even accept the construal of authority in medicine proposed in this essay, but argue that what is lacking is a wider community and/or morality sufficient to sustain and support such a medicine. This response probably would be apropos, but it is important to understand why.

As suggested earlier, physicians like Cassell insist that one of medicine's tasks is to teach us how to die. This task is drawn from the authority of the body. But in the absence of any consensus of what an appropriate death morally involves, how can any profession be entrusted with such an important task? It is no wonder that in the absence of such consensus or community the medical profession is tempted to become a self-protective interest group which tries to secure unwarranted power over our lives by claiming to be in possession of a knowledge peculiar to itself. It tries to justify its power by being what it cannot – a science that frees us from, rather than teaching us, the limits of our bodies. This is not really the result of increasing technological power. Instead, increasing technological power is an attempt to maintain the moral coherence of medicine in a morally incoherent society – that is, medicine gains its moral coherence by drawing on the fear of death, the one thing people still seem to have in common. As a result, rather than a profession which provides assistance in living with the body, medicine becomes the modern analogue to the gnostic heresy.[29]

Put differently, a medicine which assumes that its first task is educative in the sense I suggested here cannot help but appear as a sectarian community and challenge to a pluralistic society. This point can be illustrated by calling attention to the difficulty as well as necessity of physicians avowing their fallibility. That such an avowal is necessary is implied in the commitment to care for individual patients. This commitment involves contingent judgments which in principle exclude certainty.[30] Of course, some judgments can be more assured than others, but in principle physicians know they are making judgments for which they cannot claim infallibility.[31] Therefore, the physician's pledge to the patient (or perhaps more appropriately, the *covenant* that the physician and patient enter) does not include a guarantee of errorless judgment, but rather a pledge of steadfast presence and care.

The avowal of fallibility required of physicians is also necessitated through their commitment to learning how better to care for their patients, which is not the same thing as the growth of medical knowledge. Good patient care, as well as good science, depends on the willingness to expose what does not work as readily as that which works. Failure is actually more important than success. Consequently, what is good for medicine as a profession may be disquieting to the patient who sees the physician as savior. Patients have to learn that they cannot put themselves under the care of physicians and in doing so assume that such care can be without error.[32] Indeed, patients must face the possibility that the best possible medicine of the day may be the wrong thing for them.[33] This is no reason to reject the care the physician can offer, but it does change decisively the attitude with what care should be approved.

Yet as this essay suggests, the practice of fallible medicine cannot help but appear as a sectarian alternative in our society. Medicine as a profession only exists because it is also supported by an equally sectarian community formed by essential convictions. Such a community must not presuppose that the task of medicine is to keep illness and death at bay as if such a task were an end in itself. Rather, the community should recognize that medicine involves those skills which allows its members to continue pursuing the goods of that community. These benefits naturally will be offset by some members suffering from illness and finally dying. Thus, a fallible medicine is sustained not only because this medicine serves the common good, but also because participation is a form of service for the whole community.

The absence of such a community in actuality, however, has meant that medicine (as MacIntyre suggests) increasingly has been forced to take the form of a contract between patient and physician. Contracts are the moral substitutes for modern society's lack of shared moral tradition. Of necessity medicine continues to insist that it is a self-sufficient institution, at least in part as an attempt to preserve its past commitment to the service of individual patients. As a result:

> ... it develops and maintains in the profession a self-deceiving view of the objectivity and reliability of its knowledge and the virtues of its members. Furthermore, it encourages the profession to see itself as the sole possessor of knowledge and virtue, to be somewhat suspicious of the technical and moral capacity of other occupations, and to be at best patronizing and at worst contemptuous of its clientele. Protecting the profession from the demands of interaction on a free and equal basis with those in the world outside, its autonomy leads the profession to so distinguish its own virtue from those outside as to be unable to even perceive the need for, let alone undertake, the self-regulation it promises ([8], p. 370).

Until now the only solution to this dilemma has been to demand more patient "autonomy", that is, to use the disease to try to cure the disease. This strategy is doomed to fail since the contract between physician and patient can never be "voluntary" in that the very condition which encourages patients to seek their physicians' help is coercive. Physicians are also bound to this contract by the fact that in their state of submission, patients expect the impossible. Once physicians fail, as they inevitably will, patients will blame them.

There seems to be little possibility of breaking this vicious cycle of false expectations and correlatively distorted forms of authority and power. At least for awhile the practice of medicine probably will remain better than critics of medicine allege. MacIntyre suggests that one possible strategy would be to work with "those with whom one does share sufficient beliefs to rescue and to recreate authority within communities that will break with the pluralist ethos. In medicine it means working for a variety of new forms of medical community, each with its own shared moral allegiance. With these the notion of authority could again begin to find context and content" ([12], p. 212).

This strategy might also have the unexpected effect of aiding in understanding the relationship between religious and medical communities. Ironically, the appropriate sense of the authority of medicine probably is not unrelated to the authority of the priesthood mentioned at the beginning of this essay. The ability of a community to sustain a fallible medicine, a medicine that understands its first task to be mediating between us and our bodies, is ultimately dependent on convictions about goods that set the task of medicine within a larger framework. When these goods are not seen to exist, or at least can be safely ignored, medicine is tempted to become an end in itself. It thus becomes a pseudo-salvific institution.

In other words, medicine requires the existence of another institution to be able to keep its extremely significant, but limited, task *limited*. This does not mean that religious convictions should be supported in order to sustain medicine. Indeed, such functional justifications of religious beliefs are ill-advised. (If religious beliefs are false, then they should not be entertained no matter what good results they might engender.) Yet the fact that medicine as a practice requires convictions and institutions beyond itself to sustain its activity at least helps us understand why we are constantly tempted to ask too much of medicine in our secular times.

University of Notre Dame

NOTES

1 Aspects of modern medicine correspond to each of Weber's types, but this should not be surprising since as "types" they are not meant to be mutually exclusive. For an analysis of medicine that draws more directly from Weber's theory of monopolization, see Berlant [2].

2 One of the difficulties with this topic involves how one should draw the distinction between authority *in* medicine and authority *of* medicine. Most of the current discussion is concerned with the latter, but the former is possibly more important. The question of authority in medicine seems to involve organizational and procedural questions internal to the profession, while the latter concerns questions of the profession (and its representatives) over those who are recipients of medical care. Questions about the nature and legitimacy of each kind of authority are certainly different, but not unrelated. The authority *of* medicine depends for its legitimacy on claims about how authority functions *in* medicine. It becomes evident that part of the issue involving the authority of medicine is whether medicine ever has been the sort of practice capable of maintaining internal authority or whether, even if it once had the capability, it still is able to maintain that authority. For a fascinating depiction of how authority functions in medicine, see Bosk [4]. Bosk contends that the authority of attending physicians over their subordinates in surgery is not ultimately based on technical skill (though that must surely be present), but rather resides in their moral commitment:

> The professional's last line of defense is a moral one because it is a proper moral performance alone that substantiates a claim to proper technical performance when events mock such a claim. Moral error breaches a professional's contract with his client. He has

not acted in good faith. He has done less than he should have. Such conduct is not honest and defensible but undercuts all the presumptions on which the professional-client relationship is based. For this reason moral errors are treated more seriously than technical ones. Hence the control of technical performance is subordinated to the control of moral performance; without the overarching moral system, the technical system is not amenable to control ([4], p. 171).

Bosk's study as a whole is an impressive counter to the often-made claim that physicians receive almost no ethical training; he documents well that "post-graduate training of surgeons is above all things a technical training" (p. 190). Thus, technical error can be forgiven, but not moral error.

[3] See, for example, Nisbet [14] and Sennett [16]. One of the fascinating aspects of recent discussions of this topic is how similar the analysis of this social "problem" is from those on the political left and right.

[4] ([3], p. 67). Blum's book is meant to be a guide to help the doctor better "manage" the patient, but in fact it is an extremely useful account of the kinds of skills required if medicine is to be a legitimate practice. Thus, Blum argues that "the physician who fails to act as educator will be opening up the floodgates of disaster, both for himself and for his patient. Proper management of the relationship requires that the patient be an informed treatment partner of the doctor, one who knows what the basic assumptions of the profession and practice of medicine are, and one who knows something about the general content and limits of knowledge about the human body" ([3], pp. 287–88). Of course Blum fails to note that such a patient might prove difficult to "manage".

[5] Thus, Eliot Freidson maintains that "by virtue of being the authority on what illness 'really' is, medicine creates the social possibilities for acting sick. In this sense, medicine's monopoly includes the right to create illness as an official social role. It is part of being a profession to be given the official power to define and therefore create the shape of problematic segments of social behavior" ([8], p. 206). Freidson is not denying that disease involves biophysical processes, but that when it is defined as an illness by medicine it is changed: "Thus, when a veterinarian diagnoses a cow's condition as an illness, he does not merely by diagnosis change the cow's behavior: to the cow, illness remains as an experienced biophysical state, no more. But when a physician diagnoses a human's condition as illness, he changes the man's behavior by diagnosis: a social state is added to a biophysical state by assigning the meaning of illness to disease" ([8], p. 223).

[6] See, for example, Berlant's compelling analysis of the development of medical ethics from Percival's code to the present day as a study of the legitimation of medical monopolization ([2], pp. 64–127).

[7] For a good example of the political implications of this supposition, see Dahl [7]. What proponents of such a view often fail to realize is that autonomy itself is a form of authority which can be as destructive as paternalism. For a sensitive discussion of autonomy as a form of authority, see Sennett ([16], pp. 84–121). Sennett suggests that the stress on autonomy forces all human relationships to be understood as forms of manipulation to maintain dominance. He states that

... when a person is needed by others more than he needs them, he can afford to be indifferent to them. If the bureaucrat ignores the distress of the welfare client filling out complicated forms, if the doctor treats his clients like bodies rather than persons, these very acts of indifference maintain dominance. In the complex form of autonomy, keeping cool when others make demands on you or challenge you is a way of keeping the upper hand. Of course, few people set out to be rude or callous. But autonomy removes the necessity of dealing with other people openly and mutually. There is an imbalance, they show their need for you more than you show your need for them. This puts you in control ([16], p. 86).

Sennett thus argues that appeals to autonomy as a way to legitimize certain relations is an illusion, because such appeals disguise the fact that one side holds more power. This imbalance often goes unnoticed, though, because it is assumed that in an autonomous relationship there is no power present – or if present, it is legitimate since it is exercised "impersonally" ([16], pp. 104–116).

[8] I certainly do not intend my argument to be an apology for everything done in the name of modern medicine. If applied consistently, the position developed in this essay would require some profound changes in the practice and institutionalization of medicine. However, I have tried to present my argument in a positive manner since what we need is not another diatribe about what is wrong with medicine, but some sense of what constructively needs to be done. Criticizing modern medicine is a little like continuing to criticize the failings of the church – it is fun, but finally not very interesting intellectually. For example, Beauchamp and Childress certainly do not attempt to make autonomy the only value by which medical care is ethically evaluated, but it is nonetheless true that it is one of their central commitments ([1], pp. 56–96, 201–227). They explicitly deny that autonomy qualifies all claims to authority, but still maintain the latter is only legitimate when it is "autonomously accepted" ([1], p. 61). As a result they fail to appreciate that "autonomy" has in fact become their overriding authority – only it is not independently justified. From such a perspective the primary issue for physician-patient relations is whether they are paternalistic and how such paternalism can be avoided. By offering a different account of authority I do not mean to deny many of the valuable criticism made against the medical profession by those who assume "autonomy" is the litmus test for all authority.

[9] MacIntyre suggests that this understanding of scientific authority is very similar to some accounts of church authority – particularly in relation to questions of doctrinal development. I suspect he is right and that the analysis of the similarities and differences would prove to be an extremely fruitful enterprise. For an attempt to understand the authority of scripture in a similar manner, see Hauerwas ([9], pp. 53–71). The analogy of science and theological development may not be entirely happy, however, as it tends to suggest that tradition always grows in a positive direction. That is by no means the case. In fact, one of the remarkable things about Scripture is the inclusion in the text itself of the mistaken directions tradition has taken. Even more importantly, Scripture does not make clear in itself which were the mistakes and which were the successes. This makes it necessary for each new generation to struggle with and continue the arguments begun in Scripture itself.

[10] I simply do not have the competence to state, much less defend, the epistemological assumptions underlying this claim. I assume, with Aristotle, that ethics deals with "matters that can be other," and that such is the case is not an epistemological liability except for those who assume that necessary knowledge is paradigmatic of truth. Moreover, I assume that much of our knowledge, such as that in medicine, involves knowledge

that is more like moral knowledge than certain epistemological theories assume. That this is so, however, does not entail that such knowledge is any way deficient or false.
[11] ([12], pp. 199–200). Bosk points out that there are

> ... two competing systems of legitimation for medical authority: clinical expertise and scientific evidence. These systems are not of equal importance: in the case of discrepant opinion, arguments based on clinical expertise override those based on scientific evidence. Such a system of legitimation concentrates power in the person of the attending physician. On the one hand, he is the active creator of the most recent scientific evidence: in some specific cases the attending physician is literally the last word on the subject. On the other hand, by virtue of his clinical experience, he knows when scientific findings are not appropriate for charting a course of action. He knows the rules and their exceptions. The subordinate is learning the rules; he does not yet have enough experience to recognize the exceptions ([4], p. 85).

That is why medical training inherently requires apprenticeship to a master, since it is only through the master that one can acquire the experience necessary for the training of judgment.
[12] MacIntyre defines a practice as

> ... any coherent and complex form of socially established cooperative human activity through which goods internal to that form of activity are realized in the course of trying to achieve those standards of excellence which are appropriate to, and partially definitive of, that form of activity, with the result that human powers to achieve excellence, and human conceptions of the ends and goods involved, are systematically extended. Tic-tac-toe is not an example of a practice in this sense, nor is throwing a football with skill; but the game of football is, and so is chess. Planting turnips is not a practice; farming is ([11], p. 175).

Practices have standards, of course, though they are not immune from criticism. It is still true, however, that we cannot be initiated into a practice without accepting the authority of the best standards to date for that practice. That is why it is essential to note that practices have a history, as they are not constituted by goals fixed for all time, but the goals themselves are transmuted by the history of the practice. MacIntyre's analysis of practice is crucial for his understanding of virtue since the latter is "an acquired human quality the possession and exercise of which tends to enable us to achieve those goods which are internal to practices and the lack of which effectively prevents us from achieving any such goods" ([11], p. 178).
[13] Furthermore, there is the question of whether medicine is a practice. MacIntyre clearly identifies it as such and I think he is correct to do so.
[14] See also Simon ([18], pp. 144–194). Simon's theory of authority is dependent on his theory of prudence, or moral judgment. It is fortunately soon to be published in English [19].
[15] ([7), p. 8). It is very interesting to note that Dahl's example of the "criteria of competence" as a qualification of the "criteria of choice" is that of medicine.
[16] There are further issues involved in MacIntyre's view that can only be mentioned in this context: the question of the relation of a practice to an institution and the problem of the unity or possible conflict between the virtues. In terms of the first question, MacIntyre maintains that practices must not be confused with institutions since the

latter are characteristically concerned with external goods. No practice can survive without institutions, as they characteristically form a single causal order; yet, that such is the case means a practice is constantly open to distortion. That is why the virtues are essential, since without them a practice cannot resist the corrupting power of institutions ([11], p. 181). Against Plato, MacIntyre maintains the possibility of the conflict of virtues. That is why our "situation is tragic in that we have to recognize the authority of both claims. There is an objective moral order, but our perceptions of it are such that we cannot bring rival moral truths into complete harmony" ([11], p. 134). That is why we require a community capable of maintaining the necessary conversation between practices, each of which we may need, but which are in potential if not actual conflict. Moreover, the very need for specialization assumes added importance from this perspective because often the specializations reflect different virtues which society needs, but which may be in conflict. Accordingly, a morally healthy society may well be one that is able to sustain the necessary tension between professions.

[17] ([12], p. 207). I am not denying, of course, that physicians' expertise is irrelevant to their authority. Rather, I am suggesting that this expertise is relevant only within a more determinative moral framework.

[18] However, Blum documents that most patients attribute authority to physicians today primarily because they are considered such "experts" ([3], pp. 81 ff.). This is part of the reason attempts to define a "profession" are so inconclusive. A profession is inherently a normative concept denoting service to the basic goods which a particular community thinks are essential for its moral identity. The reason many specializations which require perhaps even more skill than the traditional professions still are not professions is because they are not essential to the community's moral purpose – though they may be to its physical survival.

[19] For a more extended analysis of this point, see Hauerwas ([9], pp. 111–127). I cannot pretend, however, to have dealt sufficiently with all the issues raised by suggesting that a relation is capable of being qualified by a virtue.

[20] See, for example, Eric Cassell's claims in this respect ([6], pp. 87, 113). Of course, I am not denying that various illnesses involve normative judgment, but I am suggesting the idea of "health" as a clear and distinct idea is a chimera. Health is an activity with a shifting meaning. The current attempt to limit the province of medicine by developing a firm definition of health is thus doomed to failure.

[21] From this perspective one of the most overlooked aspects of our current situation is how medical schools continue to function as schools of virtue. They are among the few institutions in our society that have coherent enough purpose that enables them to form character. I only wish we could exhibit the same kind of self-confidence in our seminaries.

[22] This fact may be one of the reasons that medicine and religion are always interrelated. Each deals with the same subject, but in different ways. Both are tempted to deny the special task of the other in hopes of being the sole authority. In truth, neither can be helpful without the other.

[23] For a particularly compelling account of the notion of "embodiment" and its implications for medicine, see Richard Zaner [21]. Zaner's analysis is particularly helpful in suggesting how bodies are at once "mine" and yet "not mine," but nonetheless not an object that can be placed over or against a person.

[24] Again the church provides a useful illustration in this respect. The more specialized

the function of the priest became from that of the layman, the more the potential for the delegitimation of the priesthood itself. The more laymen viewed their priests' roles as foreign to their own lives, the more likely it became that the roles of the priests would be associated with magic and/or arbitrary power. This would result finally in either rejection or legitimacy, the latter by making Christianity a mystery cult. With rejection laymen are no better off because too often priestly authority is rejected in the name of an equally destructive authority which offers a bogus salvation. The technological form of contemporary medicine involves many of the same dangers. The more laymen are prevented from understanding what is being done to them in the name of science, the more likely they are to turn to alternative forms of care. Quackery and purely technological medicine are but two sides of the same coin. From the laymen's perspective they are judged by the same criterion – results.

[25] Cassell's examples are not just illustrations – they are the argument, and rightly so. Contrary to the most contemporary accounts of argument, I assume that good arguments cannot be separated from the context that makes them intelligible in the first place. It would take me too far afield to develop this point, but stated briefly it involves the contention that there exists no foundational point on which arguments as such rest. Rather, all arguments begin in the midst of things and are proved true or false exactly by how plausibly they display the narratives on which they depend. For a more thorough defense of this view, see David Burrell [5].

[26] No doubt Cassell means that when people are faced with illness or death they exhibit what they want and what they are. But I think it wrong to suggest this is a challenge to social convention, since what we really want and are is itself a convention. Conventions are sometimes lies but they are also just as likely to be the way to truth.

[27] For further reflection on this idea, see Hauerwas [10].

[28] Cassell's way of putting this is an interesting case of someone's insight fighting against its own expression. Although Cassell uses the word "soar", the very examples he uses (polio victims' struggles to retain some control over their bodies) suggest that "soaring" is really more a matter of learning to live at peace with the body. The same kind of problem occurs in Cassell's defense of the importance of the "omnipotence" of physicians for helping patients recover their own omnipotence. Yet Cassell's own critique of the dangers of such omnipotence for physician and patient alike suggests that the control patients seek is not so much omnipotence as simply the power to make their lives their own ([6], pp. 142–145).

[29] Gnosticism was not only a Christian heresy, but a widespread and extremely complex phenomenon in the ancient world. No simple generalization can be sufficient to characterize gnostic beliefs or practices. By suggesting that some aspects of modern medicine bear close analogy to gnosticism I mean no more than: (1) medicine, like gnosticism, is often seen, at least implicitly, as offering a form of salvation; (2) that such salvation is obtained through esoteric knowledge possessed by those who have a special training; and (3) that the salvation offered is basically an attempt to free us from the limits of our bodies.

[30] ([15], p. 124). Actually, Bosk [4] presents the most complete analysis of error in medicine. He distinguishes between *technical errors*, which are expected to happen to everyone and which must thus be quickly reported, *judgmental errors*, which involve clinical judgments, and *normative* and *quasi-normative errors*, which involve a failure to fulfill the moral expectations of the physician's role. In medicine the former must be

exposed and forgiven, since only in that way can the failure be prevented from happening again ([4], p. 128). Thus Bosk notes that Grand Rounds and Mortality and Morbidity Conferences are actually elaborate rituals "the entire congregation of surgeons have evolved for witnessing them [errors], resolving the confusion they create, and incorporating them into the group's history and the individual's biography" ([4], p. 121).

[31] Their account of clinical judgments is particularly worth reading, as is their argument for the necessity of discretionary space in professional judgments ([15], pp. 155–169). For a particularly biting critique of the model of the clinician as requiring personal judgment to justify the "autonomy" of the physician, see Freidson ([8], pp. 346–349). However, Bosk's study of how medical students are trained to assume the moral role of "professional self-control" at least qualifies Freidson's critique. Bosk points out, "The problem is not, as some have claimed, an absence of any socialization, controls, or ethical sense in the profession; the problem is rather a system which celebrates individual conscience as a control while ignoring corporate responsibility. The profession of medicine needs to develop structural remedies – or structure socialization – in a way that brings into balance both the corporate and the individual dimensions of control" ([4], p. 188).

[32] I have not discussed the implication of my analysis of the authority of medicine for the specification of and/or relation between the various roles in medicine – i.e. physician, nurse, counselor. I think no *apriori* formula exists by which this can be done. Different roles develop historically as part of medicine's conversation with itself or are governed by changing needs of patients. However, the current dominance of the physician, in part justified by their technical expertise, or the attempt of the physician to usurp all other roles, is dangerous for the physician as well as the patient. If the physician is "first among equals," he is so because of the need to have someone morally responsible, not simply because of his expertise.

[33] It is interesting that Bosk only treats the necessity of surgeons to expose errors among themselves – he does not ask if error should also be exposed to the patient and, if so, what would be the implication of such exposure.

BIBLIOGRAPHY

1. Beauchamp, T. and Childress, J.: 1979, *Principles of Biomedical Ethics*, Oxford University Press, New York and Oxford.
2. Berlant, J. L.: 1975, *Profession and Monopoly*, University of California Press, Berkeley.
3. Blum, R.: 1960, *The Management of the Doctor-Patient Relationship*, McGraw-Hill, New York.
4. Bosk, C. L.: 1979, *Forgive and Remember: Managing Medical Failure*, University of Chicago Press, Chicago.
5. Burrell, D.: 1981, 'Argument in Theology: Analogy and Narrative', *Journal of the American Academy of Religion: New Dimensions in Philosophy of Religion* (forthcoming).
6. Cassell, E.: 1976, *The Healer's Art: A New Approach to the Doctor-Patient Relationship*, J. B. Lippincott Company, Philadelphia.
7. Dahl, R.: 1970, *After the Revolution*?, Yale University Press, New Haven.
8. Freidson, E.: 1970, *Profession of Medicine*, Harper and Row, New York.

9. Hauerwas, S.: 1981, *A Community of Character*, University of Notre Dame Press, Notre Dame.
10. Hauerwas, S.: 1978, 'Religious Conceptions of Brain Death and Associated Problems', *Annals of the New York Academy of Science* **315**, 329–338.
11. MacIntyre, A.: 1981, *After Virtue: A Study in Moral Theory*, University of Notre Dame Press, Notre Dame.
12. MacIntyre, A.: 1977, 'Patients as Agents', in H. T. Engelhardt, Jr., and S. F. Spicker (eds.), *Philosophical and Medical Ethics: Its Nature and the Significance*, Reidel Publishing Company, Dordrecht, Holland, pp. 197–212.
13. May, W.: 1977, 'Code and Covenant or Philanthropy and Contract?', in W. Curran, A. Dyke, S. Reiser (eds.), *Ethics in Medicine: Historical Perspectives and Contemporary Concerns*, MIT Press, Cambridge, pp. 65–76.
14. Nisbet, R.: 1975, *Twilight of Authority*, Oxford University Press, New York.
15. Pellegrino, E. D. and Thomasma, D. C.: 1981, *A Philosophical Basis of Medical Practice*, Oxford University Press, New York.
16. Sennett, R.: 1980, *Authority*, Alfred Knopf, New York.
17. Simon, Y.: 1980, *A General Theory of Authority*, University of Notre Dame Press, Notre Dame.
18. Simon, Y.: 1951, *Philosophy of Democratic Government*, University of Chicago Press, Chicago.
19. Simon, Y.: *A Critique of Moral Knowledge*, R. MacInnerney (tr.), University of Notre Dame Press, Notre Dame (forthcoming).
20. Weber, Max: 1958, 'The Social Psychology of the World Religions', in H. H. Gerth and C. W. Mills (eds.), *Max Weber: Essays in Sociology*, Oxford University Press, New York, pp. 295–301.
21. Zaner, R.: 1978, 'Embodiment', in W. Reich (ed.), *Encyclopedia of Bioethics*, Free Press, New York, pp. 361–365.

RICHARD E. FLATHMAN

POWER, AUTHORITY, AND RIGHTS IN THE PRACTICE OF MEDICINE

Power, authority, and rights are edgy, adversarial notions. They come into play primarily where there is disagreement and incipient or at least latent conflict. Exploring these somewhat contentious ideas (whose home ground of politics is an arena in which we expect contention) in the context of the practice of medicine might seem marginal if not alien. The argument of this essay is that an image of a kind of constrained disputation or conflict – an image at once suggested by and conducive to the use of "power", "authority", and "rights" – is in fact appropriate to much of current medical practice. As might be expected of a political theorist, this argument will be presented in part through models and analogies familiar from political thought and practice. But the matters before us are sensitive. For this and more specifically analytical reasons that will emerge as we proceed, it will be well to seek perspective by first giving attention to the venerable and apparently more comfortable notion that medicine forms a practice.

I

The concept of a practice is a tolerably rich and variegated notion which in several guises has been put to considerable service in nineteenth- and twentieth-century thought.[1] Of its salient aspects or dimensions, two will particularly repay attention in the present context.

The first dimension is the notion of a rule. We commonly speak of medicine and law as practices; anthropologists comment on the practices characteristic of societies and cultures; and we say of groups and even individuals that they do or do not "make a practice" of this or that activity. These locutions predicate order and pattern, regularity and predictability, of the activities in question. These characteristics, however, while discernable by observers who do not themselves participate in the activities, are not to be understood on the model of the regularities detected in nature by physicists, chemists, and their ilk. There are rules in the sense of observable regularities in both cases, but in practices rules further involve regulations or norms that practitioners knowingly and intentionally follow because there is some sense in which (it can be any one of a considerable number of senses) the rule requires

George J. Agich (ed.), Responsibility in Health Care, 105–125.
Copyright © 1982 *by D. Reidel Publishing Company, Dordrecht, Holland.*

that they do so. To mention but one example, in the practice of medicine there is a rule that communications from patients to doctors must be kept confidential. This requirement is firmly established in the practice and doctors have an obligation to adhere to it. It might even be said that the rule is one of the constitutive features of the practice and that knowing and following it is a feature of the status of practitioner.

If we focus on the salience of rules in the practice of medicine, the concepts of authority and rights are likely to assume a comfortable and even a prominent place in our thought about it. I have argued elsewhere that *authority* and *rights* are practice-dependent notions and that rules are the features of practices on which they most directly or immediately depend ([4], pp. 64–120; [5], pp. 13–90). I have argued for the same view in respect to *power*, albeit with important modifications ([5], pp. 126–167). Patients (or their lawyers) who believe that a physician has violated their rights often partially support their claim by citing rules that they think establish the rights in question. In response to such claims, physicians often try to show that their actions were within their authority as defined by other established rules and norms.

It is frequently the case that the existence of a rule requiring a particular mode or pattern of conduct betokens disagreement or conflict. It is plausible to think, for example, that the confidentiality rule is needed because the often intimate nature of medical care could readily lead to abuses or at least the suspicion thereof. The existence of a firm rule defining the scope of a physician's authority and establishing a patient's rights gives a degree of needed assurance to both parties. The salience of rules in the practice of medicine itself suggests the presence of authority and rights and further suggests that these obtain and are in fact employed in a setting of latent if not actual conflict.

Rules or their role in medicine cannot be adequately understood without considering the second feature of practices. Prominent students of rules and rule-following (such as Max Weber, Ludwig Wittgenstein, and Ronald Dworkin) have emphasized that rules actually govern or guide conduct only when there is acceptance of values, beliefs, and ways of thinking and acting which are more encompassing, or of wider relevance and significance, than the rules themselves.[2] These values and beliefs provide participants with a basis for thinking it is valuable to have at least some rules and for the view that on the whole rules ought to be followed or obeyed. These are understandings that logically cannot be part of the formulation of any particular set of rules. (For example, legislatures do not pass laws requiring people to obey laws.) In this respect, the notion that practices involve accepted beliefs and values wider than rules sets constraints upon – but is not inconsistent with – the inferences drawn thus far from the salience of rules in practices. The writers just mentioned nonetheless contend that there must also be a consensus concerning general objectives and purposes. This consensus yields understandings in terms of which to decide upon and to interpret the content of the rules. A pertinent example of both these points is the Hippocratic Oath, which would be incomprehensible to persons who do not accept the notion that some conduct ought to be governed by general and prospective norms and who do not share at least some beliefs concerning human benefits and harms, well-being and suffering. When consensus about such values and beliefs diminishes, the particular imperatives of the Oath become difficult to interpret, to follow, and to enforce.

The idea of a consensus on beliefs and values has been introduced as a presupposition of rules and of rule-dependent phenomena such as authority and rights. Focusing attention, however, on this second and wider characteristic of the practice of medicine might have a quite different effect: it might suggest that power, authority, and rights have little or no place in medicine. There are two possibilities here. If there is in fact an effective consensus concerning the values and beliefs basic to medicine, then rules, and authority and rights defined by rules (and power and the fear thereof that prompts the desire for and promulgation of these), will be marginal and perhaps even superfluous. Participants in the practice will simply act on, will relate to one another directly in terms of, the values and beliefs they share.

It may help in focusing this idea to recall Rousseau's contention that a political society whose members had accomplished the sort of moral transformation and achieved the sort of moral community imagined in the *Social Contract* would act in accordance with the General Will. Rousseau seems to suggest that in this circumstance there would be little power and little need for authority, law, punishment, rights, and the rest of the apparatus of government and its rule. Recall also Marx's expectation that government and law would wither away under communism. On the other hand, if there is little or no consensus, if there are few values and beliefs shared among participants, there may indeed be power but it would be impossible to formulate, apply, or enforce rules. As a result, claims to authority and rights would be mere show. Consider in this connection the view that authority and rights (and indeed anything other than blatantly coercive imposition) presently are impossible in societies such as Haiti, El Salvador, Lebanon, and

Uganda. As much as these societies seem to be in need of rule, they are unable to generate or to sustain it.

II

It might appear from these considerations that our initial effort has been a failure. I sought perspective on issues of power, authority, and rights in medicine by looking to the notion that medicine constitutes a practice. But the notion of a practice does not yield a single, unified approach to these issues. In fact, consideration of two of the elements fundamental to practices has suggested competing – indeed conflicting – understandings of the place of power, authority, and rights in the practice of medicine. This outcome is instructive. The alternative understandings that have emerged correspond to and will help identify conflicting images or models of physician-patient relationships. Two of these models will be examined before paying further attention to the concept of a practice. In this way the conflicts between the two models may be easier to assess and reconcile.

The first model concerns an image of medicine that corresponds to the notion of practices as *consensual* – consensual to a degree that excludes power and renders authority and rights superfluous if not anomalous. It is a model whose general characteristics are familiar from communitarian thought about political societies and that, *qua* model of medicine, owes a good deal to a traditional, perhaps nostalgic and romanticized conception of the general practitioner as family physician. Physicians of this image do have specialized training and knowledge; they are expert concerning questions about which their patients know less. But these physicians are not thought of as wielding power over patients and certainly are much more than experts concerning medical science. If they are *good* physicians they have a close, perhaps even an intimate, knowledge of their patients – knowledge extending well beyond their medical histories. Physicians know their patients' tastes and preferences, interests and concerns, successes and disappointments. Along with this further knowledge, physicians have a concern for the well-being of individual patients, a concern that may approach the encompassing solicitude that is often associated with friendship and with relationships among members of communes and imagined utopian communities. The physician-patient relationship is pictured as reciprocal in that patients know their physicians well and have concern for them as persons. Patients may reciprocate not only the concern but the "care" their physicians offer, perhaps by providing them with expert services as lawyers, mechanics, stock brokers, or the like. Patients trust physicians in respect to those matters about which physicians are expert. Physicians reciprocate that trust in their relations with patients *qua* experts in law, car repair, or investment.

It requires no detailed analysis of rights to see that this notion has, at most, a subordinate role to play on the traditional model of the physician-patient relationship. The point is not so much that patients do or do not "have" this or that right. Rather, it is that questions about rights, cast in the always implicitly adversarial language of rights, is out of place on this model. Physicians and patients share values and beliefs, concerns and objectives; their thinking and acting are informed by these commonalities and the concern and trust they engender. Their thinking is *not* informed by the understanding that they are pursuing competing interests or engaged in some kind of power struggle. Good health, cure, and recovery are matters of mutual gratification. Illness, injury, and unsuccessful treatment are occasions not for recrimination or legal action but shared disappointment and a continuing search for more effective measures.

Because authority is a more complex notion, its place in the traditional model cannot be identified without noting some basic distinctions:

(a) Presidents and policemen are *in* authority by virtue of holding an office that is invested (and that invests its occupant with) authority over some other persons;
(b) Charles Goren holds no such office and hence no such *in* authority. Rather, by virtue of his exceptional knowledge of and skill at playing the game of bridge, he is *an* authority for people with an interest in that game;
(c) My real estate agent may or may not hold an office of *in* authority on the Realty Board and may or may not be *an* authority concerning housing patterns in my city, but my *authorization* gives him authority to show my house to potential purchasers;
(d) To my knowledge, Edmund Hoyle never held an office and is in any case long since deceased, but play "according to Hoyle" continues to be *authoritative* among players of poker and numerous other games.[3]

On the model under consideration, physicians are rarely if ever *in* authority over their patients. Although people sometimes speak of the office they hold, the orders they give, and even the sanctions suffered by those who disobey them, these are metaphors. In fact, physicians must have an authorization from their patients to conduct tests, give advice, prescribe medicines, regimens, etc. – an authorization that in principle can be withdrawn at the patients' discretion. (If the physician-patient relationship conforms to this model, though, such authorization is not apt to be withdrawn.) Patients themselves are likely to believe that their physician is *an* authority concerning medical science. This belief probably took its origin from opinion widely enough shared to be authoritative in the community and one that is sustained by the community's experience with the physician's care. Of course no single patient will be able to assess in detail the merits of all of a doctor's diagnoses, prescriptions, etc. A patient competent to make such assessments would have little need for a physician (although he could possibly have use for a surgeon!).[4]

Physicians' expertise in medical science, their standing as *an* authority concerning a body of technical knowledge and skill, partly explains and justifies their distinctive role in physician-patient relationships. But all patients judge the effects of their physicians' performances on them. Various patients have some of the technical knowledge necessary for further assessments; and, of course, physicians judge physicians and physicians are judged by those many non-physicians (nurses, paramedics, etc.) who themselves play roles in medical practice. Thus even in their technical aspects, the substance of physicians' decisions and actions is subject to scrutiny. The more important point, however, is that on the consensual model patients judge whether the physician's conduct is consistent with, or gives expression to, a set of beliefs and values accepted in the community. These beliefs and values provide the criteria for distinguishing good from bad physicians. As *an* authority concerning medicine, the decisions and actions of good physicians enunciate (in part through performances with a technical dimension) the beliefs and values of the community which accords them authority.

III

Power and rights, then, as the most explicitly and sharply adversarial of the three concepts presented, have little or no place on this consensual model of the physician-patient relationship. On the other hand, attributes and relationships which are commonly included in authority find a significant place. Anyone wary of authority and attracted to the view that it should be hedged by rights therefore will regard this model with suspicion. The notion of authority has as its basis the idea that if Baker concedes Able's authority in respect to X, that in itself is reason (albeit not a conclusive, all things considered, reason) for Baker to accept, go along with, give credence to, obey, etc., Able's judgments and decisions in respect to X. However well-justified Able's authority may be, this elementary fact seems to put Baker at risk in various ways. At the least, prudence commends the thought that Baker – or rather the Bakers of the practice – should insist on certain rights against the Ables.

The consensualist or communitarian understanding under consideration, however, depicts physician authority in ways that deflect patients from this stance. Having himself authorized the ministrations of physician Able, patient Baker may therefore be less likely to look warily upon Able's judgments and prescriptions. This, however, is not the important point in the present context. What matters more is that the Bakers of the practice authorize Able's treatments *because* they have reason to be confident of Able's professional competence and above all of Able's concern for them. The authorization is given in a setting of authoritative beliefs and values and established patterns of interaction that encourage confidence and trust. Able's standing as *an* authority, his standing as someone eligible to be accorded such an authorization, depends upon a continuing congruence between his decisions and the beliefs and expectations established in the community of which Able and Baker are members. The authority relations between Able and Baker are cushioned – that is, they lose what might otherwise be their threatening quality – because of the setting in which they occur. Even individuals who generally are wary of authority in the manner of much liberalism and all anarchism might agree that medical authority is tamed by the practice itself and hence that those subject to this authority do not need the further protections afforded by rights. Individuals who are favorably disposed to communitarian conceptions might take the still more affirmative view that rights – and the rights mentality – would disrupt communitarian relationships and impede realization of the distinctive benefits that can be generated by a practice of medicine on this model.

The second model of medical care relationships takes a very different view of these matters. In this model the contention is that the authority and power of physicians necessarily distance them from their patients, put physicians in an at least partly adversarial relationhip with them, and allow physicians to have significant advantages over them. Accordingly, it insists that patients must have protections – preferably the protections of enforceable rights – against physicians. Rights are necessary if the medical well-being of patients is to be protected and if their freedom, autonomy, and dignity are to be preserved. Before turning to this second model, however, it is important to give closer consideration to conceptual questions, particularly those concerning authority and power, that are crucial to both models and to the normative positions implicit in each.

It was noted earlier that Able's continuing standing as *an* authority eligible to be accorded Baker's authorizations is grounded in congruence between Able's decisions and beliefs and values that have authoritative standing in Baker's community. *An* authority and authorizations are dependent upon the content and the substance of the *authoritative* as it is understood by those over whom (or with respect to whom) these types of authority are held and exercised. This dependence and continuing congruence assures that the decisions and action of authority serve the common good of the community and are compatible with the well-being, freedom, and dignity of the Bakers.

Since Thomas Hobbes, a number of students have denied that phenomena with these characteristics should be regarded as instances of authority. Michael Oakeshott ([7], [8]) in particular has insisted that authority can have nothing whatsoever to do with Able's knowledge, expertise, or wisdom; nothing to do with the content or merits of Able's decisions, choices, and directives; and nothing to do with the beliefs, values, or opinions held by Baker or the members of Baker's community. Properly understood, the concept of authority should be restricted to relationships or arrangements in which Baker's responses to Able's directives are formulated entirely without reference to Baker's assessment of their content. Baker must know what that content is so that he can conform to the directives. He may or may not form an assessment of the merits of that content. But if he forms one and allows his actions to be influenced by this assessment, he has transformed his relationship with Able from one in terms of Able's authority to one in which he receives Able's directives, advice, or counsel but acts, as we might be tempted to put it, on his own authority. Thus, if the assumption is correct that Able's standing as *an* authority for Baker depends on the congruence between the content of Able's prescriptions and the content of the beliefs and values that Baker accepts, then Oakeshott contends that Able's authority is not so much softened or tamed by the setting in which it exists, but rather that there is no authority in that setting at all. "*An* authority", "authorizations" grounded in the belief that Able is "*an* authority", and beliefs and values that are "authoritative", become spurious or bogus notions. They are species of authority only by virtue of abuse of the term.[5]

However it is assessed, Oakeshott's position helps in grasping the issues posed by the informed concern-mutual trust model of the practice of medicine. On his understanding, insofar as there is genuine, encompassing consensus as to what, substantively speaking, ought and ought not to be done in a practice, there is no work for authority to do. If authority enters, it does so just because disagreement and conflict either prevent action on questions which cannot be sidestepped or postponed or lead to impositions by those powerful enough to achieve their ends despite disagreement. The members agree to establish offices of *in* authority and commit themselves to abide by the *intra vires* decisions of the office-holders regardless of their merits. If members insisted on assessing and acting on their assessments of the merits of the decisions, they would simply recreate the difficulty that induced them to establish authority. Alternatively, if there is partial consensus on substantive issues, and if views which express or enunciate the partial consensus are accorded authority for that reason, then authority becomes nothing more than power – power exercised by those who share in the consensus over those who do not. Christening the contested views with the name *authority* adds nothing to the evidence or reason in favor of the content of those views. If labelling them in this way indicates anything more than confusion, it signals the willingness of those who already accept the views to require dissenters to go along with them. Failure to convince dissenters of the merits of these views, coupled with failure to win the assent of the dissenters to authority in the proper sense, causes those individuals who accept the contested views to force submission upon the dissenters through a variety of pressures and threats.

Applying this analysis to medicine, if patient Baker agrees with the substance of Dr. Able's prescriptions, calling Able *an* authority adds nothing to understanding the relationship between them. Baker is convinced that Able's view is correct and Baker has acted on a conviction that he holds. If Baker disagrees with Able and refuses to follow the latter's "orders", any authority that Able may claim has failed and Baker's actions must again be explained in terms of the views Baker holds. Finally, if Baker disagrees with Able but "goes along" with Able's directives, then Baker has submitted to something other than the (so-called) *an* authority of Able. That "something" might be a desire to be cooperative, a wish to sustain the relationship with Able, to avoid the disapproval of other members of the community, or to sidestep any number of other unpleasant consequences. *Power* may be regarded as the intentional use by A of threats or threatening inducements to force B to do something that he would not otherwise (in the absence of the threats) do or to avoid doing something that he would otherwise do. By this definition, in many instances it is appropriate to say that Baker has submitted to power. Authority thus has a place in medicine only to the extent that patients follow physician's orders in order to maintain the practice of medicine despite disagreement about the correct resolution of medical questions.

Applying this analysis to the consensual model of medicine, three possibilities emerge. If the model were descriptively accurate or were regarded as an ideal to be pursued, authority would in fact have little if any place in the practice of medicine or would be regarded as a blemish to be eliminated in the progression toward an ideal practice. The third possibility is less agreeable. Recall that the consensual model of medical practice implies that physicians have a kind of authority to which patients should submit, but also that patients (as such) should not infer this to mean they have rights over physicians. Thus, through subsequent misunderstanding, conspiratorial intent, or a combination of the two, the consensual model is employed when there is a disagreement on important questions and when at least some participants dissent from widely received values and beliefs, norms and rules. To the extent that this third possibility is realized, the consensual model at once generates and is a cloak for power. This power may be dangerous to the medical well-being of patients and is certainly obnoxious to their freedom, autonomy, and dignity.

In summary, Oakeshott does not deny that there could be a practice of medicine that conformed to the consensual model. If there were such a practice, however, *all* of the concepts under consideration would be excluded. When combined with the fact that the physician is commonly regarded as *an* authority, his argument gives reason to suspect that practices viewed in this way involve a good deal of power. This suspicion in turn prompts the thought that patients would be advised to follow the example of citizens in their relations to the power of the state and establish enforceable rights against physicians.

IV

Setting these primarily conceptual issues aside for the moment, the most casual observer can think of empirical characteristics of contemporary medical practice which put the consensual model into question and encourage acceptance of the alternative model. The extraordinary achievements of medical science and technology have greatly increased the salience of the expertise of physicians and other medical professionals. These same achievements (made more noteworthy in that laypersons have such difficulty maintaining a competent understanding of them) have created an inequality between physicians and patients (and between physicians in one medical specialty and those in others) which makes it extremely difficult for patients to assess their performances. The highly technical and rapidly changing knowledge that physicians must acquire and maintain has also thrust them out of traditional patterns of interaction with patients and into relationships with other specialists – physicians, life scientists, bio-medical engineers – and indeed with big government, big industry, and big insurance and finance.

In most instances, patients must still authorize their physician's treatment, but this process may take the form of a blanket consent signed when entering a hospital or subscribing to a health care plan. The notion that patients choose one particular physician over another, or that patients realistically can terminate their physicians' care should they become dissatisfied, while still viable in certain respects, is of decidedly limited applicability. Moreover, for both patients and physicians, recent achievements have transformed the sense of what is at stake in medical care and hence in relations with medical professionals. Patients have always looked to physicians in matters concerning health and sickness, life and death. Once medicine could offer only partial symptomatic relief for whole classes of diseases, defects, and injuries. Now it can often cure and make whole and good. Where so much can be hoped, fear that the hope will be disappointed becomes inhibiting if not paralyzing. Patients with enough expertise to ground their doubts about their physician's judgment and positioned to act effectively on those doubts nevertheless may be reluctant to hazard an expression of their views.[6]

The elements of an alternative to the consensual model readily emerge from these considerations. Various kinds of authority are highly visible in medical practice, but authority is not now exercised in the reassuring setting of informed concern and reciprocal trust. The knowledge and skills of the medical profession are highly valued and the services of its members avidly sought and richly compensated. Physicians are seen not only as distant and impersonal, but also as wealthy and powerful. The admiration accorded to them therefore is alloyed with suspicion and fear of the sort commonly engendered by dependency on the high and the mighty. The expertise of physicians must be available, but their authority and power must be kept in check. Accordingly, patients readily think and talk not only of their dependence upon doctors but of their rights against them. The question is not whether a rights mentally is appropriate. Rather, it is what the rights should be and how they can be asserted effectively without jeopardizing the highly-rated benefits of expert medical care.

This alternative view could be termed a *constrained disputation* or even a *constrained conflict* model of the relationship between physician and patient. Physicians have substantial authority and power and thereby are in a position to do good and harm in distinctive measure. Patients seek to avail themselves of the good by submitting to the care of physicians while attempting to avoid the harm by insisting upon rights against them. The model depicts the relationship as cooperative and mutually advantageous at the same time as it is adversarial.

Although this model may be descriptively accurate and normatively appropriate given its descriptions, there is neither the evidence nor the space here to defend such a judgment. Like the consensual model, the constrained conflict model seems sufficiently accurate and influential to repay exploration.[7] This assumption presents a number of important questions. Largely because of the central place it accords to rights, the conceptual relationships that make up this model are more complex than those of the consensualist image. In part for the same reason, the model depicts the practice of medicine as making conflicting and perhaps irreconcilable demands on practitioners. Practice appears sharply adversarial, indeed frequently antagonistic – so much so that one wonders how it can hold together. Exploring these apparent implications of the constrained conflict model will involve further consideration of those elements of practices with which the discussion began. Examining Oakeshott's understanding of authority and power again will provide the basis.

As shown earlier, Oakeshott contends that all authority is *in* authority. It might appear that in the constrained conflict model physicians are invested with just such authority. Patients subscribe to the *in* authority of physicians in order to sustain a practice they value. This interpretation is suggested by two prominent facts: a) patients are severely restricted in their capacities to judge the substantive merits of decisions made by their physicians; and b) patients nevertheless commonly accept and conform to those decisions, sometimes even regarding it as a kind of obligation to do so. This interpretation also yields a definite – albeit narrowly circumscribed – place for patients' rights. Patients do not and could not have rights to good medical treatment if this is taken to mean treatment that actually improves the patient's health or medical well-being. Formulating, interpreting, and exercising rights of this kind would require consideration of substantive questions that are the province of physicians. But the concept of *in* authority always involves procedural rules and norms ("adverbial" rules as Oakeshott calls them) that specify and thereby limit the manner in which those invested with *in* authority are authorized to act.

Oakeshott himself does not use the language of rights in connection with these rules, but it is perfectly appropriate to think of violations of them as abusing the rights of those who have subscribed to the authority which the rules define. There is nothing anomalous or conceptually peculiar, for example, about the confidentiality rule or the notion that this rule establishes patients' rights. There could be a considerable number of rules-*cum*-rights – such as patients' rights to be informed of treatments they are to receive and of costs involved; or the necessity of a physician consulting with at least one other physician before initiating certain treatments; or insistence that physicians prescribe only those medicines and employ only those procedures which have been tested and certified in certain specified ways. As with such constitutional provisions as the prohibitions against bills of attainder and searches and seizures without judicial warrants, these procedural rules differentiate between *intra* and *ultra vires* action by physicians and constitute a bill of rights for patients. Malpractice consists in *ultra vires* action and gives patients moral standing to object to physician's actions and often legal standing to sue to protect the rights violated by those actions.

This interpretation would help in understanding how a practice fitting into the constrained disputation model could sustain itself. The *in* authority of the physicians affords the practice what in political vocabulary is called legitimacy. Patients accept and conform to the decisions of physicians not because they agree or approve of them, but because they have subscribed to the physicians' *in* authority to make them. In short, we understand how the practice holds together in the same way that we understand how some diverse, pluralistic political societies manage to hold together despite disagreement on numerous questions of public policy.

It is clear, however, that neither Oakeshott nor anyone else would accept the foregoing as an adequate interpretation of medical practice under the circumstances posited by the constrained conflict model. Leaving aside the general difficulties intrinsic to Oakeshott's view, the patients of this model are not likely to take the view that it is conceptually or otherwise *improper* for them to assess the merits of physicians' decisions or to act on such assessments. Patients will not regard themselves as debarred from such assessments or actions by the fact that they have subscribed to *in* authority on the part of physicians. They may believe that they have procedural rights such as those mentioned above and they may (certainly they should) value such rights highly. The distinctive standing of physicians, nonetheless, will continue to depend on their expertise and skill as medical professionals, on their reputations as *an* authority concerning a subject matter and an activity. Patients are likely to *regret* their *de facto* inability to understand and assess the substance of the decisions of physicians; they will be anxious to extend the notion of malpractice to include unnecessary, incompetent, and injurious treatment and to enlarge their rights so as to make such performances actionable. Whatever may be the case with governments (it cannot be as Oakeshott suggests as will be apparent soon), it is clear that on this model medical authority is primarily *an* authority and questions about authority and rights will be understood to extend to questions of substance, not just of procedure.

As already suggested, there is no reason to think that Oakeshott would dissent from this contention. On his view this contention is true not just about a model but about reality, and this truth specifies the sorry state into which we have fallen in regard not only to medicine but to much of life in the contemporary world. *An* authority and the authoritative are not species of authority at all but terms employed inappropriately in talking about beliefs and values shared among members of communities and groups. By accepting them as genuine species of authority, people afford a bogus but dangerous legitimacy to "experts". They have put themselves under what in political thought has always been regarded as despotism. Society's despots are physicians (and any number of other experts). These despots may or may not be benevolent in their intentions and the effects of their "rule" may or may not be beneficial to health, longevity, peace of mind, and the like. One thing, however, is certain. Through a commitment to conform to prescriptions concerning matters of great substantive significance, prescriptions about which they are not likely to agree, people have forsaken their dignity. Each person who accepts and acts on this understanding has become an "individual manqué" [7].

There *is* much to lament. Our relations with physicians are but one of the more dramatic instances of our dependence upon experts whose decisions and actions we can judge primarily in respect to (and frequently only after the fact of) the gross consequences of those decisions. Nor is Oakeshott alone in thinking that this circumstance – or rather this circumstance on anything like his Hobbesian understanding of it – leaves a choice between the despotism just discussed, loss of the benefits the experts can bestow, or perhaps unconstrained, destructive conflict.

It is not clear, however, that the situation, at least in respect to medicine, is as desperate as Oakeshott's analysis suggests. It is unclear, to say the least, that Oakeshott's analysis of authority and power perspicuously identifies the precise character of the difficulties encountered. It would take a veritable panglossian to deny that there are both despotic and destructively conflicting features in contemporary medical practice. Yet the practice continues and some of its achievements excite the admiration – nay the wonder – of many. Much remains to be accomplished with respect to the rights of patients; sharp disagreement and no doubt considerable conflict can be anticipated in this regard. But improvements have been effected and there is intense interest in the issues involved. For these reasons, perhaps an attempt to amend the analysis under consideration would be profitable.

V

It is manifest that a good deal turns on the notions *an* authority and the authoritative and their relationship to rights. It is idle to object to the terminology. "*An* authority", "authorization", and "the authoritative" are usages at least as well established as "*in* authority". The issue of consequence is whether Oakeshott has correctly identified the conceptual differences that distinguish the four notions. Much of this issue turns on the idea of "surrender of judgment", the notion that Baker's subscription to Able's *in* authority entails that Baker forego action on his judgments (if any) of the merits of Able's actions that are within Able's authority. To adapt a phrase from John Rawls that gives pointed expression to this idea, *in* authorities issue rules and commands to be obeyed, not propositions to be believed or disbelieved or judgments to be approved or disapproved.[8] For example, when one obeys a law or conforms to the decision of an umpire or referee, one does not thereby indicate agreement with that decision.

As the examples indicate, this explication appears correct at least for *in* authority. The explication also appears to be entirely mistaken about *an* authority, the authoritative, and authorizations grounded in them. To say, seriously and sincerely, of Dr. Able that he is *an* authority on heart disease just is to say that in my judgment Able's statements and judgments on the subject are (as a generalization and perhaps by comparison with the statements of other persons) true, cogent, worthy of approval, and the like. Similarly, to say in my own name that a belief or value, a norm or way of doing things, is authoritative, or to act in the ways that express this view, is just to announce that I believe and accept them. Moreover, saying or showing that I hold these beliefs often carries quite definite implications for my action. If in the course of a serious discussion of heart disease I allow that Able is *an* authority on that subject, I thereby commit myself to giving respectful attention to his statements concerning it. If I instead proceed to dismiss his views out of hand, it will appear that I have contradicted myself and others will expect an explanation. Again, if Dr. Able allows that the confidentiality rule has authoritative standing but then uses Baker's consulting room statements as a basis for gossip at cocktail parties, worse than a contradiction will occur. Thus, it appears that my first person present tense uses (as opposed to mentions) of "*an* authority" and "the authoritative" involve a commitment to act in the very ways Oakeshott claims are categorically excluded by *in* authority relationships.

These distinctions, however, as important as they are, cannot be drawn in the manner Oakeshott suggests. Subscription to *in* authority, as with all human conduct, is informed by, is literally incomprehensible apart from, beliefs and values, objectives and purposes accepted by the actors or agents in question. Oakeshott himself has provided an acute general analysis in this regard, which in fact is exemplified by his discussion of the most important case of subscription to *in* authority.[9] His *cives* or citizens subscribe to the authority of the state *in order to* "abate" somewhat the "contingency" that is at once the condition and, if entirely unabated, the deadly enemy of their liberty.[10] An actor who cared not for his liberty, or who did not believe that subscription to authority is necessary to it, could not make such subscription. In a society lacking a broad, more or less encompassing consensus on these beliefs and values, authority would be what it presently appears to be in Lebanon and Haiti – an impossibility.

Moreover, "abating contingency" is a portmanteau objective that requires a good deal of elaboration and interpretation if it is to yield guidance in formulating, applying, and obeying or disobeying the rules and commands of the state. These processes will of necessity be informed by any number of more specific beliefs and values. Where there is no consensus on some set of such further beliefs and values, these processes – and hence, relations in terms of *in* authority – cannot be sustained. Interpreting and acting on beliefs, values, rules, and commands informed by them and so forth necessarily involves the exercise of judgment; the "surrender" of judgment, so far from being required by *in* authority, is incompatible with it.

On the other hand, *in* authority shares with *an* authority and with authorizations a dependence upon the authoritative and judgments grounded in the authoritative. To adapt the language taken from Rawls further, if there are no propositions that are believed, no judgments that are approved, there can be no authority. The other side of this relationship between *in* and *an* authority is at least as important for present purposes. Relations involving *an* authority and the authoritative themselves entail restrictions on the exercise of judgment, restrictions that do not obtain in interactions with non-authorities and that do not obtain in thought and action concerning the non-authoritative.

To begin with, the judgment that someone is *an* authority and the conviction that a belief or value is authoritative are not made or reached whimsically or on the basis of mere caprice. I cannot simply decide, for no reason at all or for entirely idiosyncratic reasons, that Billy Graham is *an* authority on heart disease or that the beliefs and values of Zen Buddhism are authoritative throughout the United States. Further, if I have reason to regard Dr. Able as *an* authority on heart disease, I therefore respond quite differently to his or her diagnoses and prescriptions from the way I respond to the opinions of my neighbor on this subject. Similarly, I respond differently to the claim of my opponent that his proposed play is according to Hoyle than to his view that he will find the game more enjoyable if he is allowed to make that play. In neither case am I debarred, logically or in any other way, from questioning and disagreeing.

My questioning, however, must be cognizant of the standing of the statements in question. The considerations that I may adduce in forming and defending my judgments are restricted by the subject matters of those judgments. These several restrictions on the exercise of judgment make *an* authority relations and relations involving the authoritative more closely analogous to *in* relations than Oakeshott allows.

If these last remarks are well-founded, it follows that the prominence of *an* authority and the authoritative in medicine does not itself entail the grim conclusions canvassed here. Acceptance of the physician as *an* authority and of beliefs and values as authoritative requires judgment on the part of participants in the practice. Hence, the prominence of genuine *an* authority and genuinely authoritative beliefs and values would in fact be a barrier to "despotism". At the same time, such acceptance restricts the manner in which judgment may be exercised. For this reason, the presence of *an* authority and authoritative beliefs and values serves to constrain disagreement and conflict and hence to sustain the practice. If the situation is anything like that described above, it is due not to the presence of *an* authority and authoritative beliefs and values but to their absence. Instead, it is due to the fact that circumstances make it difficult or impossible for individuals to make and agree upon the judgments and to sustain the relationships presupposed by *an* authority and the authoritative. By way of concluding these reflections, it is appropriate to consider their bearing on power and rights and on the two models of medical practice.

VI

The findings about authority discussed in this essay are elaborations of the general themes about practices considered initially. The discussion has brought those themes to bear on authority of the several types already distinguished. Some of the conditions found to be presupposed by all types of authority are also prominent in the consensual model of medical practice. There must be shared beliefs and values and these must inform and thereby constrain what can be termed the divisions of labor or the specializations of function characteristic of medical practice.

These findings, however, do not simply endorse the consensual model. Certainly they do not support the view that the consensual model specifies the conditions necessary to and sufficient for a viable (or a defensible) medical practice. Rather, the consensual model posits so inclusive and so detailed a consensus that the divisions of labor characteristic of medicine appear to be largely superfluous and perhaps otiose. The role or function of the physician becomes unnecessary in much the same way that authority becomes unnecessary in communitarian thinking about politics. Authority presupposes rules and rules presuppose consensus. But authority and rules also presuppose differentiation of function and at least the possibility of disagreement and conflict.

These considerations have an immediate bearing on power and rights and hence on any model of medicine that includes them. If power is something other than brute force, the A's who employ it must have a notion of the kinds of threats and threatening inducements that will bring the B's against whom it is employed to do the bidding of the A's. This notion must prove correct at least some of the time. That is, there must be some occasions on which the B's regard the threats as sufficient reasons for doing what the A's want them to do. A parallel proposition holds for rights. As with power, rights are adversarial. They presuppose disagreement and the possibility of conflict. But the concept of a right loses its meaning if the A's against whom the rights are claimed and asserted do not sometimes, or rather as a general rule, treat those rights as sufficient reasons for acceding to the claims that the B's advance.

Just as with all types of authority, then, power and rights presuppose a combination of agreement and disagreement, consensus and conflict. There must be agreement at some levels or in some regards, disagreement at other levels and in other regards. By denying the disagreement, the consensual model excludes power and makes rights unnecessary. Because the combination of agreement and disagreement can be made to appear implausible or even impossible, the constrained conflict model can be made to look unrealistic or unworkable. Knowing as we do, however, that there are societies and practices in which power, rights, and the several types of authority are present and more or less effective, we know that this combination is not an impossibility. Arguments that the combination is impossible misconstrue the concepts, fly in the face of the facts, or both.

Is some version of this combination possible in contemporary medicine? At this juncture, there are two connected issues: one conceptual, the other empirical. The conceptual issue concerns the undoubtedly problematic relationship between *an* authority and rights. Able's authority depends on the correctness, wisdom, skill, and so forth of his decisions and actions. Mistaken or foolish decisions, clumsy or inept actions, seemingly would not violate Baker's rights against Able *qua an* authority. Rather, they would simply terminate that authority. It would seem that rights go easily with *in* authority because both the rights and the authority can often be defined procedurally. Thus, there understandably have been fewer difficulties with the notion of patients' rights when we have been able to separate our primarily procedural elements in the activities of physicians and to define the rights of patients by relation to them. The judge who denies me counsel both violates my right and retains his office of *in* authority; the physician who does not inform me of the cost of removing my cataracts violates my right but remains *an* authority on eye disease. If patient rights are extended to include medically effective or beneficial treatment, the very notion of *an* authority becomes threatened.

These remarks bridge both the conceptual and empirical issues in question. As with any discussion of authority, the procedural-substantive distinction is unstable. When the distinction seems clear and firm, that appearance reflects especially encompassing and detailed agreement on what from a stance outside the consensus will be seen as highly substantive questions. Consider, for example, the procedural requirement that police abjure searches and seizures without judicial warrant. The existence and efficacy of this requirement reflects a broad consensus on fundamentally substantive questions about law and order and its relation to individual liberty. As every student of the Fourth Amendment knows, applying the requirement in novel or difficult cases all but invariably raises substantive questions and tests the consensus concerning them. If there turns out to be sharp and widespread disagreement, the rulings and the rights they define will be difficult to enforce. If such disagreement recurs over a wide range of issues, the system of *in* authority will be put in jeopardy.

The empirical question, then, can be stated as follows: Can agreement be reached and maintained concerning the objectives and purposes of medicine sufficient to sustain authority, power, and rights – no less than all three –

in medical practice? I have no answer to this question. My claim for the foregoing discussions is no more than that they show the question to be properly and appositely posed.

The Johns Hopkins University

NOTES

[1] In my judgment the single most important treatment of the elements fundamental to the practice concept is by Ludwig Wittgenstein, who only rarely used the word itself ([11], [12]). Wittgenstein's "language games" and "forms of life" express many of the ideas that inform my understanding of practices. His great influence on contemporary philosophy has extended these ideas throughout much recent philosophical work. A more explicit treatment of "practice", closely akin to Wittgenstein's (despite the fact that each proceeds from different philosophical assumptions) is in Michael Oakeshott's *On Human Conduct* [7]. As Richard Bernstein has shown (without using the "practice" terminology), there are also important analogues and parallels to these ideas in pragmatism, phenomenology, and some strands of Marxism and critical theory ([1], [2]). My own most extended discussion of practices is in Chapter One of *The Practice of Rights* [4] and I rely heavily on the practice understanding throughout *The Practice of Political Authority: Authority and the Authoritative* [5].

[2] Max Weber is at least implicitly concerned with rules and norms throughout his work. The most explicit and immediately pertinent discussions are in the treatments of rational-legal and traditional authority in *Economy and Society* [10]. The topic of rules and rule-following recurs throughout Wittgenstein's later work, often explicitly, frequently in the guise of discussions of "knowing how to go on". The most closely focussed discussions are in *Philosophical Investigations* ([11] paras. 85–91, 14–243) and *On Certainty* ([12] paras. 21–33, 43–50, 61–65, 93–100, 139–40, 309, 493–98, 519). For Ronald Dworkin's discussion, see *Taking Rights Seriously* ([3], esp. Chapters 1–4).

[3] These distinctions owe much to the discussions of Michael Oakeshott [7] and to Richard B. Friedman [6].

[4] Or rather, such a "patient" would need a physician only in the respects in which, even on this model, the physician has authorizations from sources other than the patient – for example, those *in* authority who license physicians to prescribe drugs, use hospital facilities, and the like.

[5] These and the following discussions of Oakeshott's views are based on *On Human Conduct* [7]. He has a more detailed treatment of the relationship between authority and power in "The Vocabulary of the Modern State" [8]. My assessment of his views is stated more fully in *The Practice of Political Authority* [5].

[6] Of course there have been definite limits on patient consent for a long time. To mention an obvious case, the anesthetized patient on the operating table is not well placed to refuse or withdraw consent to treatment. The developments mentioned in the text only complicate and intensify a difficulty inherent in much of medical practice.

[7] I have not done the kind of investigation necessary to determine how widely this or

the previous model of medical practice is accepted. Anyone disposed to dismiss it as without influence on actual thought and action would have to deal with some obvious facts. Perhaps the most striking fact is the burgeoning phenomenon of malpractice suits. Each of these legal actions presents the claim that patients have definite rights and each asserts that a physician, a hospital, or some agent or agency of the medical care profession has exceeded the limits of authority. Again, the fact that individuals increasingly resort to lawyers and courts to enforce rights certainly signals a belief that physicians and health care agencies are too powerful to be controlled by patients themselves. Dependent and relatively powerless patients must seek assistance about rights from experts and even from the government itself – which many people consider the ultimate authority and power in society.

To take a piece of evidence that is perhaps less dramatic but closer to home, consider for a moment the phenomenon of this conference itself – namely, the popularity of subject matters such as medical law, medical ethics, and the politics of medicine.

8 John Rawls used this phrase in his early essay, "Legal Obligation and the Duty of Fair Play" [9].

9 Oakeshott's general analysis of "conduct" is in the first essay of *On Human Conduct* [7]. His discussion of *cives* and their conduct in subscription to authority is primarily in the second essay in the same volume.

10 For the discussion of abating contingency, see ([7], p. 74).

BIBLIOGRAPHY

1. Bernstein, R.: 1971, *Praxis and Action*, University of Pennsylvania Press, Philadelphia.
2. Bernstein, R.: 1978, *The Restructuring of Social and Political Theory*, University of Pennsylvania Press, Philadelphia.
3. Dworkin, R.: 1977, *Taking Rights Seriously*, Harvard University Press, Cambridge.
4. Flathman, R. E.: 1976, *The Practice of Rights*, Cambridge University Press, New York.
5. Flathman R. E.: 1980, *The Practice of Political Authority: Authority and the Authoritative*, University of Chicago Press, Chicago.
6. Friedman, R. B.: 1972, 'On the Concept of Authority in Political Philosophy', in R. E. Flathman (ed.), *Concepts of Social and Political Philosophy*, The Macmillan Company, New York, pp. 121–146.
7. Oakeshott, M.: 1975, *On Human Conduct*, The Clarendon Press, London.
8. Oakeshott, M.: 1975, 'The Vocabulary of the Modern State', *Political Studies* **23**, 197–219, 409–414.
9. Rawls, J.: 1964, 'Legal Obligation and the Duty of Fair Play', in S. Hook (ed.), *Law and Philosophy*, New York University Press, New York, pp. 3–18.
10. Weber, M.: 1968, *Economy and Society*, G. Roth and C. Wittich (eds.), Bedminister Press, New York.
11. Wittgenstein, L.: 1953, *Philosophical Investigations*, The MacMillan Company, New York.
12. Wittgenstein, L.: 1969, *On Certainty*, Basil Blackwell, Oxford.

ROBERT M. VEATCH

MEDICAL AUTHORITY AND PROFESSIONAL MEDICAL AUTHORITY: THE NATURE OF AUTHORITY IN MEDICINE FOR DECISIONS BY LAY PERSONS AND PROFESSIONALS

The nature of authority in medical decisions is a subject of current controversy. In their analyses of medical authority, Richard Flathman in "Power, Authority, and Rights in the Practice of Medicine" and Stanley Hauerwas in "Authority and the Profession of Medicine" have contributed to advancing the debate. In spite of their apparently diverging analyses and proposed solutions, they share much in common. Both are acutely aware that the authority of the medical professional has seen hard times recently. Both recognize that historical notions of physician authority grounded in technical expertise and skill are not an adequate basis for authority. Both appear compelled to salvage some residual element of legitimate professional medical authority. And both make interesting attempts.

I am convinced that the salvaging operation is worth pursuing. In the end, however, I fear that what each in his own way has dredged from the submerged wreck of the traditional notion of medical authority is not the golden treasure of a workable model of authority, but a hulk that will need refurbishing and remodelling.

I. TWO CRITICAL DISTINCTIONS

I fear that for both Hauerwas and Flathman, the salvaging operation may have started in the wrong waters by their failure to make clearly two distinctions: the distinction between medical authority and professional authority and the distinction between authority on medical facts and authority on medical values.

Medical Authority vs Professional Authority

Both Flathman and Hauerwas insist that medicine is a practice governed by rules and a system of beliefs and values. At times they seem to recognize that the practice of medicine is not limited to behaviors of physicians or even of health professionals. Hauerwas, for example, says that medicine is a practice that includes both physicians and patients. Both recognize that practices are relational, communal activities.

George J. Agich (ed.), Responsibility in Health Care, 127–137.
Copyright © 1982 by D. Reidel Publishing Company, Dordrecht, Holland.

Certainly, most medical decisions are made by lay people. When I decide to take aspirin for a headache, I practice medicine. When I diagnose my son's injured finger as a sprain not requiring a physician's attention, I practice medicine. When I choose a lifestyle in part based on its impact on my health, I practice medicine. Any notion of authority in medicine will have to be broad enough to encompass these as well as professional decisions. Yet both Flathman and Hauerwas often lapse into a narrower thinking, in which they assume that the main question concerns professional authority rather than medical authority. Medicine is, however, an institution – an organized, complex set of practices of which only a fraction are engaged in by professionals. There is a legitimate place for *professional* authority, but it is much more limited than the notion of *medical* authority. My vision, then, is one of the patient as the leader of the health care team.

Technical Authority vs Value Authority

Both Hauerwas and Flathman fail to distinguish adequately between authority related to judgments of medical fact and authority for judgments related to medical values and behavioral recommendations based on those values.

The fact/value distinction is undoubtedly simplistic on at least two counts: certain values, such as ethical values, can be considered in some meta-ethical frameworks as a particular kind of fact (empiricists speak of moral facts, for instance) and any statement of facts necessarily incorporates a system of beliefs and values (at least insofar as reporting facts requires selecting what is *significant* or *valuable* from an array of data). Still, it is unclear how the question of authority in medicine can be analyzed adequately without an initial – even if simplistic – working assumption that the authority for the essentially non-evaluative factual elements of medical decisions potentially will differ from the authority for the evaluative aspects. Since every medical decision necessarily requires an integration of both facts and values, both kinds of authority will be necessary. Hauerwas and Flathman, however, seem to emphasize the moral dimensions of authority so much that the residual significance of the professional's technical authority is overlooked. Hauerwas, in fact, states boldly that the medical professional's authority cannot derive from scientific or technical skill. A reformulation of the notion of medical authority therefore seems to be in order.

II. A RECONSTRUCTION OF THE NOTION OF MEDICAL AUTHORITY

A reformation can begin with a consideration of Flathman's consensual model. Flathman argues that a necessary condition for the practice of medicine in the consensual model is agreement on the beliefs and values among those engaging in a medical interaction. But he also claims: "if there is in fact an effective consensus concerning the values and beliefs basic to medicine, then rules, and authority and rights defined by rules . . . will be marginal and perhaps even superfluous" (p. 107).

Technical Authority

This view seems correct only to the extent that we appeal to professionals in the medical relationship as a way of resolving the questions of what we ought to do – of what ought to be prescribed and what behaviors are appropriate. We may, however, have a very different objective in mind. Even though in some medical relationships, there exists a consensus on the beliefs and values, the medical lay person still may not know what to do because he does not have the non-evaluative facts. In a medical relationship, then, we may still need someone who is *an authority* on the non-evaluative facts – on diagnosis, pharmacology, impacts of diet, and the like.

To use Flathman's language, it seems plausible to talk about someone who is *an authority* on non-evaluative facts. In fact, we who lack adequate knowledge do so all the time in various areas of our lives. Health professionals are, among other things, plausibly taken to be authorities on some portion of the relevant non-evaluative facts needed for medical decisions by lay people. They are of course not experts on all the non-evaluative facts. One would need in addition to know about law, psychology, economics, aesthetics, personal preferences, and spiritual matters before making any definitive choice, but one does need medical facts. Health professionals are, as a class, authorities in these matters. Such authority in medicine, however, is radically different from the authority Flathman speaks about when patients follow a physician's orders despite disagreement about the correct resolution of medical questions. This kind of case is not a matter of naked power causing Baker to yield to Able even though he disagrees. It is rather Baker yielding to Able's authoritative technical knowledge once they agree on the beliefs and values. This seems to be the model of medicine that dominated during the glorious era of medical ascendency of the 1940s and 1950s. During that time we had substantial agreement about the beliefs and values relevant to medical decisions, but desperately needed someone who was an authority on the facts. If we were suffering from pneumonia, there was little disagreement about the values: we wanted to live. We thought the minimal risks of treatment were worth accepting if the treatment would be safe, simple, and sure. We simply wanted to know the name of the right drug. If an authority could tell us it was penicillin, we were quite happy. In fact, since rightly or wrongly we believed that indiscriminate use of penicillin could not be tolerated, we turned to the physician as someone *in* authority, licensed by the state to control access to the drug.

Thus Flathman is not entirely correct when he says that physicians are rarely if ever *in* authority over their patients. They are licensed by the state to the office of gate-keeper over the nation's pharmaceutical armamentarium. They are *in* authority to control access to hospitals, to legal surgery (including abortions), and to Medicaid reimbursement. As public health officers, they have the right to quarantine us against our consent. That is a substantial degree of authority, of Flathman's *in* authority variety. Still, it rests upon a substantial consensus about beliefs and values. The authority recognized is one rooted in technical competency or at least the belief that people in the publicly recognized health professional role are much more likely to have technical competency than the rest of us. The authority is rational in the Weberian sense. We should be aware, however, that even judgments rooted in this technical authority incorporate beliefs and values, but often it is reasonable to assume sufficient consensus on those beliefs and values to proceed as if the judgment were purely technical.

Value Authority

We are all, however, uncomfortable with the notion of authority as stemming from mere technical competency for at least two reasons. Hauerwas suggests the first reason. Just as medicine is more than mere technical proficiency because it requires a set of beliefs and values, so likewise medical professionals hold a set of beliefs and values about what they are doing. (Hauerwas seems to imply that medical professionals are legitimate authorities on the beliefs and values of medicine.) There is a second, somewhat contradictory reason why we are uncomfortable with the notion of professional authority stemming from technical competency. Increasingly, the modal problems in medicine do not follow the 1950s model of pneumonia where everyone agrees on the basic beliefs and values and the problem is one of technical facts. Increasingly, the dominant problems in medicine are ones in which the beliefs and values themselves are at stake.

The two dominant medical problems in Western society today are cancer and heart disease. Together they account for a substantial percentage of deaths. Both conditions are subject to medical manipulations, but the manipulations are such that we are far from a consensus on whether the manipulations are worthwhile. For cancer we can operate, radiate, and expose the patient to toxic chemicals. We can recommend changes in diet and work environment. In many cases these will produce statistically significant changes in the probability of dying in a particular way at a particular time. Yet the real question is whether the treatments are worthwhile. For heart disease we can operate, transplant, medicate, and change basic life style, and once again, the question is whether it is worthwhile. That question, however, is a matter of fundamental beliefs and values and not a matter of technical competence.

With regard to the example of heart disease, Flathman misses this distinction when he says that he would respond quite differently to a physician's diagnoses and prescriptions than he would to the opinions of his neighbor. It is obvious that for descriptive matters such as diagnosis, authority on the non-evaluative facts is necessary, and the heart specialist should be regarded differently from a neighbor. Thus, if he says I have simple vessel occlusion of the cardiac vessels, I give that judgment about the facts substantial weight in comparison to that of my neighbor. If he goes on, however, to say I should have coronary bypass surgery, he is saying something quite different and more complex. He is predicting outcomes with and without the surgery, an area in which he still is exercising technical authority. He is also making a normative judgment, however. He is saying that the predicted outcome with surgery is preferable to that without.

Suppose he tells me that the outcome, based on current evidence, is that the surgery will lead to decreased morbidity, but increased short-term mortality with questionable impact on long-term mortality. If he then recommends surgery, he is in effect recommending that an increased risk of short-term mortality is worthwhile in order to decrease pain and suffering. That, of course, is a decision that will be influenced by moral judgments about the duty to preserve life as well as questions of personal preference, life-style, and life-plans. There is no necessary reason why the physician should be regarded as an authority on the question of my duty to preserve my own life or on the question of how great a risk of death is justified to reduce future pain and suffering. In fact, my neighbor may be a more authoritative counsel in this area than my physician. What is critical is that at the level of prescription, the judgments are necessarily evaluative. They involve choices requiring moral and other evaluative inputs.

Virtually every other major cause of death today and every medical problem worth worrying about is of this same character. We have some half-way effective interventions, but given our beliefs and values we are not sure whether they are worthwhile. To solve these new dilemmas in medicine, a very different kind of authority than the authority needed to treat pneumonia is needed. Technical authority may be relevant, but only after we have settled the much more difficult problems of belief and value. The oncologist may tell us that three years on the combined four-drug chemotherapy regimen will add five percent to our survival probability and make us nauseated, bald, and anemic. What we really need to know, however, is whether the marginal increase in survival chance is fitting given our system of beliefs and values. What we really need is an authority on the right beliefs and values.

Flathman uses the example of confidentiality and assumes that it is obvious that a physician should keep confidential any information about a patient learned in the course of practice. That rule, however, is one of the most debated in medical ethics. Lay people and professionals, at least until very recently, have drawn on different sources of authority to reach different conclusions. Consider the case of a physician who knows that his patient has rare attacks of grand mal epilepsy, but is also a commercial truck driver endangering the lives of himself and others if he continues driving. The interesting dispute is not over the calculation of the medical risks. That could be done easily using technical authority. The real issue is over the ethical limits to the principle of confidentiality. Should the goal be to serve the patient's interest as Hauerwas and the Hippocratists claim, to serve the social welfare as utilitarians claim, or to hold to a deontological commitment to non-disclosure, regardless of the consequences, as Flathman suggests? Different authorities provide different answers. There is no reason to assume the professional answer is the right answer. In fact it may be systematically wrong. Anyone who blindly cedes to health professionals moral authority over such questions would have to face the very difficult task of justifying such a move in the first place.

Flathman's constrained conflict model is one which lends itself to situations like this, in which the values as well as the technical facts of alternative interventions are in dispute. The question being pressed by both the libertarians and by Hauerwas is whether there is a legitimate authority for resolving questions of belief and values. Hauerwas clearly believes there is; the liberals answer that no one beyond the individual patient can be so identified.

Hauerwas's intriguing reinterpretation of Alasdair MacIntyre and Yves Simon goes so far as to claim that authority of the type related to beliefs and values is necessary for social interaction. His conclusion is remarkably similar to Flathman's, that our plight "is due not to the presence of *an* authority and authoritative beliefs and values but to their absence" (p. 121).

For the purpose of discussion, I am going to accept this view. Some legitimate authority in the sphere of beliefs and values is necessary for medical interactions between lay person and professional, and this requirement is not necessarily incompatible with individual freedom. The critical question, however, which neither Flathman nor Hauerwas answers adequately, is whether medical professionals can hold that authority.

I am convinced that Hauerwas is on the right track in seeking an alternative to liberalism. Raw contracting between utterly isolated free individuals is not enough to provide a foundation for the physician-patient relationship. There must be some authority undergirding the relationship upon which to base the interaction. The question is: what is that authority to be? At this point, Hauerwas makes a critical mistake. He assumes that medicine – mistakenly equated with medical professionals – professes the authority of the body. He argues that it is necessary to establish a philosophy of medicine in which the professional is viewed as the priest of the cult of the body. The physician in Hauerwas's scheme of things is the custodian of the virtues related to our bodies. He cites with approval MacIntyre, who says: "The good of health is entrusted to the medical profession with its concomitant virtues."

Hauerwas recognizes that there are many values and virtues to which people are loyal. One of them is health. In fact, many go so far as to say that it is one of our duties. "The body is the temple of the Lord" is the way one dominant religious traditions has expressed it, implying our obligation to care for it properly. The task of physicians, according to Hauerwas, is to function as priests to preserve this value, to teach it to us, and to support the life projects of patients insofar as those projects involve a well-functioning body. The physician's overriding commitment, therefore, is to care for individuals who come to them with complaints of illness. The authority of the physician thus derives from the intrinsic value of the body and our duty to preserve it when possible.

I concede that health is a legitimate value. I even concede that medical professionals should be the priests of that value. I submit, however, that no one in his right mind would conclude that those who are custodians of a particular value should bear the authority for resolving disputes over the relation of that value with other values leading to one's integrated wholeness.

Consider the following medical problem faced by lay people: Should I risk my health by eating nutritionless junk food? We first recognize that there are empirical problems raised by the question, such as: Does junk food really constitute a risk to my health? I assume that physicians are legitimate technical authorities on that question (although I recognize that there are significant dangers of having apparently value-free factual judgments such as these clouded by the biases or by the inevitable and legitimate system of beliefs and values of the technical authority). That turns out not to be the interesting question, however. The important question is this: Assuming junk food will hurt my health, will it make me happier than all alternatives, and if it will, should I feel a moral obligation, on balance, to avoid this kind of happiness in order to preserve my health?

In such questions about beliefs and values, the health professional has no legitimate authority. Assuming that health professionals are committed to the special values of preserving the health of the body, it is likely that the health professional would give the answer that is now being given by those physicians who are evangelists for better nutrition, less smoking, and more healthy lifestyles. Grant for the moment that these are values worth pursuing. The problem is how to relate these values and obligations to other values and obligations in one's life. Rational persons would not always choose the courses that made them healthiest. No one would always opt for the value that Hauerwas has claimed is the medical professional's special concern. No one would say that, regardless of the circumstances, he wants always to be made well when he is ill or kept well when he is well. No rational patient would always want the physician to do what the physician thought was in the patient's medical interest. That would not only sacrifice the patient's autonomy (the liberal's problem); it would also sacrifice all other values and obligations.

Anyone who subordinates his being to the body ends up being a subscriber to Mr. Atlas body-building programs, a jogging freak, or a victim of medical professional domination. Rational people may well need a center of authority to resolve problems such as these. I am not objecting to a person who turns to his religious tradition and learns that the body is a holy temple. To learn whether the body is a value, however, one should not simply turn to the authority of those who are charged with the preservation of the value of the body.

Hauerwas's argument goes something like this: Liberalism is wrong. There must be some center of authority for resolving the problems of beliefs and values in medical decision-making. Therefore, physicians, as custodians of the value of the body, should have that authority. If that is his conclusion, it is dangerous and irrational.

Flathman views things somewhat differently. Full consensus is no longer possible, if it ever was, since it requires a non-existent agreement about beliefs and values. It makes important division of labor superfluous and perhaps otiose. The relationship cannot be totally adversarial and conflict-ridden, either. His resolution is Hegelian, a combination of agreement and disagreement. Perhaps I do not understand him here, but it seems unclear how he envisions combining the two. I sense a half-hearted, half-trusting amalgam of faith and suspicion, authority, power, and rights.

III. AN ALTERNATIVE MODEL FOR MEDICAL AUTHORITY

My own solution is somewhat different. It involves several steps in the recognition of legitimate medical authority. First, I concede that there is limited, legitimate technical authority that should be ceded to all *in* authority professionals. That authority comes not from their unique commitment to the value of health, but from their technical competence. In those increasingly rare cases in which the beliefs and values at stake are beyond legitimate dispute or where the value differences are trivial in comparison with the need for technical expertise, the authority of the physician is legitimate and deserves respect. When a patient is brought to the emergency room bleeding and unconscious, a value judgment is required to know that he wants the bleeding stopped, but we can generally agree on that. In such cases, we only need someone who knows how to stop the bleeding.

Second, I concede that increasingly medical decisions – made by lay people as well as professionals – involve questions where matters of belief and values are in doubt. Different systems of belief and values will lead to different answers.

Third, I concede that some authority for resolving questions of belief and value is needed. For that authority we turn to those individuals (if any) we acknowledge to be experts on beliefs and values. If religious, we turn to the church; if not, we turn to the secular surrogates for the church – the civil liberties union, the feminist movement, the Communist Party, the John Birch Society, or the Masons – whatever happens to serve as the authoritative illumination for problems of this sort. Some authoritative community is available to every person. If we especially should want to hear the case for the wisdom of the body, physicians should be among those able to provide it.

Fourth, I concede that if we as lay people want medical professionals to draw on their technical authority and combine it with a moral authority that we acknowledge, we shall have to find professionals who share a faith in the same beliefs and values we have. We must recognize, however, that as professionals in the medical sphere, they do place unique value on the maintenance of the health of the body and be on guard against that. Even though they share a committed loyalty to the same community of moral authority, they will deviate from it somewhat because of this unique role-specific moral duty. That will lessen their moral authority in our eyes somewhat, but if both we and they remain true to the more global, integrated vision we strive for – the one which sees medical values as one among many, oftentimes competing values – their moral authority will not be lessened too severely by this deviation.

It would be irrational, however, to entrust in an evangelist for body worship the primary authority for deciding the proper mix of values. Do not misunderstand. This will not lead to a breakdown of trust between lay people and professionals. I am not talking about the kind of challenge that Flathman envisions in the more crude form of his conflict model. Rather, loyalty of lay person and professional to a common, legitimate community of authority provides a real, legitimate basis for a trusting relationship. We still should not entirely trust the physician to choose our beliefs and values and to integrate complex combinations of conflicting beliefs and values. No autonomous person should cede such authority. I would no more trust my physician to choose the beliefs and values that are the basis of critical decisions about my medical future than I would trust my clergyman to do my income taxes. It is not because I do not trust my clergyman, but rather because trust is inappropriately placed when placed in this way. Mutual commitment to a common community of authority, however, provides a real basis of trust where it is appropriately placed: for example, when I need to trust my physician's technical authority, when emergency decisions must be made, when the logic of the choice excludes lay participation, and when the ideology of a system of beliefs and vlaues must be incorporated into the professional's behavioral choices.

The result is a system in which technical authority will rest with various professionals who have various skills and commitments, but in which moral authority rests in some community having a more balanced, integrated set of beliefs and values. Strangely enough, the Oral Roberts Medical Center, the Jehovah's Witnesses, and the Seventh Day Adventists become the ideal model for medical authority. At least they are ideal in form, if not in substance. Although these groups have very bizarre visions generating what to most people are unacceptable systems of beliefs and values, they at least share in common the notion that an integrated vision of authority combines medical values with religious, economic, aesthetic, gastronomic, and intellectual ones. Medical authority, insofar as it is moral authority rather than mere technical authority, rests not with the medical professional. Rather, medical professional and medical lay persons alike find their authority in some common community of beliefs and values.

Thus, Hauerwas is on the right track when he makes use of the metaphor of a sectarian community. He has the metaphor confused, however. It is not that the entire group of medical professionals will appear to the rest of the world as a single sectarian community. Rather, sectarian communities – literal religious communities such as the Seventh Day Adventists and metaphorical ones such as the women's health collectives – will provide a theological, ethical, and cultural foundation for making medical decisions for their members. They will identify certain individuals from their belief system to be trained for specialized ministries to promote the value of the body and to preserve health according to the belief system of the sect. The core source of moral authority for medical decision-making, however, will be the belief system of some common community shared by lay person and the professional who is the functionary of that community.

For many of us, that common community of moral authority will look very different from that of the religious groups that have made health an integral part of their value system. It will look more like the system of beliefs and values of the liberal Anglo-American West, the mainstream churches, or their secular equivalents, but it will be an authority for beliefs and values that extends well beyond the Aesculapian authority of the physician as priest for the worshippers of the body. Both medical professional and medical lay person will find their authority as they find their freedom – in a mutually acceptable integrated moral community. Authority in medicine that has any other basis cannot be legitimate.

Georgetown University

SECTION III

ETHICS OF CONSULTATION AND INTERPROFESSIONAL RELATIONSHIPS

MARK SIEGLER

MEDICAL CONSULTATIONS IN THE CONTEXT OF THE PHYSICIAN-PATIENT RELATIONSHIP*

There is widespread agreement that the physician-patient relationship is changing and remains in a state of flux. This assertion is incontestable with the proviso that the physician-patient relationship is changing more for some patients and physicians than for others. The traditional paternalistic medical model, characterized by the patient's trust in and dependency on the physician, has been replaced in many cases by a more equal relationship in which patient autonomy and self-determination is emphasized. While this newer model certainly has many advantages, there are times when patients' rights and physicians' responsibilities conflict. When this happens, an adversarial relationship may develop between physician and patient which could negate the cooperative, reciprocal, mutual, voluntary, and goal-oriented engagement essential for both parties.

An analysis of the rights of patients and the responsibilities of physicians may be beneficial in understanding why these conflicts arise and how they may be prevented. For this reason I have chosen to examine the physician-patient relationship in the complex but fascinating setting of medical consultations.[1] (The complexity may be partly responsible for the paucity of either medical or ethical literature on the subject of medical consultations.) An attempt will be made to describe medical consultations as they currently operate in medicine, to distinguish them from other forms of physician-patient encounters, and to indicate the remarkable spectrum of possible interactions that can be described properly as medical consultations.[2]

An understanding of the rights and responsibilities of individuals within the arrangement referred to as medical consultation requires a preliminary understanding of what medical encounters qualify as consultations. The term *medical consultation* as it is used here and in contemporary American medicine is defined as the evaluation of a patient by a physician-consultant for the purpose of providing the primary care physician with additional information which will assist him in the care of the patient.[3] The situation described is one in which Dr. A requests that Dr. B evaluate Patient C and render an opinion or perform a diagnostic or therapeutic procedure on Patient C. As used here the term consultation involves three persons – two physicians and a patient – and thus differs in profound ways from the

George J. Agich (ed.), Responsibility in Health Care, 141–162.
Copyright © 1982 by D. Reidel Publishing Company, Dordrecht, Holland.

standard two-person physician-patient encounter that characterizes much of medical practice.[4]

Even when this narrow definition is used, the consultation situation remains extremely complex. It implies a prior and continuing relationship between a primary physician who requested the consultation and the patient who agreed with the primary physician that such a consultation should be sought. Any analysis must relate the rights and responsibilities of the three parties involved in a medical consultation (patient, primary physician, and consultant) to those of the two parties (patient and primary physician) in the original relationship. In turn these analyses must be related to the nature of medicine itself – its goals, practices, and organization. Since the decision to seek a medical consultation can best be understood as a specific application of the general rules guiding decision-making within a morally acceptable relationship, the consultant's responsibility will depend in large measure on the procedural adequacy and moral acceptability of the patient-physician relationship which generated the consultation in the first place. In other words, the ethical standards for medical consultation must be based upon an ethically acceptable model of both the physician-patient relationship and of decision-making in medicine, which will finally depend upon an understanding of the nature and limits of medicine itself.

I. MEDICAL CONSULTATIONS: WHAT THEY ARE AND ARE NOT

Any commentary on the rights and responsibilities of individuals involved in a medical consultation is impossible without understanding what constitutes a consultation and what does not. In efforts to discern what actions in medicine are morally acceptable, description ought to precede prescription and empirical observations ought to be a precondition to ethical analysis. Without this priority, ethical analysis lacks a firm connection with the realities of medical practice.

There are numerous types of physician-patient encounters which need to be distinguished from medical consultations. Four of the most common are: principal or primary care physician-patient relationships, care provided by health care teams, independent primary physician-patient relationships, and referrals. A brief description of each of these encounters seems in order.

First, *principal or primary care relationships* involve continuing and comprehensive care. They necessitate a long-term commitment by a physician with the consent of the patient to provide health care, including diagnosis, treatment, advice, education, and health counseling. Primary care physicians may seek the opinion of one or several medical consultants and then incorporate such opinions in providing for their patients' total health care needs. In contrast, medical consultation is episodic rather than continuous and usually is limited in scope. Today, most consultants have expertise only in their own fields (for example, surgery or internal medicine), often only in a particular subspecialty (for example, thoracic surgery or endocrinology), and often only in a particular organ system (for example, the eye, the heart, or the liver).

Second, consultations differ from the *care provided by health care teams*. As Theodore Brown points out in his essay, "An Historical View of Health Care Teams," although the health care team may be composed of individuals who represent various disciplines and have different expertise, their interaction does not resemble that of a medical consultation and is not called a consultation. The hierarchic nature of such teams and the leadership role typically accorded the physician resolves the inherent ambiguity of the inter-relationships of team members. However, even on teams composed primarily or exclusively of physicians (cardiologists and cardiac surgeons who work together in the management of open heart surgery cases, or a group of physicians who jointly direct a bone marrow transplant unit), the relationship among these physicians is not considered to be a consultation. This may be because the physicians involved have an equal status and enjoy equal and comparable relationships with the patient. Alternatively, since none of the physicians on a team enjoys a primary physician-patient relationship with the patient, the situation is one in which the concept of consultation simply does not apply.

Third, many patients are followed in the outpatient setting by more than one physician simultaneously (for example, by an internist and an ophthalmologist or by an internist and a psychiatrist). Furthermore, many patients are followed by more than one primary care physician simultaneously (for example, by an internist and a family practitioner or by an internist and a gynecologist).

These situations, which may be called *multiple independent primary physician-patient relationships*, are quite different from medical consultations. In such cases the physicians often act independently and do not serve as consultants to each other. They might only learn of the existence of the other if the patient chose to communicate the fact. The patient retains almost total control over the exchange of information between the physicians and might only encourage an exchange by asking Dr. A a question such as: "Would you check with Dr. B to find out if the medicine you want to place me on can be taken safely along with the medicine he is giving me?" No one would choose to describe the relationship between Doctors A and B as that between a principal physician and consultant.

A fourth common physician-patient encounter is a *referral*. The distinction between a medical consultation and a referral and the relationship between consultations and referrals is important – and one not often appreciated even by physicians. As opposed to a medical consultation, a referral usually means that a patient is sent by a primary physician to a new physician (perhaps a "consultant" physician) for medical care.[5] In this case the "consulting physician" now becomes the patient's new primary care physician.

Referrals may be partial or complete. An example of a partial referral would be a situation in which an internist refers a patient to a surgical colleague for an operation. The referral is partial if the internist and patient plan to continue their previous relationship after the resolution of the surgical problem. It must be noted that with any referral, in contrast to a consultation, the primary physician at least temporarily relinquishes decision-making in the patient's medical care to another physician. Despite this fact, in partial referrals the primary physician remains "involved".

In a complete referral, the responsibility for the patient's care is shifted permanently to another physician or institution. One reason for this may be that the patient's medical needs have changed (for example, a patient with chronic diabetes who has been followed by an internist develops renal failure and requires a nephrologist to manage chronic hemodialysis). Another reason may be that difficulties have arisen in the primary physician-patient relationship such that either the physician or the patient now prefers to sever the relationship. The physician then makes a complete referral to a new physician.[6]

In considering the distinction between consultation and referral, it is important to realize that a consultation often may be a prelude to a long-term referral. Furthermore, in contrast with a consultation, a complete referral generates a new physician-patient relationship, a new two-person relationship. A consultation or a partial referral maintains a triangular relationship among a patient and two physicians. These are quite different situations and they generate quite different ethical conflicts.

A major point differentiating a consultation and each of the other physician-patient arrangements is that consultations are characterized by a three-way engagement in which each of the participants – patient, primary physician, and consultant – has multiple and divided obligations to each of the other two persons and to himself within the boundaries of the medical encounter. The patient's loyalty may be divided between the primary physician and the consultant. The primary physician has an ongoing commitment to the patient, but he also has obligations arising out of collegial and professional tries to the consultant. The consultant of course is divided in his loyalties and responsibilities between the physician who invited him to see the patient and the patient for whom he is now partly responsible.

By contrast, standard physician-patient relationships, multiple independent physician-patient relationships, or complete referrals retain the essential features of a two-person encounter. Team medicine often generates its own tensions, but they differ from the specific tensions created by the triangular relationship characteristic of consultations.

II. THE SPECTRUM OF MEDICAL CONSULTATIONS

After distinguishing medical consultations from other types of physician-patient encounters, it is essential to attempt to describe the many types of situations which may generate consultations and the specific details of individual consultation arrangements. The ethical questions raised regarding medical consultations and their resolution are dependent upon the details and specifications of consultation arrangements. There will be no attempt here to analyze how the details of the consultation modify the responsibilities of the various parties. Nevertheless, the description of the range and heterogeneity of medical consultations should provide a clinical framework and the necessary background to enable others to pursue the kind of systematic ethical analysis required.[7]

There are numerous factors which modify consultation arrangements and which should influence any understanding of obligations in the consultation process. The most prominent of these factors are listed below:

The Decision to Seek Consultation

Who initiated the consultation, the patient or the physician? Did the other party agree? If it was the physician's decision to seek a consultation, did the patient have the capacity to express a preference for or against the consultation?

The Selection of a Consultant

Who selected the specific consultant? Who decided what type of specialist should be chosen? If there was disagreement, how was the matter resolved? For example, consider a situation in which a patient wanted to see a cardiologist for chest pain which he feared was of cardiac origin, but his physician suggested a thoracic surgeon to evaluate the patient for the repair of a hiatus hernia, which the physician believed was causing the patient's chest pain. It would be important to note which consultant was called in and how this arrangement was negotiated between the physician and the patient. Furthermore, which of the parties – the primary physician or the patient – assumed responsibility for the consultant's skill, competence, personality, charges, and for the outcome of the consultation?

The Type of Specialist Consulting

What type of specialist has been called in? Both the special area of expertise of the consultant and the specialty training of the primary physician will have a profound effect on the nature of the consultation process. The entire dynamics of the consultative process depends on what type of specialist is seeking a consultation from what other type. Consultations to internists and surgeons differ in many respects from those to psychiatrists. To add to the complexity, consultations requested from a particular service (for example, from psychiatry) will differ according to which primary service (for example, cardiac surgery) is requesting the consultation. There are many reasons for these differences, including the nature of the medical problem, the training of the consultant, and the severity of the patient's condition.

The Severity of the Illness

How severe is the patient's illness? The answer in any particular case modifies many aspects of the consultation arrangement just as it modifies many aspects of the primary physician-patient relationship. For example, a critically ill patient may be seen by one or several consultants in an emergency situation without consenting to these arrangements and often without even being aware of them.

The Setting of the Consultation

Is the case in question an inpatient or outpatient situation? Consultations on inpatients are different from those on outpatients, and consultations in university hospital settings often differ from those in community hospitals.

The very fact that inpatients require hospitalization implies that they generally are sicker than outpatients. Hospitalized patients often have their care paid for by some form of third-party insurance. Consultants are more available in the hospital than in the outpatient setting, but there may be more rules and administrative requirements to obtain their services. Finally, there is more scrutiny of care in the inpatient setting than in the office. For these reasons, inpatient consultation differs from the office setting. In general, hospitalized patients are less free to choose whether to see a consultant, who the consultant will be, or whether to reject the consultant's recommendation.

The details of the consultation process will probably differ depending on whether the patient is seen in a university medical center or in a community hospital. The latter has the single mission of providing care for community residents. The university center engages in the triple mission of providing care, educating students and houseofficers, and generating new knowledge through research. Furthermore, the university hospital is often staffed with a large number of medical specialists ("consultants"), and medical practice in such university centers is often dominated by these specialists.

In addition to the factors already discussed, it is important to recognize that in a decision to seek medical consultation, the primary physician and the patient may be pursuing different goals. The most frequent goal sought in obtaining a consultation is *technical expertise*, either for diagnostic purposes (such as when a radiologist is called in to perform and interpret a CT scan) or for therapeutic purposes (such as when a plastic surgeon is called in to resect a skin lesion). When a consultation is sought to obtain technical expertise, the consultant may accept or decline the request to participate in a case, but otherwise there is not much latitude for the consultant to modify the primary physician's diagnosis or treatment plans. If the consultant declines to perform the diagnostic or therapeutic service, the primary physician must seek the assistance of another expert. In general, technical experts are interchangeable.

Another goal in consultation may involve the need for *clinical judgment*. The primary physician may call in a consultant not because the latter possesses a special technical skill, but because he wishes another opinion from someone whose clinical judgment he respects.[8]

There also may be *medical-legal reasons* for obtaining a consultation.[9] For example, a physician may be concerned about missing a condition for which he could later be sued. This is sometimes referred to as "defensive medicine". Or, he may wish to show good faith in searching for the correct diagnosis in a difficult case. In another situation the physician may wish to countermand an unwelcome recommendation from a previous consultant by getting a contrary opinion. Occasionally, consultations are sought as a means to avoid or defer taking action. Sometimes the patient is the one who calls for a consultation and the physician may feel obligated legally and morally to act on this request.

Furthermore, the physician may be required to request a consultation for *administrative reasons*. For example, some hospitals require that all patients over a certain age who are scheduled for elective surgery must be "cleared for surgery" by a cardiology consultant. In another situation, compliance with certain third-party insurance requirements may necessitate a "second opinion" before elective surgery.

Other reasons why a physician might seek a consultation are *personal*. For example, he may wish to solidify his reputation with colleagues, to reciprocate for previous referrals, to assure a patient "everything is being done," to share responsibility and potential liability for unforeseen results, or to punish a patient for non-compliance. Finally, in *preparation for a referral*, a physician may seek consultation in situations in which the disease has changed or the patient is a "problem patient".

In summary, the ethical obligations of the parties to a consultation – the patient, the primary physician, and the consultant – vary according to the specific details of the consultation itself. Therefore, the search for a single solution to the range of ethical dilemmas and conflicts which could arise in the context of medical consultations would be naive. On the basis of the preceding observations, it should be clear that the consultation process is superimposed on an existing and continuing physician-patient relationship. In contrast to many other medical engagements, it involves three persons enmeshed in a complex network of relationships. The presumptive obligations of the consultant, then, ought to coincide with the basic goals of medicine – to attempt in an ethically appropriate way to improve the health and well-being of patients, most of whom present themselves voluntarily to physicians in seeking care. As a consequence, consultants should fulfill their ethical and clinical obligations to patients by serving as exclusive agents neither to the patient nor to the primary physician, but rather *by serving the original physician-patient relationship* from which the request for consultation originated.

In practice, the consultant's presumptive obligation to serve the physician-patient relationship in order to provide the best medical care for the patient is achieved by conforming to the traditions and current modes of medical practice as regards consultation. This usually means that the consultant reports his findings to the primary physician and not directly to the patient.

In communicating to the primary physician, the consultant will be improving the stability of the underlying physician-patient relationship and the quality of health care provided the patient. To repeat: the consultant generally helps the patient achieve the goals which the patient and primary physician established by serving that original relationship rather than by serving either of the individual parties.

III. THE PHYSICIAN-PATIENT RELATIONSHIP AS THE MORAL CENTER OF MEDICINE

As suggested earlier, a proper understanding of medical consultations as distinguished from other forms of physician-patient encounters logically implies the prior existence of a primary physician-patient relationship. Medicine is an institution with ends and purposes related to caring for persons who voluntarily seek help in the care of their health. The physician-patient relationship historically has been the central means by which such care is provided. Thus, a well-constructed physician-patient relationship remains the clinical and moral center of medicine ([6], [8]).

A properly constructed physician-patient relationship should involve two persons who negotiate a voluntary, consensual, non-coercive, and mutual accommodation aimed at achieving the health care goals of the patient while remaining consistent with the conscientious beliefs of the physician both as an individual and in his role as a physician. These days there are many types of primary physician-patient relationships, many of which are neither long-standing nor stable. Some involve temporary accommodations between patient and physician limited to the details of a specific clinical situation. The strength of a physician-patient relationship depends upon the patient, the physician, the quality of their interaction, the setting in which they meet, and the nature of the patient's illness.[10]

In the gradual achievement of a long-standing, stable, primary physician-patient relationship, many issues such as patient rights and arrangements for truth-telling, decision-making, and even for the way in which consultations will be handled, may have been discussed and negotiated between the physician and the patient. These discussions and negotiated arrangements provide an ideal and morally acceptable basis for medical practice.

Medical consultations, however, resemble transient accommodations between physician and patient, and they differ profoundly from well-established, stable physician-patient relationships. The consultant cannot hope to achieve the same degree of voluntary, consensual, non-coercive, and mutual accommodation as has been developed over time between the primary physician and the patient. Duties in medicine and duties in general derive from relationships. In respect to truth-telling, the duties of the primary physician to the patient differ from the duties of a consultant.[11]

The physician-patient relationship is the moral and clinical center of medicine, and decision-making within this accommodation is the central event of the medical enterprise. The decision to seek a consultation, like any other medical decision, is made in this context. Most clinical decisions in medicine begin with the delineation of the medical goals being sought by the patient and the acquiescence by the physician to these goals. These goals might include restoration of health, relief of symptoms (physical and psychological), restoration of function or the maintenance of compromised functions, the prolongation of life, or increased knowledge about a medical problem and its prognosis. Based upon the specific goals being pursued, the primary physician's central responsibility is to use his medical expertise to respond to the patient's request for help in the care of his health by proposing a medically-indicated course of action which appears to be the best approach to the patient's problems and health care goals.

The first step in the decision-making process involves the physician's recommendations. The physician normally proposes a diagnostic or therapeutic course or suggests that nothing be done. One recommendation that a physician might make is that the patient be seen in consultation by another physician. In deciding on a specific recommendation, the primary physician will take into account the technical aspects of the case (its severity, acuity, its potential for improvement, the risks involved either in doing nothing or in taking this or another action), and also the psychological and social needs of the patient. At this point, the physician normally proposes a diagnostic or therapeutic course or suggests that nothing be done.

Chronologically, the second stage in the decision-making process is the patient's reaction to the physician's clinical suggestion. Competent patients may either accept or reject physician's recommendations. In this regard, patient preferences are the weightiest ethical consideration in decisions reached within the physician-patient relationship. If the physician proposes a consultation for medically indicated reasons, the patient is free to accept or refuse the suggestion. In the normal course of events, the patient will usually accept this recommendation. If, however, the patient rejects a recommended consultation, several events could occur. The physician might modify his recommendation and decide differently. If he chose not to do so and substantial disagreement remained, the relationship could be severed because the physician might feel that his ability to care adequately for the patient was compromised.

On the other hand, if the patient and physician were to agree to seek a consultation, the consultant would be serving them jointly and his allegiance should be to the relationship which generated the request for his services. This situation is analogous to other decisions in medicine unrelated to consultation which are made mutually, consensually, non-coercively, and voluntarily by physician and patient, but which require the services of third parties to be implemented.[12]

An Empirical Claim

The goals of medicine are achieved better and more efficiently through primary physician-patient relationships with their traditional interactions with medical consultants than by alternative arrangements which essentially by-pass the primary physician-patient relationship. This claim is empirical and thus far has not been proven by any compilation of data.[13] Nevertheless, this claim seems intuitively correct to many physicians actively practicing medicine either in ambulatory or in-patient settings. By and large, patients who have sound, well-established physician-patient relationships get better outpatient and inpatient care than do patients who are practiced upon by teams of consultants in the hospital or whose interactions in the ambulatory setting are episodic, disjointed, and involve many consultants. There are several reasons why this is so. First of all, the relationship between physician and patient in a primary healing relationship seems to be the most effective way to provide care and to achieve the goals of medicine. This primary relationship between patient and healer also appears to have historical and transcultural validation [11]. Even with all the changes in the health system which serve to undermine long-term primary physician-patient relationships, those relationships which rely as much on trust and confidence as on technical expertise are regarded both within the profession and by patients as useful and desirable.

Another reason stems from the belief that the primary care or principal physician should assume responsibility for continuous and comprehensive health care for patients. Such care should be not only technically competent and humane, but also should be directed at the entire person rather than at some isolated organ system. A principal physician should also serve as his patient's friend, advisor, and advocate within the health care system. This latter responsibility includes guiding the patient through the maze of hospitals, laboratory services, and *consultants*.

A well-established physician-patient relationship also promises better care because the primary physician cares for his patient by collating and integrating the opinions of various consultants, thereby generating a comprehensive approach. By contrast, the consultant may present a recommendation that is not appropriate in terms of the patient's total health care needs or personal wishes. The principal physician would have taken account of the whole person – his disease, personality, history, fears, wishes, beliefs, and finances. On the other hand, too many consultants have a tunnel-vision perspective in which they see the patient as a "liver" or a "heart" wrapped in human form or as a "subject" to be catheterized or biopsied or operated upon.

The primary physician should be the spokesman for all physicians involved in a particular case. This role should lessen patient confusion when several contradictory or apparently contradictory reports are presented by various consultants. (Both good news and bad news, but particularly the latter, should not be transmitted to the patient by a consultant whom the patient has met once and may never see again.)

Alternatives to the Traditional Relationship

Some individuals might prefer to negotiate arrangements with their primary physicians so that a consultant could discuss findings and suggestions directly with the patient rather than with the primary physician. If such arrangements between patients and primary physicians are reached in a voluntary, consensual manner, there should be no moral objection to this plan. As mentioned earlier, though, there remains the real concern that patient care might be compromised by such a plan.

Other individuals might prefer to bypass the entire system of primary care relationships and traditional medical consultations in favor of alternative arrangements such as multiple, independently-negotiated accommodations with numerous physicians. These individuals might refer to such arrangements as "consultations" ("I will seek a consultation from the famous surgeon, Dr. A"), but as shown earlier, those schemes more closely resemble free-standing, dyadic physician-patient relationships than the three-part arrangement characteristic of consultations.

In modern American medicine, an individual who can pay for health services may enter into multiple, voluntary, and consensual arrangements with physicians even when such arrangements bypass a preliminary primary physician-patient relationship and the model of consultation described in this essay. Although patients have such license, it seems doubtful that this policy should be universalized in that society's general interest would suffer, particularly with respect to increasing health care costs. More importantly, it would limit the opportunity to achieve the goals of medicine. The policy of multiple independently-negotiated physician-patient accommodations tends to be adversarial, contentious, time-consuming, costly to patients and physicians, counter-productive in regard to medical goals, and probably would not generate additional liberty and freedom, which already exists in properly negotiated primary physician-patient relationships. The same policy would also thwart the development of trust, confidence, and hope upon which the success of the medical encounter depends [5].

Although the presumptive obligation of the consultant is to serve primarily the physician-patient relationship, a variety of circumstances could encourage the consulting physician to override this presumption and to deal directly with the patient. For example, a consultant who realizes that a true medical consultation (the three-party relationship) is not occurring, but rather that either the physician is referring the patient permanently or that the patient is seeking a second opinion independently, probably will conclude that the patient's medical interests will be served best by open and direct communication. It can also happen that the consultant may decide conscientiously that he would serve an individual patient best not by strengthening the primary physician-patient relationship but by encouraging its disruption. In this case, there would be an obligation to act accordingly. The consultant's grounds for such action might be based upon the technical inadequacies of the primary physician or upon his perception that the primary physician-patient relationship was not a morally sound arrangement. For example, if the primary physician proved incompetent or physically or emotionally impaired, and if these deficiencies could not be corrected within the framework of the institution or the profession, the consultant would be obligated to inform the patient that medical care should be sought from another, more competent physician.[14]

Another reason why a consultant might choose to deal directly with a patient would be if the basic goal of medicine were compromised. For example, if the consultant and the primary physician have irreconcilable technical differences regarding a treatment plan, and if private discussions prove unsuccessful in resolving these differences, the consultant may either confront the patient directly or announce to the patient that he is forced to withdraw from the case because of a serious difference of opinion with the primary physician. (In the latter case, the consultant should suggest to the patient that another consultation opinion be sought.)[15]

IV. ADDITIONAL VIEWPOINTS ON RESPONSIBILITIES OF CONSULTING PHYSICIANS

Besides the views discussed thus far, two additional models of the responsibilities of the consultant can be distinguished: a paternalistic model and a contractual model.

In medical practice, a paternalistic interpretation of the responsibilities of medical consultants has emphasized the primary responsibility of the consultant to the physician who asks the consultant for an opinion. If disagreements arise between the primary physician and the consultant, they usually are resolved without involving the patient in the discussions.

This paternalistic model of medical consultation is represented well in the writings of Philip Tumulty, a distinguished consulting physician at The Johns Hopkins University School of Medicine. Tumulty has written: "Obviously, the role of consultant is to help the patient by aiding his primary physician and is not to supplant him or override him or to push him aside . . . " ([9], p. 45). He is concerned that some consultants make it difficult for the primary physician to play an essential role in the care of a patient. One way consultants do so is by giving information directly to the patient or family, or by making suggestions regarding diagnosis in treatment without first getting approval from the primary physician. Tumulty believes that under no circumstances should the consultant give to the patient or his family any specific information relating to diagnosis, treatment, or prognosis unless directly requested to do so by the primary physician. Tumulty notes that when this rule is violated, " . . . doubts may be planted and confusion may begin to grow. The primary physician may start to lose control of his own patient's management . . . " ([9], p. 45). In an effort to avoid this situation, Tumulty suggests the following strategy:

> If, after examining the patient, the consultant is backed into a corner by members of the family, who insist upon getting an opinion from him, it is always possible to gracefully put them off by saying something to the effect that . . . it is essential to review certain aspects of the problem with Dr. Blank before forming an opinion ([9], p. 46).

Tumulty's attitude toward medical consultation is presented explicitly with his statement that the consultant should be ever mindful of the difficult problems encountered in the everyday practice of medicine, and he should therefore make a deliberate effort to buttress the position of the primary physician ([9], p. 45).

There are several problems with Tumulty's suggestions regarding consultations. First, he emphasizes the relationship between the consultant and the primary physician almost to the exclusion of the relationship of either to the patient. This focus on collegial relationships between medical professionals is more a matter of medical etiquette than medical ethics. Tumulty acknowledges that the ends being sought in a medical consultation are health care benefits for the patient, but he stresses that the consultant serves the patient's medical needs best by serving the primary physician. Tumulty argues that in situations of serious disagreement between primary physician and consultant, the consultant should strive to resolve these matters in discussions with the physician and not involve the patient in such disagreements. Even in the "worst case" scenario, when negotiations between the primary physician and consultant collapse, the protocol outlined by Tumulty again stresses primary physician-consultant actions and again minimizes discussions with the patient.

Tumulty notes that in situations in which the responsible physician persists in a manner which the consultant believes to be harmful, the consultant should explain to the patient or family that he must withdraw from the case because he can no longer be helpful to them ([9], p. 48). Tumulty further indicates that it should be made clear to the patient and family that the central matter is one of failure to agree: "They should *not* [italics in text] be told by the consultant that he is necessarily right and the other physician is wrong. It should again be stressed that medical problems are like all other problems; there is room for disagreement" ([9], p. 48). A final problem with Tumulty's analysis of medical consultations is its unabashedly paternalistic attitude, which argues that the physician knows what is best for the patient.[16] Although the ends being sought are the health of the patient, such a paternalistic stance understates the mutual, voluntary, consensual, and non-coercive arrangements between physicians and patients, which ought to be the moral basis of medical practice.

Another model of consultation emphasizes the "rights" and "freedom" of patients. On this model, the patient is squarely at the center of the encounter and all communication and decision-making is carried out with the patient. By contrast, the two physicians have only limited or minimal obligations (or perhaps no obligations to each other), and both are primarily responsible to the patient. Any disagreements which arise between primary physician and consultant are brought directly to the attention of the patient, who then makes a choice of alternative programs of management. This model might be referred to as a *contractual model* of medical consultation.

This view of medical consultations, at least with reference to liaison psychiatry, has been defended by H. Tristram Engelhardt, Jr., and Laurence

McCullough [2]. With respect to confidentiality in psychiatric liaison consultations, Engelhardt and McCullough have suggested that the consultant physician's duty is to the patient and that any "qualification of confidentiality can be made only with the permission of the patient." In their analysis, the consultant is free to divulge information to the primary physician only when given permission to do so, and the canons of explicit informed consent must be followed to insure that the patient's consent to release information about himself or herself is informed and voluntary. Engelhardt and McCullough observe that if the patient refuses to give informed consent:

> ... one will have paid one of the prices for respecting persons; less that optimal treatment. ... Acknowledging such freedom is central to treating patients as autonomous agents. Moreover, it allows the resolution of the morally ambiguous position of the consultant through the patient's determining the extent to which the consultant will be an agent of the patient, i.e., determined by the patient's interests.

Their contractual and libertarian model of consultation is stated explicitly:

> We have here suggested that the choices [among the duties and goods the consultant seeks] should be made in favor of respect for patient autonomy both out of regard for patients as well as in order to establish a practice which supports public liberty. Such a choice, however, is made only with the loss of other goods, in particular those that would be achieved through more paternalistic practices regardless of patient wishes, i.e., divulging information to third parties insofar as communication of information is in the best interests of this patient ([2], p. 412).

Although Engelhardt and McCullough's essay concerns the specific issue of confidentiality in liaison (consultative) psychiatry rather than consultations in general, the view developed in this particular setting offers a different model of consultation. Whereas many forms of psychiatric consultation closely resemble traditional medical and surgical consultations, some psychiatric consultations, particularly those imposed upon a patient without consent – for example, as a precondition for commitment proceedings – differ in profound ways from routine medical and surgical consultations. It appears that in their analysis Engelhardt and McCullough focus on involuntary, coerced "consultation" which must be regarded as an aberration of the traditional medical model and not as its standard. As a result, Engelhardt and McCullough avoid dealing with the practical and ethical complexities of consultations by proposing a model which bears little resemblance to consultations as they currently exist or as they have been understood traditionally in medical practice.

The physician-patient encounter as described by these authors is not a consultation in that a three-person relationship does not appear to exist. In their model, there is no presumptive obligation on the part of the consultant to communicate with the primary physician or indeed to have any interaction with that physician at all. The depicted model more closely resembles a situation in which the patient has entered into several entirely independent relationships. This model ignores the primary physician and the circumstances which generated the initial physician-patient relationship and from which the decision to seek a consultation was made.

The most serious problem with this model, however, is that by depicting autonomy and rights of the patient as the highest goal of medicine and by characterizing ethics as representing "an alternative to force", the authors describe an essentially adversarial view of medical practice.[17] This adversarial vision requires contractual guarantees to protect patients entering the medical system. The goal of medicine and in particular the human needs which encourage a patient to seek help from a physician are ignored ([5], [6]).

Consultations in medicine are the result of decisions taken in pre-existing physician-patient relationships. If these original relationships were developed in accordance with the moral principles of mutuality, consensuality, voluntariness, and non-coerciveness, and if the decision to seek consultation was made in accordance with morally sound procedures, then the issues of patient "freedom" and "rights" will all have been negotiated prior to the consultation. Thus, in the absence of serious disagreement, it remains the responsibility of the consultant to try to settle differences within the context of the enduring physician-patient relationship rather than in the transient setting of the consultant-patient relationship.

V. CONCLUSION

The model of responsibility in medical consultations proposed in this essay recognizes the voluntary, mutual, consensual, and non-coercive agreements of all parties to both the consultation process and to the physician-patient relationship which generated the request for a consultation. Any party could withdraw from the consultative arrangement (or for that matter, from the physician-patient relationship) at any time and thus change what was originally a consultation to another form of physician-patient encounter.

This view rejects the position advocated by Tumulty, which supports the primary physician and attends mainly to issues of medical etiquette in the physician-consultant relationship. It also rejects the thesis advanced by Engelhardt and McCullough that consultants have a primary obligation to patient "autonomy" (thus focusing primarily on the patient-consultant relationship). Their thesis essentially ignores the original context of care in which the consultation was sought. In practice, the view advocated here suggests that the loyalty of the consultant and of the primary physician interacts directly. Such interactions both serve and preserve the primary physician-patient relationship – the technical and moral center of medical practice. If the decision to seek a medical consultation was arrived at in the context of a morally acceptable patient-physician relationship, the consultant would act most properly by dealing mainly with the primary physician and not directly with the patient. However, when the patient's health care and health will be ill-served by the perpetuation of an ineffective or destructive (and thus morally unacceptable patient-physician relationship), it then becomes the obligation of the consultant to so inform the patient in order that the goals of medicine – the health care and health of the patient – might be better achieved through another arrangement. In general, this approach also maximizes patient benefit and permits consultants to adhere to the collegial requirements of the medical profession.

University of Chicago

NOTES

* Work on this paper was supported in part by an Interdisciplinary Incentive Award (OSS-8018097) from the Ethics and Values in Science and Technology (EVIST) Program of the National Science Foundation.

[1] I have been interested in the question of how to establish the rights of patients and the responsibilities of physicians at a time when a societal consensus no longer exists. This paper in some ways continues the work Ann Dudley Goldblatt and I did in the Ninth Trans-Disciplinary Symposium on Philosophy and Medicine [7]. We noted in the earlier paper that a morally and technically acceptable model of the physician-patient relationship would take account of the specific clinical circumstances in which doctor and patient were interacting. Thus, we described profound differences in the physician-patient relationship between situations of acute, critical illness and those of chronic, non-critical outpatient care.

As mentioned, this essay will explore the physician-patient relationship in the context of medical consultations. An earlier version of this paper was entitled "Medical Consultations: Divided Loyalties and Uncertain Responsibilities." That title reflected the commonly held view that the central ethical dilemma in the consultation process is the consultant's divided loyalties and responsibilities to both the patient and the primary physician. The issue is sometimes framed as a question: Is the consultant primarily an agent of the attending physician or is he an agent of the patient? I believe this is an oversimplified – and possibly even a wrong – rendering of the issues involved in medical consultation. Framing the question in this way ignores the historical preconditions and negotiations within the physician-patient relationship that enabled a medical consultation to occur in the first place. In this paper, I will examine the issue of the responsibility of consultants not as an isolated event, but as an interaction which is best understood within the general context of physician-patient relationships which occur within our system of medicine [1].

2 This paper will not present an historical or anthropological analysis of medical consultations. Nor will it examine consultations in systems of health care different from that of the United States. For example, the relationship of general practitioners to "consultants" in the British National Health Service is a fascinating subject and was the focus of a recent book [3]. Finally, no attempt will be made to formulate new ways to practice medical consultations: rather, an attempt will be made to describe medical consultations as they are currently practiced.

3 On occasion, physicians seek assistance from health professionals such as social workers, chaplains, dieticians, occupational therapists, etc. These requests for assistance are often described as consultations. Thus, one might say: "I will obtain a social service consultation." For reasons of simplification, in this paper I will restrict my analysis to physician-physician consultations. Many of the points made in this paper should be applicable also to non-physician health professional consultations.

4 Some medical analysts, often contractarians who believe medicine can be reduced easily to the buying and selling of a product – rather like shopping for a used car – might prefer to use the term "medical consultation" to describe what they do when they seek second or third opinions or when they go "doctor shopping". Thus, such individuals might say: "Dr. A. told me I had hypertension and should be treated; I will obtain a 'medical consultation' from Doctor B." I have no quarrel either with the wish of such individuals to seek additional medical opinions or with their peculiar use of the term "medical consultation", rather than "medical opinion" or "second opinion" to describe their activities. Such activities, however, more closely resemble the establishment of multiple primary physician-patient relationships rather than medical consultations as the term is commonly understood in medicine.

Another possible use of the term "consultation" would be to describe an opinion rendered by a specialist, a so-called consultant, at a time when the specialist was interacting with the patient in a role as a primary physician and not in the role of a consultant. The differentiation between this use of the term and the way I choose to use it relates to whether the second opinion was sought by a patient independently (thus, not a true consultation) or whether the second opinion was sought within the context of a physician-patient relationship. The former situation involves two persons; the latter situation, the true consultation, involves three persons.

5 It should be noted that the term "refer" may be used to describe either the seeking of a consultation or the making of a true "referral" in the sense of sending a patient away to be cared for permanently by another physician.

6 Referrals are frequently made at the patient's request or because a patient is dissatisfied with the primary physician. In a study by Williams *et al.*, about one-third of cases of referral from a primary physician's office to a medical center were at the request of the patient [10].

7 I will suggest, however, that an analysis of responsibilities within specific consultation situations in medicine ought to take account of the three factors noted later in this essay which begin to explicate the moral basis of consultations:

(a) the relationship of medical consultations to the original physician-patient relationship which generated the request for a consultation and the moral soundness of that original physician-patient relationship [6], [8];

(b) the adequacy of the procedural standards which generated the decision within the physician-patient relationship to seek a medical consultation [4];

(c) the likelihood that the central goal of medicine – improvement in the health care and health of the patient – will be achieved as a result of the consultation.

8 It should be noted that the skills of consultants who possess keen analytic ability and discriminating clinical judgment are not interchangeable in the way in which those of technicians are. Many aspects of their medical knowledge, interpersonal and interprofessional skills, and their success as consultants, are very special and are not transferable to another individual. In many respects, this is our generic impression of what a consultant is and what he does.

9 I am distinguishing between the *goals* and *reasons* for a consultation. I am using the term *goals* to describe decisions arrived at jointly by patient and physician based upon legitimate medical indications. By contrast, the *reasons* for seeking a consultation may be based upon medical indications, but usually also relate to non-medical factors – legal, administrative, personal – and usually are determined by the physician without patient participation. This distinction between the *goals* and *reasons* for obtaining a consultation represents a preliminary effort at the important task of describing the broad range of consultations and why they are obtained.

10 [6]. Too many commentators tend to have an apocalyptic vision of medicine in which all patient illness is regarded as life-threatening. Such a viewpoint colors analysis of the physician-patient relationship, because the patient is invariably regarded as weak and helpless in the face of critical illness and the physician is regarded as powerful and controlling. This vision is quite different from the real world of medical practice in which most patients do not have acute, critical illness, but rather come to physicians with a complaint or for the care of non-critical, chronic diseases.

11 For example, among the many duties which primary physicians owe to patients is the duty of veracity. If a patient develops a grave disease such as colon cancer, it is the obligation of the patient's physician to inform the patient at the proper time, in the proper manner, and in conformity with the patient's wishes. It would be outrageous and unethical if a patient were informed by a radiology consultant who performed a barium enema or by a gastroenterology consultant who performed colonoscopy that a colon cancer had been detected. Rather, the consultant's obligation was to provide a report of the consultation to the primary physician who would act on such information based upon prior agreements between himself and the patient on how matters such as these would be handled in their relationship. The special quality of the primary physician-patient relationship would mandate that a consultant work through that relationship and not outside of it in providing information to a patient. It is the difference in the quality and depth of relationships between patients and primary physicians, as contrasted with relationships between patients and consultants, that reinforces the point that the presumptive obligation of consultants is to function with the framework of the existing primary physician-patient relationship and to act in ways which maintain that primary relationship.

12 For example, imagine a situation in which after considerable discussion and negotiation, the physician and patient decide that the patient should try a dangerous, but

potentially beneficial, drug treatment. A prescription is written by the physician and taken by the patient to a pharmacist. The presumptive obligation of the pharmacist is to dispense the medication, although he may wish to warn the patient of its potential side-effects and even perhaps telephone the physician to confirm the prescription and dosage. In general, it would not be appropriate for the pharmacist to refuse to fill the prescription or to intrude into the physician-patient relationship which resulted in the mutual decision to use this particular medication. The pharmacist would be deviating from his appropriate role as a pharmacist if he intruded into the decision which had been arrived at jointly by the physician and patient. Similarly, consultants have been invited into a case as a result of a mutual decision reached in the context of a morally acceptable physician-patient relationship. In this situation, the consultant's obligation should be to the physician-patient relationship which generated the request.

[13] My claims in this section of the paper regarding the value of primary physician-patient relationships are empirical ones and should be subjected to experimental verification. Nevertheless, I believe that the medical relationship has been organized traditionally around primary physician-patient relationships, and therefore it remains the responsibility of those who wish to argue in favor of alternative arrangements (such as multiple independently-negotiated physician-patient accommodations) to marshal data to support their proposed innovations.

[14] It should be noted that this last general obligation of the consultant to intrude into unsuccessful physician-patient relationships is a more stringent and different requirement from those previously expected of consultants. The consultant now has a duty not only to assist the patient in the care of his health by strengthening the primary physician-patient relationship when appropriate, but sometimes to assist the patient by encouraging the disruption of that relationship. The consultant may now be required to probe both into the benefits of the existing physician-patient relationship for the patient and into its potential weaknesses. There is a great risk of officiousness here.

[15] These examples of consultant-patient interaction inevitably raise the question of whether the consultant should work to reinforce the primary physician-patient relationship or to intrude upon it. Although the presumptive obligation should be to enhance the primary relationship, circumstances such as were noted here might lead a consultant to the opposite conclusion. This conclusion and many other medical decisions are reached by a process of clinical discretion [4]; others have called this process clinical judgment. Essential to this process is discretion, the ability to draw relevant distinctions, to discard extraneous facts, to penetrate to the heart of the matter, and to make choices of one course of action as the better among many possible ones. That choice can be defended as "better" not in some absolute sense but because, given the available facts and their interpretation, judicious reflection suggests it fits the actual situation more adequately than other available options. Good choices about how to provide patients with the best medical care require clinical discretion.

[16] Tumulty's paternalistic approach to medicine is evident throughout his excellent book [9]. Interested readers in particular should examine the Introduction and also Chapter I.

[17] This adversarial vision of medicine is understandable if one accepts as the standard medical encounter a situation in which a consultation is being obtained in order to restrain a patient involuntarily. Of course, this is a limited and inaccurate portrayal of most medical and psychiatric consultations.

BIBLIOGRAPHY

1. Cassell, E. J.: 1976, *The Healer's Art: A New Approach to the Doctor-Patient Relationship*, J. B. Lippincott Company, Philadelphia and New York.
2. Engelhardt, H. T., Jr. and McCullough, L. B.: 1979, 'Confidentiality in the Consultation-Liaison Process: Ethical Dimensions and Conflicts', *Psychiatric Clinics of North America* **2**, 403–413.
3. Honigsbaum, F.: 1979, *The Division of British Medicine: A History of the Separation of General Practice from Hospital Care, 1911–1968*, St. Martin's Press, New York.
4. Jonsen, A. R., Siegler, M., and Winslade, W. J.: 1982, *Clinical Ethics: A Practical Approach to Ethical Decisions in Clinical Medicine*, Macmillan Publishing Company, New York.
5. Kass, L. R.: 1980, 'Ethical Dilemmas in the Care of the Ill: What is the Physician's Service?', *JAMA* **244**, 1811–1816.
6. Siegler, M.: 1981, 'Searching for Moral Certainty in Medicine: A Proposal for a New Model of the Doctor-Patient Encounter', *Bulletin of the New York Academy of Medicine* **57**, 56–69.
7. Siegler, M. and Goldblatt, A. D.: 1981, 'Clinical Intuition: A Procedure for Balancing the Rights of Patients and the Responsibilities of Physicians', in S. F. Spicker, *et al* (eds.), *The Law-Medicine Relation: A Philosophical Exploration*, D. Reidel Publishing Company, Dordrecht and Boston, pp. 5–31.
8. Siegler, M.: 'On the Nature and Limits of Clinical Medicine: An Essay on the Doctor-Patient Accommodation', in E. J. Cassell and M. Siegler (eds.), *Changing Values in Medicine* (submitted for publication).
9. Tumulty, P. A.: 1973, *The Effective Clinician*, W. B. Saunders Co., Philadelphia.
10. Williams, T. F., White, K. L., Fleming, W. L., and Greenberg, B. G.: 1961, 'The Referral Process in Medical Care and the University Clinic's Role', *Journal of Medical Education* **36**, 899–907.
11. Young, A.: 1980, 'An Anthropological Perspective on Medical Knowledge', *Journal of Medicine and Philosophy* **5**, 102–16.

CHRISTINE MITCHELL

INTEGRITY IN INTERPROFESSIONAL RELATIONSHIPS*

The concept of integrity is of particular importance to health professionals because it lays bare moral tensions inherent in health care which are not immediately obvious in the usual debates involving such concepts as justice, rights, utility, or the quality of life. These concepts are applied most often in an effort to discern the duties and moral obligations owed to others by health professionals. The strain and conflict which these duties cause health care workers, however, has largely gone unconsidered. Integrity, on the other hand, directs attention to the moral agency of the health professional.

Integrity is a fundamental moral concept because it intimately involves the concept of self as well as the self in relation to others. We speak of an individual, such as a nurse or physician, as having integrity and thereby express a judgment of character. We may also speak of a collective or group, such as a health care team, as having integrity, and thereby make an important observation about its unity as a community. An analysis of integrity in health care will bring to the surface moral tensions which health care workers experience in themselves, in relationships with other health professionals, and in relationships with health care institutions, which are not fully revealed in sociological and psychological analyses or even in standard medical ethical analysis. Attention to integrity, therefore, serves as a reminder that ethical conduct is linked ineluctably to the formation of moral character and community in health care as elsewhere.

It seems appropriate to begin with a brief discussion of the common usages of the word *integrity* and a categorization of the main meanings employed in ethics. This categorization will then be applied to health care, in particular to bring to the fore the moral conflicts faced by nurses. Nurses will be the main concern because their position in the social structure of health care and the role relationships open to them are paradigmatic for non-physician health professionals. The conflicts they experience will be illustrated by a case discussion which will permit analysis of the competing and incompatible conceptions of health care which contribute to nurses' compromised integrity. Finally, the essay will conclude with an examination and evaluation of some main arguments against allocating a high priority to integrity as a virtue for nurses.

George J. Agich (ed.), Responsibility in Health Care, 163–184.
Copyright © 1982 by D. Reidel Publishing Company, Dordrecht, Holland.

I

Integrity is derived from the Latin *integritas*, meaning unimpaired condition, soundness, health, honesty, uprightness. Several different usages of the word "integrity" are evident in English language usage and literature: moral integrity, physical integrity, structural integrity, aesthetic integrity, professional integrity, and psychological integrity.[1] Of these usages, moral integrity is more germane in the context of this essay, though the other aspects of integrity are clearly related. At least five aspects of the meaning of moral integrity can be distinguished on the basis of usage in the ethics literature: truthfulness, fairness, pureness, fittingness, and wholeness.

First, integrity etymologically means *truthfulness* or honesty. Having integrity in this sense means that an individual is truthful on two levels – with others and with himself. On one level, an individual with integrity is described as one who does not lie or deceive others, but speaks instead with sincerity ([14], p. 191). For example, we speak of the integrity of businessmen when seeking to establish that they are honest and that their claims are truthful ([12], p. 114; [17], p. 210). On another level, integrity applies to individuals – in the sense that persons who are not honest with themselves do not have integrity ([4], p. 25n). Benefactors who are blindly convinced of their own virtuous goodness, but who are actually motivated by selfish considerations which they are unable to acknowledge to themselves, are said to lack integrity. Thus, both individuals who deceive others and self-deceptive individuals can be said to lack integrity in this sense.

Second, integrity as *fairness* refers to being unprejudiced, unbiased and impartial. Integrity in this sense is employed normatively as an ethical standard regarding obligations to treat others fairly. Furthermore, it has a self-transcendent quality in that it requires the overcoming of selfishness and partiality. Integrity as fairness means being upright, acting with probity, and strictly adhering to the moral demands of justice. It is in this sense that we speak of the integrity of a judge who regards all equally and, without favoritism, gives each individual a fair hearing.

Third, integrity as *pureness*[2] refers to being uncorrupted, undefiled, without impurities or foreign admixture. In this sense we may think of integrity as analogous to pure water wherein every drop is as consistent and as unpolluted as another. Every belief and action of an individual with integrity reflects a consistent and uncorrupted spirit. When we speak of a politician's integrity being corrupted by a bribe or the integrity of a leader being corrupted by a lust for power, we have perceived that their vows to serve the people were polluted by selfish motives. On the other hand, persons of moral integrity are consistent. They do not say one thing and do another; they do not behave in a certain manner one time and in a diametrically opposed fashion another time.

The fourth aspect of the moral meaning of integrity is *fittingness*, which emphasizes the formal requirement of interdependence and harmony among the integral parts of a unit. Integrity as fittingness is often invoked in remarks about the integrity of a person's life, where convictions, commitments, and projects all fit coherently together across the life span ([16]; [32], pp. 108–118). We may also speak similarly of the integrity of a system, such as the judicial system with its laws, courts, and prisons, in which all of the parts fit harmoniously within the whole, thereby contributing to the unity of the system.

The fifth and most common meaning is integrity as *wholeness*. Here integrity refers to solidarity and completeness: solid in the sense of undivided, and complete in the sense of lacking nothing essential ([20], p. 26). On a personal level, one who is divided within himself cannot act with integrity. Similarly, on an interpersonal level, a group which is divided within itself, or which lacks essential elements, cannot function with integrity. There is an inherent threat to integrity in any system or chain of command with a weak link which can be pulled and pushed, drawn this way and that until it snaps, drops out, and leaves a gap, thus disabling the whole.

The foregoing discussion makes it clear that moral integrity involves a richness of meaning. Perhaps the most important feature of the concept of integrity is that it refers simultaneously to the self in terms of character and the self in relation to others as a group or community. At the simplest level, the individual with integrity is thought to cultivate an honest consciousness; to control tendencies toward unfair partiality; to develop an internally consistent and uncorrupted set of beliefs; to nurture dimensions of the self which fit together and which are fitting for a particular time, place, and profession; and finally, to manifest a wholeness and solidarily of self which signifies individuality. It is in action and in interaction, however, that individuals express their selves. Thus, in relation to others, the individual with integrity acts honestly and fairly, behaves with consistency through time, and fulfills an essential function in interdependent interaction with the parts of the whole. Finally, a group or institution may manifest an integrity which, though primarily formal, also has moral overtones. Thus the health care system may be said to have integrity if it represents itself truthfully, treats its own and others fairly, is uncorrupted and acts with consistency, exhibits a fittingness among the component parts, and expresses a wholeness wherein all essential elements contribute to the complete system.

An examination of health care reveals that integrity is compromised at each of these levels. The individual nurse is severely handicapped in acting with integrity. Nurses' interprofessional relationships with physicians come into direct conflict with their relationships with patients. Consequently, the integrity of the whole health care system is threatened.

II

It is one thing to speak of the meaning of an ethical concept and ideal and quite another to face the concrete and the real. In order to reveal the moral strains within the health care community, a case illustrating the problem of integrity facing nurses will be used. At the outset, however, several caveats are in order. Situations, issues, and problems are rarely only moral in nature. Rather, in addition to moral considerations, a complex intermingling of psychosocial, professional, and historical factors are usually involved. This point will be evident in the analysis of the following case. Although the case could be discussed in terms of patients' rights, informed consent, quality of life, or autonomy (patient and/or professional), remarks have been restricted to those relevant to the concept of integrity. To this end, some of the case information not crucial to a discussion of integrity has been omitted.

While this case highlights the plight of the nurse, it is obvious that nurses are not the only health professionals who experience and are affected by moral conflicts involving integrity. Psychologists, various kinds of therapists, chaplains, social workers, and physicians – as well as moral agents not involved in health care – face questions of integrity. For purposes of this essay, however, only the moral predicament of the nurse will be considered. Other considerations will be subordinated to an analysis of the conflicts contributing to the nurse's compromised integrity. Although this case may tend to elicit sympathy for the nurse's position, it is the nurse's position, not the sympathy, which is significant. Regardless of any agreement or disagreement with the moral judgments made in the case, it should be evident that the nurse faces a problem of integrity partly as a result of her position in health care. Hence the crucial question becomes: How important is the nurse's integrity in health care?

* * *

Sharon Andrews was the primary nurse for two severely neurologically damaged young men – Joe and Bill. Both patients had been involved in automobile accidents and were brought to the acute care ward of the neurological unit in a large teaching hospital. Twenty-one year old Joe had been driving while intoxicated and had crashed into a tree. He sustained multiple lacerations and a spinal cord compression at the sixth cervical vertebra which was unrelieved by attempted surgical decompression. He was completely paralyzed except for gross motor movement of his arms and head. Although he could not speak because he was on a respirator, he was fully alert until shortly before his death.

Doctor Samuels, a neurosurgeon attending the case, instructed Nurse Andrews that Joe was not to be coded, meaning that in the event of an emergency, which was likely to occur in the unstable course of Joe's condition, no resuscitation efforts were to be made to save Joe's life. When Nurse Andrews questioned the order, the neurosurgeon said, "I don't code my quads." ("Quads" is shortened medical vernacular for quadriplegics – those who are paralyzed from approximately the neck down and are thus unable to make voluntary movements of their four extremities.) Nurse Andrews was unable to convince the physician to change this order, which he later entered in Joe's record.

The other patient was Bill, an eighteen-year old, who had stormed out of the house following a family argument, driven away in the car, and lost control of the automobile on a corner not far from his home. As a result of the accident, he sustained severe head and spinal cord injuries which had left him in a coma. Bill was completely flaccid, with fixed and dilated pupils, and unresponsive to all language and touch except some painful stimuli. He did not, however, have a flat electroencephalogram, which is often used as a criterion for brain death. Bill's physician did not order "no code" and Bill was resuscitated several times before the final failure to restore and sustain his heartbeat.

A comparison of the physician's and the nurse's writing on Joe's case is telling. Nurse Andrews charted the usual technical data regarding vital signs, intravenous infusions, respirator, settings, and so forth. She also wrote: "Patient extremely agitated and upset. Makes frequent attempts to attract attention. Flails arms frequently. When given pen, and a pad of paper held by the nurse, writes 'my mouth hurts.'" Doctor Samuels wrote: "NS" (meaning "normal sinus," the usual rhythm of the heart) "Awake. Intubated" (meaning that Joe was attached to a respirator to assist breathing). Three days later the nurse noted, "Is able to communicate needs by drawing letters in the air with his hand." The physician wrote, "Quadriplegic as before. No code." He wrote new orders for respiratory care designed to progressively wean Joe from the respirator. If successful, the respirator would not be reinstituted during a respiratory crisis under the no-code order. The nurse indicated that Joe did not want to be left alone. She stated that during times when he was off the respirator he flailed his arms, wildly mouthing, "Help me". The physician ordered morphine sulfate to be administered as necessary for restlessness.

In discussing this case several months after Joe's death, Nurse Andrews clearly recalled Joe's pride in those first simple words which he wrote and the nurses recognized. She said, "The letters were shaky but they were easily made out by the staff. Joe did seem rather proud of himself for that accomplishment." And she vividly remembered his look of terror during periods of asystole when his heart would temporarily stop beating. Clearly he knew something was wrong and nothing was being done about it. Nurse Andrews told what it was like on the evening he died:

> I stayed with him until his heart finally stopped for good. He had been pretty much alert until the day before he died. He knew he was getting worse and seemed scared. His family was in and out. They knew he was going, and I guess they found it hard to stay and watch. I tried to talk to him that night, but you know how hard it is to talk to patients who don't respond at all. I don't know if he could hear me or not. After awhile I just took care of him and held his hand. I remember I kept thinking, "Joe, we could have saved your life." I think he really wanted to live. I know Doctor Samuels thinks no one would want to live that kind of life, and three-quarters of the staff felt that Joe's death was better than his being alive as a quadraplegic. Still, he tried hard to exercise and always cooperated with the cough and deep breathing routine after we told him how important it was. He didn't want to die. He fought all the medications we used to sedate him, trying to stay alert, as if fighting for his life. After awhile I don't think he trusted any of us, and you can't blame him. It's no wonder he was terrified. The funny thing is, my other patient during that time was a quad too, much worse than Joe. But he was Doctor Rossi's patient, and we coded him quite a few times. I remember, that night, looking over at Bill while I was standing at Joe's bed. And I asked myself, "Why do we keep saving his life, and we let you die?"

* * *

Nurse Andrews was morally troubled. Her integrity was compromised. This claim may be examined in the light of the meanings of integrity – integrity as truthfulness, fairness, pureness, fittingness, and wholeness.

First, the nurse was not completely truthful toward Joe. She may indeed have been hopeful in encouraging Joe to exercise and to write, to understand

and to participate in the world around him. Nevertheless, it could not have been easy (if even possible) to be genuinely sincere in offering such encouragement when she knew that she would withhold the crucial action of saving his life. Nurse Andrews, therefore, was guarded. Although integrity might require spontaneity and candor, and while she might have wished she could simply say to Joe, "Look, your doctor has written an order that means we will not try to save your life in an emergency," she was simply not that truthful. In their interactions, she was not spontaneous, but guarded, in order to prevent Joe from asking unsettling questions (such as "Am I going to die?" or "Can I depend on you to help me?"), which she felt constrained from answering fully and which would force her to face the fact that she was not completely truthful with him.

Some would say that Nurse Andrews should simply have told Joe the truth – the whole truth. After all, it is a patient's right to know the full nature and extent of his illness and the prospects afforded by health care. But is it the nurse's right to inform the patient? A tradition of respect for and deference to the physician-patient relationship, bolstered by legal rulings and institutional norms which support the primacy of that relationship, leaves the nurse who does not follow orders – particularly in a moral matter where patient and professional competency are in question – vulnerable to legal action at the worst and to severe censure from medical colleagues at the least.

Many health care professionals, including most nurses and physicians, would say: "Of course, the nurse can be honest." If Joe had asked her if he was going to die, these professionals might argue that she should have said everyone dies sooner or later; that Joe would probably die sooner than others his age because he was so seriously ill and injured; and that neither nurses nor physicians can know exactly how soon anyone will die. Nurse Andrews should have suggested, they would say, that Joe talk with his physician about this matter. Such an answer, however, is itself guarded and guileful. In fact, it is outrightly evasive and deceptive. The message is clear: "This topic is highly sensitive; don't ask me." Joe could not depend on the nurse to face the topic in a forthright manner – even though as his nurse she probably knew him better than did any other member of the health care community. Had she made such a response, the nurse would have implied that there was nothing untoward in Joe's case. She would have concealed from him the information he needed in order to ask the right questions. Joe probably did not know what a "code" is. He might not have known that every patient does not routinely receive the most extensive efforts of all health care personnel to save his life. Because the nurse could not behave and speak truthfully, she cannot be said to have acted with integrity. Paradoxically, she is kept from acting truthfully by the requirements to support the physician-patient relationship and to perform her role according to physician's orders.

It is clear that these two patients did not receive equal treatment, that the same efforts were not made to save their lives or to let them die. The nurse who participated in the resuscitation efforts for Bill and did not respond to the asystolic episodes of Joe was not nursing them both impartially. She lacked integrity in the sense of fairness. It is difficult not to be partial to the patient with a demonstrated desire to live and improve. Nurse Andrews probably wanted to help Joe, who clearly acted as if he wanted to be helped, to live, and to get better. Recognizing her moral and professional obligation to treat all patients fairly and impartially, she also sought to give Bill equally good nursing care. In the instance of nursing care to be provided during a life crisis (such as when the heart develops an irregular rhythm or stops), however, Nurse Andrews had been ordered to give nursing care to Bill and not to give nursing care to Joe.[3] Thus Bill's nursing care involved a partiality on the side of life and Joe's nursing care involved a partiality on the side of death. Furthermore, the ordered partiality was out of line with the felt partiality. Nurse Andrews violated her own sense of fairness in giving nursing care in this manner, and thereby compromised her integrity.

These events also illustrate the meaning of integrity as pureness. The nurse's position cannot be maintained without some sort of moral schizophrenia. It might be helpful here to indicate what regularly occurs over a period of time in a nurse's professional and moral experience. Like other moral beings, the nurse has a strongly felt need to maintain coherence between what she thinks should be done and what she is doing. She must act in situations, though, in which several different physicians decide what should be done with different patients. For example, if Doctor Smith writes orders for vigorous medical management of a living fetus from an abortion which was performed too late, the nurse is expected to share underlying values, such as a belief in the "sanctity of life". Yet when Doctor Jones decides to provide minimal medical intervention for another brain-damaged and deformed infant, the nurse, in turn, must find a belief that fits the situation, perhaps a belief regarding "quality of life". She is rarely able to maintain a single set of values in her work. Different, oftentimes conflicting beliefs are needed and are collected over a period of time in the attempt to salvage some sense of integrity while caring for patients, cooperating with physicians, and functioning within the system. Thus, an incompatible mixture of beliefs becomes an essential component of the strategy to maintain at least a minimal coherence between beliefs and acts in specific instances. Along the way, however, the nurse abandons consistency across time and so sacrifices integrity as pureness.

The moral crisis involving integrity is thus best illustrated when the nurse has two similar patients at the same time whom she is expected to care for differently. As the cases are proximate and concurrent temporally, an error in moral reasoning painfully emerges. Nurse Andrews may have attempted to achieve coherence in one case by believing in the lifesaving goal for Bill and acting to give him assiduous nursing care. Similarly, she may have tried to believe in the rightness of Joe's "no code" status (as apparently three-quarters of the staff did), and to enact that belief by not taking the usual emergency measures to stimulate his heart. The inconsistency between the two beliefs and between the two actions is especially blatant when not separated by time. In this situation, the nurse is handicapped in determining how to act morally because she lacks integrity as pureness. She has a history of choosing coherence between beliefs and actions in each case sequentially, and relinquishing consistency among beliefs and actions across cases and time. Thus she cannot rally all the forces of herself scattered among incompatible beliefs and actions, and bring her integral self to bear with precision and strength upon the present moral problem caused by the orders to give different care to similar patients.

This point suggests that the nurse's integrity is compromised in the aspect of fittingness as well. Not only do her beliefs and actions not fit together coherently, but her practice does not demonstrate fittingness with her profession as a nurse – one who seeks to comfort the suffering, care for the sick, and safeguard the rights of the afflicted.[4] Moreover, attempts to diminish the inner conflict by bringing it into the open are likely to meet with recrimination, alienating the nurse from her medical colleagues, and threatening the unity and harmonious functioning of the health care community.

The nurse, then, is left divided within herself and troubled by the threat to community solidarity which would occur if she were to resolve her conflict by maintaining consistent beliefs and actions across time. The problem of integrity as wholeness deeply touches the nurse's sense of self and also involves interprofessional relations within the health care community. For example, Nurse Andrews might have sought to avoid inner conflict and maintain individual integrity by trying to change one of the orders, by finding a new belief to morally justify her different actions, by refusing to follow orders she believed to be morally wrong, or by removing herself from the situation.

The specific complexities of these alternatives are worth noting. Nurse Andrews was unable to convince Joe's physician to change the no-code order.

Although she apparently complained to other physicians, they were unwilling to insert themselves, uninvited, into another physician's case. The problem might have been solved if the nursing supervisor or director had been willing and able to convince one of Dr. Samuels's medical superiors or a hospital administrator to intervene. As it was, the supervisor suggested that some other nurse who could follow the physician's order be assigned to these patients. It might well be argued that the supervisor should have supported Nurse Andrews. That, however, would only have solved *this* case, but not address the generic issues presented by the situation, namely, the problems involving integrity which occur when physicians make moral decisions which nursing personnel are expected to carry out. Participation of nurses in moral decision-making in health care is rare and occurs mostly when the nurse disagrees and is willing to take considerable professional risks to express that disagreement. Any remedy designed to protect and enhance integrity must provide for the full participation of those who carry out the moral decisions involved.

Another alternative available to the nurse seeking to salvage individual integrity would be to find a new, higher principle to justify her seemingly contradictory actions. It is enlightening to examine, for example, the way in which this technique may be employed in resolving other moral contradictions. Many health professionals now honor the wishes of terminally ill patients regarding the remainder of their foreshortened lives. A patient who says, "Nothing fancy, just let me go," may receive nursing care and comfort with little if any medical intervention designed to lengthen life. On the other hand, a similar patient who says, "Do everything," may encourage the physician to institute interventions intended to prolong life until the illness finally overwhelms every effort to allay it and death occurs. The moral decisions may be consistent in each case, *and* across cases and time, if the health professional endorses the priority of a principle of patient autonomy. For, in both of these examples it was the patient who decided what amount and kind of health care was appropriate.

When the patient cannot express an autonomous will, as in the instance of children and incompetents, the health professional faces a problem more truly like that of Nurse Andrews. The health professional who is confronted with one set of parents who wants to let their imperfect infant die and another set of parents who wishes to save the life of their similarly imperfect infant must determine on what basis each decision should be made. If the health professional cannot endorse a principle of parental autonomy over other relevant moral principles (such as non-maleficence), then that professional faces a problem of integrity. Parental autonomy may be an important norm for a variety of reasons, such as the fact that parents must live with, care for, and pay for their child. These reasons may be morally compelling, so much so that parental autonomy becomes a principle which influences decision-making. If it is not the first principle or a higher-order principle, however, other moral principles may come in direct conflict with that of parental autonomy. Thus, a principle of parental autonomy only aids the health professional in maintaining integrity if it overrides other principles.

Similarly, the nurse could resolve her crisis of integrity by resorting to a higher-order principle of "physician authority" – that is, the principle that physicians, and not nurses, have the authority to make moral decisions in health care. But "physician authority" is a socio-professional rather than a moral principle. Using it to resolve the problem would give a social and professional norm priority over moral principles such as truthtelling, beneficence, and so forth. This contradicts the very nature of moral principles if, as Richard Hare has argued, "it is characteristic of moral principles that they cannot be overridden" ([18], p. 169). The norm of "physician authority", then, is not appropriate to govern and resolve a conflict between two different moral principles, for it is not a higher-order *moral* principle.

Nurse Andrews of course might have refused to follow orders she believed to be morally wrong. Suppose she disregarded the no-code order by calling the code team and instituting vigorous emergency measures such as cardiopulmonary resuscitation and chemical or electrical cardiac correctives. The specially designated code team of nurses, physicians, and respiratory therapist would have arrived immediately and attempted to save Joe's life (assuming none of them was personally familiar with Joe's case and realized he was a "no code"). Whether Joe lived or died as a result of these measures, Nurse Andrews would have been responsible for incurring expenses she was not institutionally authorized to incur. This would be true even if she could argue that she had acted morally. If Joe died, she would have faced medical protest and supervisory requests for explanation of her behavior, bolstered by physicians' and others' observations that Joe obviously had not been helped by her intervention. Whatever arguments she could make (for example, about Joe's desire to live and the unpredictable consequences of resuscitative efforts) would have been undercut by the hindsight available to those who wished to legitimize the original order not to code by pointing to Joe's death or, perhaps, his worsened state. If Joe lived, she then would have faced the problem of obtaining new orders for his medical care from other physicians who do not customarily intervene without the knowledge and consent of the attending physician. Thus, refusing to follow the no-code order on Joe would have been difficult if Nurse Andrews had been able (albeit deceptively) to secure medical cooperation, and impossible if she had not.

The remaining alternative would be for the nurse to remove herself from the situation if she could bring herself to abandon her patients, and perhaps even leave her chosen profession. Integrity as wholeness, in its dual dimension as individual integrity and group integrity, would be shattered. The nurse seeking to salvage individual integrity – either by actively disagreeing or by withdrawing from the cases – would damage the integrity of the health care community. Her objections to orders would disturb nurse-physician relationships, her withdrawal would terminate a crucial nurse-patient relationship, and her absence would create a gap in the health care team. If, instead, the nurse were to seek to support the integrity of the health care team, then she would have to bear inner conflict. One way or the other, integrity as wholeness would be impaired. Any attempt to rectify the sharp split between the nurse's beliefs and actions would seem to splinter the solidarity of the health care team treating these two patients.

III

The problem of integrity arises out of a basic tension inherent in health care. On the one hand, the health care system is structured from the top down to carry out the medical mission of curing, healing, and saving patients' lives. The nurse is an essential participant in these endeavors. She is expected to make a technically competent contribution. The mission of the health care team, like a war mission, is conceived of as crucially important. It has top priority, and the system is hierarchically structured to best fulfill that mission with one individual in command. The mission orientation of medicine requires certain relevant nursing virtues, such as obedience, and a particular form of trust, in that the physician must be able to trust the nurse to act as directed in fulfilling the mission.

On the other hand, the health care system is conceived of as structured from the base up to meet the multiple needs of patients. These include the sensitive understanding of patients' needs, the provision of sympathetic nursing care as well as medical treatment. The nurse is the primary figure in delivering personalized care. In this system a different kind of trust is essential in that the patient must be able to trust the nurse to understand and help.

These two conceptions of health care – the mission model and the sensitivity model[5] – cannot be stably combined in a single personality. Yet the nurse has a pivotal role in each. In the mission model, it is the nurse whom the physician relies upon to carry out orders and treatments which are crucial to medical success. In the sensitivity model, it is the nurse who is the patient's daily source of comfort, support, and professional contact. On the one hand, she must share the values and aims of a variety of physicians. On the other hand, she must be responsive to the needs and goals of particular patients. Called upon to maximize first one and then the other conception of health care, the nurse is prevented from acting with integrity under either system insofar as integrity requires a formation of the self which remains consistent over time.

The nurse whose character is formed so that she fulfills the medical mission in cooperation with physicians' orders is different from the nurse whose character is formed so that she is sensitive to patients' needs. Integrity under the mission model requires that the nurse be an obedient and trustworthy instrument of the mission. In addition, this nurse must develop the flexibility necessary to respond to orders from different physicians. She may justify her action as right, even if it is not consistent, as long as it is in conformity with a mission already defined as good. Under the sensitivity model, however, the nurse whose character is formed so that she treats patients personally and holistically feels the obligation to fulfill patients' faith in her. The kind of individualized care and comfort this nurse is supposed to provide gives priority to interpersonal bonds. She must think and act with a moral imagination sensitive to patients' needs. In fact, the very nature of nursing care being offered requires that the patient be able to believe in her. No one is comforted, strengthened, or encouraged by care from someone who cannot be trusted. The problem is that these models make incompatible demands on the nurse.

Insofar as the nurse has the capacity, indeed the call, to reason from the point of view of the patient, she is potentially unreliable and so lacks integrity in performing her part in the medical mission. Insofar as she operates as an instrument under the aegis of a mission, she is never completely at her own disposal to enter sympathetically and truthfully into relationships with individual patients. She is not trustworthy under either model because she lacks integrity. It is not possible to maximize both integrity based on obedience and integrity based on sympathy, either simultaneously or sequentially. Nurses who try fail on both fronts.

While not all nurses eventually leave nursing, many do. The constraints upon nursing integrity are a major factor in the well-documented dissatisfaction and "burn-out" phenomenon noted in the nursing profession. The case discussed earlier is part of the daily experience of nurses still in practice. Although it cannot highlight every dimension of integrity, it does pose a key problem which creates a crisis of integrity: a person is expected to act in accordance with one set of moral beliefs in one situation and is expected to act in accordance with a different set of moral beliefs in a morally similar situation. In addition, the nurse experiences the competing claims of two different models of health care. As a consequence, she either seeks to salvage individual integrity by quitting or stays and sacrifices integrity. In either instance the integrity of the whole health care community is threatened. Nurses who quit leave a gap which thwarts the efforts of the entire system to provide good patient care. Nurses who stay survive precisely because they sacrifice individual integrity. In this manner the system selects nurses who consequently are unreliable under both the mission model and the sensitivity model. Health care thus is organized with an inherent flaw. By permitting – or rather requiring – that the integrity of a vital part be violated, the integrity of the whole is severely compromised.

IV

In face of this serious charge, at least four arguments have been advanced to show that integrity is not, and should not be, a critical concern. The *argument from role distinctions* and the *argument from particularity*, as they may be termed, attempt to deny that integrity is compromised. The *argument from necessity* and the *argument from utility* attempt to justify diminishing the importance of individual integrity in relation to other requirements. The common conclusion is that integrity may be ignored.

The first two arguments paradoxically are often offered by nurses themselves. At a superficial level it seems as if integrity is not a strongly held value. However, just the opposite is the case. Because integrity is a deeply felt and stringent moral requirement, nurses make every effort to believe that their integrity remains intact.

The *argument from role distinctions* accomplishes this purpose in two ways – one which involves the separation of the nursing role from other aspects of the self and one which involves separating the physician-extender aspects of the nursing role from "real nursing". In the first instance, the nurse who finds her integrity threatened in the work environment attempts to maintain integrity as a person by isolating that part of herself called "nurse" and considering it a non-essential element of the whole self. If being a nurse is not considered a crucial part of her being as a person, or is rejected as a part of the integral self, then she can claim to maintain integrity of the whole and not be concerned whether the nursing part is consistent with the rest of the self.

This strategy of keeping the nursing role distinct from the rest of the self has serious problems, however. First, it is unclear on what grounds it could be done. It would require amputating an aspect of the self which is expressed in daily action – nursing. Even if it is psychologically possible, it is morally objectionable. The person who seeks to morally separate the self who ignores a patient's pleas for help and look of terror, from the self who comes to the aid of family, friends, and some other patients, clearly violates canons of justice. If habits of action form character, as Aristotle claims, then these inconsistent actions contribute to a divided character.

A related way of solving the problem of integrity is to make a clearcut distinction between the physician's and the nurse's role responsibilities.[6] This strategy attempts to justify removing personal responsibility for those actions which fall within the realm of acting for the physician. Thus, Nurse Andrews might have argued that giving the emergency medication which would have maintained Joe's blood pressure and suppressed abnormal heartbeats was "physicianing", not nursing. In order to keep the nursing role as part of the integral self and also achieve integrity, the nurse argues that those actions which fall in the category of extending the physician's role do not count. They are actions which she performs in lieu of the physician and for which the physician, not the nurse, has moral responsibility.

This division of roles, however, is entirely *ad hoc*, generated to solve the specific situation of moral disagreement. One cannot absolve moral responsibility for one's actions by arbitrarily redefining one's role and the responsibilities which go along with it. Furthermore, the integrity of the health care community depends on the cooperative interdependent relationship between the parts of the whole. The performance of medically-ordered therapies is a vital part of nursing. Administering emergency medications in a cardiac crisis, for example, is as crucial to complete nursing practice as caring, encouraging exercise, preventing infection, feeding, monitoring fluid balance, and giving backrubs. Even if Nurse Andrews reasoned that she was not morally responsible for informing or resuscitating Joe because those aspects of his care were actually "physicianing", the other parts of the care which she competently provided nevertheless were seriously compromised by redefining and relinquishing responsibility for the physician-extender part. As a consequence, Joe could not trust Nurse Andrews.

The argument for role distinctions, then, does not solve the problem of integrity. Neither the strategy of isolating the nursing role from the rest of the self, nor the attempt to separate the "physicianing" parts from the rest of nursing practice are successful methods of maintaining integrity. While consistency may be achieved among the remaining parts, integrity is nonetheless compromised by removing an essential part of the whole.

The *argument from particularity* is similarly an unsuccessful attempt employed by the nurse to salvage integrity. It involves losing oneself in the nuances of the particular situtation and denying that there are situations so sufficiently similar as to provide reasonable precedent and require consistent action. On this view, each case is irremediably different. Since no general principles apply, no troublesome conflict between principles can occur. Joe's case is not the same as Bill's case. Not coding Joe may have been justified by the observation that he was paralyzed and the quality of his life diminished, or that his accident was the outcome of drinking while driving for which he must now bear the results of his own irresponsible behavior, or that letting Joe go would be a better decision for a family already overburdened with the financial and emotional stress of an unstable, expensive, and long-term course of rehabilitation. On the other hand, coding Bill may have been justified by observing that every effort must be made in order to avoid adding to the family's sense of responsibility and guilt already heightened because Bill's accident followed on the heels of an angry family dispute. Thus, it is the particularities of the case which justify different actions.

While this strategy seems to allow one to maintain coherence between belief and action in specific situations, it nevertheless breaks life into a series of particular cases and discrete episodes; it disintegrates the self as as actor with a history and future. Furthermore, it permits deciding each case on the basis of specially selected details and unique facts. The fact that Joe was paralyzed might have been a relevant, even determinative, factor in deciding what to do in Joe's case; while the fact that Bill was also paralyzed might not be considered a relevant factor in deciding what to do in Bill's case. The requirements of justice in relating to others, the aspect of fairness in achieving integrity of the self, come to bear heavily against the argument from particularity.

Thus, both the argument from particularity and the argument from role distinctions are unsuccessful attempts to salvage integrity by emphasizing only one aspect of its meaning. It cannot be concluded, however, that the task is simply to achieve integrity in its fullest sense, because the following two arguments – the *argument from necessity* and the *argument from utility* – are usually offered by hospital administrators, physicians, and health planners in response to nurse's complaints of compromised integrity. They suggest that such integrity interferes with the efficient functioning of a group having a mission to provide health care, and so may be justifiably compromised.

The argument from necessity concludes that the integrity of an individual or an institution may be violated because it is necessary that something be done, and "necessity leaves no choice". Used in the health care context, the argument from necessity concludes that nurses' integrity may be compromised for the sake of the orderly and conventional functioning of the health care system. There are four versions of this argument which warrant attention: the authoritative, the strategic, the moral, and the emergency aspects of necessity.

The necessity argument is often advanced with an aura of authority arising from a claim of superior knowledge regarding the complete and complex situation necessitating the specified solution. The ultimatum of necessity implies that one need not deliberate further because there is no other choice. This version of the argument often functions as a facade behind which certain other values, masked by the appeal to necessity, are being upheld. For example, it is sometimes necessary to violate bodily integrity to save a life. Or it may be considered necessary to violate a nation's integrity to preserve peace. Analogously, it may be argued that it is necessary to violate nurses' integrity in order to maintain the efficient functioning of the health care system. Some of the values underlying such violations are life, peace, and efficiency. The "facts" regarding the necessary solution are based upon values which are presumably shared or which, according to the authoritative view, should be shared. Once the underlying values have been revealed, however, the authoritative view of the situation and the necessary method of resolving it may be examined and questioned along with the assumed values and associated conception of the facts.

A particular strategy is also endorsed by the necessity argument. It does not simply state that it is necessary to do something, but rather that it is necessary to do a particular thing. For example, it is argued that health care must be organized with physicians in control of cases and the care given by other health professionals. Such organization is necessary in order to fulfill the medical mission and maintain order in a complex health care system. Nursing management of cases and independent nursing actions would erode nurses' reliability in implementing the medical regimen and would cause confusion in the orderly provision of health care. Here the argument from necessity is sometimes bolstered by the "corollary of convention" which claims that "things have always been this way" and that change would create chaos. Since physicians historically are accustomed to administrative responsibilities and nurses are not, then physicians should be in command. Similarly, physicians are not accustomed to respecting, much less soliciting, consultations from nurses.[7] Changing well-established conventions, it is claimed, would cause severe disruption of the health care system. It is worth noting, however, that this is a strategy to maintain the present situation as regards the role of physicians, rather than an argument against the claim that nurses' integrity is essential not only to nursing practice but to good patient care.

Besides the strategic dimension, there is a moral dimension to the argument from necessity. Not only is the hierarchical system of health care delivery considered necessary, but health itself is seen as a morally necessary good. Nurses are engaged in the mission to preserve a basic good – a healthy life – believed necessary for the enjoyment of other goods. Hence, the nurse should subordinate all other values to this end. The difficulty with this view is that it contains the following troublesome assumptions: that a healthy life is simply the absence of disease, freedom from pain, or the maintenance of vital bodily functions; that medical treatment is the only means or even the most effective means of achieving health; and that health is tantamount to the good life.

The fourth dimension of the argument from necessity involves emergency conditions. When under the rule of necessity, as Michael Walzer puts it, "necessity knows no rules" ([32], p. 254). In effect, this view involves the attempt to provide limits to the otherwise situational nature of the appeal to necessity. The range of justification by necessity is restricted to emergency situations, with the implication that any violation of integrity is merely temporary. Ironically, the argument from necessity implicitly acknowledges both the dubious nature of the action to be justified and the general value of integrity. Considerations of necessity in emergencies may justify violations of physical integrity – as when invasive procedures temporarily compromise bodily integrity, for example – because physical integrity presumably can be restored. It is considerably more complex to justify violations of moral integrity which seem by definition to be difficult if not impossible to restore. The argument from necessity fails because it maintains that integrity can be temporarily suspended, though the very meaning of integrity implies an uncorrupted, pure, and consistent state of wholeness.

The *argument from utility* dovetails with the argument from necessity insofar as it assumes that the good under discussion is health. The obligation to produce the greatest good, then, is an obligation to produce good health. Individual actions, by the principle of utility, should produce the largest measure of health for the largest number of patients. Both health and patients are considered quantitatively. Persons are more or less healthy, as in the case of patients with chronic renal disease who are less healthy than patients with simple hypertension, but more healthy than patients with renal failure. Similarly, patients are regarded aggregately in terms of how many receive the product, or non-moral good, called health. Under the principle of utility, it is necessary to calculate the amount of health dispensed and the number of patients treated in order to determine which actions would contribute to the greatest proportion of health to illness. The dominant view is that more health is obtained by more persons in a system organized to extend the skills of a limited number of physicians through the use of ancillary personnel. Thus, nurses and other health professionals become "physician-extenders". The role of physician-extenders is restricted to performing according to physicians' directives. They are seen as means to an end; their individual integrity may be justifiably compromised in the effort to bring about a greater good.

It is interesting to note, however, that in order to measure health as a quantity, *medical* definitions such as the absence of infection or the lowering of blood pressure have characteristically been used. Nursing priorities which are often less objective and less easily quantifiable are ignored. For example, the objectives of enhancing patients' understanding of their disease and recovery process, maintaining family bonds during stressful illness, and assuring a comfortable return to the home environment and daily routines are more difficult to measure. These are also vital aspects of good health, even though they are seldom counted in utilitarian calculations.

Even if it is possible to quantify more comprehensively the health produced, as utilitarians would undoubtedly argue could be done, the problem would not be solved. The argument from utility, as Bernard Williams points out, "cannot hope to make sense, at any level, of integrity."[8] Williams argues that individuals with integrity cannot dispense with their deepest commitments, or "projects" as he calls them, in order to obey a utility machine ([33], p. 116). A requirement to act under the aegis of utility results in alienating individuals from their own convictions and actions and represents a fundamental attack upon integrity.

Thus, both the argument from necessity and the argument from utility come to the same conclusion, namely that other factors – obedience, an orderly and conventional system of health dispersal, the extension of physicians, and producing the greatest possible measure of (medically defined) health to the largest number of persons – are more important than individual integrity. Just the opposite has been argued in this essay. The integrity of the nurse cannot be violated without sacrificing sensitive and technically competent care for patients.

Harvard University

NOTES

* I owe a debt of thanks to audiences at Southern Illinois University, the Kennedy Institute of Ethics at Georgetown University, and at Michigan State University for their helpful comments on various drafts of this paper. I am also grateful to Ralph Potter, Preston Williams, Russ Sizemore, Ed Erde, and volume editor George Agich, for their suggestions, although I accept full responsibility for the final version. Finally, I wish to express my lasting gratitude to Eunice Kennedy Shriver and the Joseph P. Kennedy, Jr., Foundation for financial support during my two years as a Kennedy Fellow at Harvard University.

1 The following indicates some of the sources which refer to these kinds of integrity: *moral* integrity is touched upon in several of the works listed in the bibliography, though rarely in depth. See especially ([2], [16], [19], [24], [27], [32]). F. M. Burnet's book, *The Integrity of the Body*, provides an excellent example of the meaning of *physical* integrity [5]. Although somewhat outdated, this volume on immunology concerns the human body, the phenomenon of "antibody", and self-recognition. For a brief discussion of *aesthetic* integrity (as well as ethical), see James Gutman's essay, "Integrity as a Standard of Valuation" [17]. *Structural* integrity is most commonly employed with regard to architecture, though it is also used to identify a characteristic of organizations. The issue of *professional* integrity in medicine comes up in Robert Lifton's article, "Advocacy and Corruption in the Healing Professions" [23]. Erik Erikson employs integrity as a psychological concept ([9], [10], [11]).

I have not separately categorized personal integrity, though the phrase is commonly found, since it seems to mean a combination of psychological and moral integrity. Although Bernard Mayo has concluded that personal integrity and moral integrity mean the same thing, I suspect moral integrity is a part of, rather than synonymous with, personal integrity [25]. I would not claim, however, that one could establish solid moral integrity without psychological integrity.

2 Admittedly a somewhat archaic term, I have used "pureness" because of its striking frequency in historical definitions and descriptions of integrity and because it conveys both the ideas of consistency and incorruptibility which are clearly contained in the meaning of integrity.

3 A "no-code" order not only prohibits medical interventions but also many associated nursing interventions. Even though a complete code requires the joint efforts of physicians and nurses, cardiopulmonary resuscitation (CPR) is often a nursing act.

4 See the "Code for Nurses" adopted by the International Council of Nurses, reprinted in ([2], pp. 296–7), and the "Code of Ethics" adopted by the American Nurses' Association, reprinted in ([3], pp. 155–157). In addition to tenets related to the nature of nurses' responsibilities to patients, Statement 10 reads: "The nurse participates in the

profession's effort to protect the public from misinformation and misrepresentation and to maintain the integrity of nursing."

5 I offer these as "ideal types" in the Weberian sense. Although physicians tend to function to a greater degree according to a mission model and nurses tend to act according to a sensitivity model, individual physicians and nurses may fall closer to one or the other ideal type.

6 Here I am using a "thin" notion of role as somewhat simplistically confined to certain specifiable tasks. For a much more detailed treatment of role responsibility, see George Agich's distinctions between task and role definitions of responsibility in this volume.

7 Note, for example, that Mark Siegler does not discuss consultations between nurses and physicians in his paper on the consultation process earlier in this volume.

8 ([33], p. 82). Williams is arguing against hedonic utilitarianism, and specifically against the problem of negative responsibility which he finds inherent in utilitarianism. Although I am discussing a principle of utility in which health, instead of happiness, is the highest good, Williams's basic argument still applies. The problem is that a person's own project is but one among many in the utilitarian calculation where the (perhaps undesirable) projects of others determine one's duty. If, for example, a nurse is deeply committed to the care and well-being of a particular patient, but the utilitarian calculation of the maximum balance of health over illness in the world involves among other things not saving that patient, then the nurse is required to modify (or abandon or never begin) her commitment to the patient. Yet the very nature of nursing is such that it requires a wholehearted commitment and an integrity which cannot be turned on and off in accordance with utility.

For an analysis of Williams's failure to confine his argument based on integrity to negative responsibility, see Harris [19]. Williams's argument nonetheless raises the general problem of sacrificing one's integrity to utilitarian calculations of responsibilities to others.

BIBLIOGRAPHY

1. Aldrich, V. C.: 1946, 'Theory and the Integrity of Experience', *The Journal of Philosophy* **43**, 379–382.
2. Beauchamp, T. L. and Childress, J. F.: 1979, *Principles of Biomedical Ethics*, Oxford University Press, New York.
3. Benjamin, M. and Curtis, J.: 1981, *Ethics in Nursing*, Oxford University Press, New York.
4. Bok, S.: 1978, *Lying: Moral Choice in Public and Private Life*, Pantheon Books, New York.
5. Burnet, F. M.: 1962, *The Integrity of the Body*, Harvard University Press, Cambridge.
6. Carr, S.: 1976, 'The Integrity of a Utilitarian', *Ethics* **86**, 241–246.
7. Curtin, L.: 1978, 'Nursing Ethics: Theories and Pragmatics', *Nursing Forum* **17**, 4–11.
8. Donnelley, S.: 1978, 'Whitehead and Jonas: On Biological Organisms and Real Individuals', in S. F. Spicker (ed.), *Organism, Medicine and Metaphysics*, D. Reidel Publishing Company, Boston, pp. 155–175.

9. Erikson, E. H.: 1968, *Identity: Youth and Crisis*, W. W. Norton, New York.
10. Erikson, E. H.: 1964, *Insight and Responsibility*, W. W. Norton, New York.
11. Erikson, E. H.: 1958, *Young Man Luther*, W. W. Norton, New York.
12. Exman, E.: 'What is the Right Thing?', in R. M. MacIver (ed.), *Integrity and Compromise*, Harper & Brothers, New York, pp. 105–115.
13. Freeman, W. W. K.: 1963, 'Training of Statisticians in Diplomacy to Maintain their Integrity', *American Statistician* **17**, 16–20.
14. Fried, C.: 1978, 'Rights and Roles', in *Right and Wrong*, Harvard University Press, Cambridge, pp. 167–194.
15. Garnett, A. C.: 1969, 'Conscience and Conscientiousness', in J. Feinberg (ed.), *Moral Concepts*, Oxford University Press, New York, pp. 80–92.
16. Garnett, A. C.: 1941, 'Deontology and Self-Realization', *Ethics* **51**, 419–438.
17. Gutman, J.: 1945, 'Integrity as a Standard of Valuation', *The Journal of Philosophy* **42**, 210–216.
18. Hare, R. M.: 1963, *Freedom and Reason*, Oxford University Press. New York.
19. Harris, J.: 1974, 'Williams on Negative Responsibility and Integrity', *Philosophical Quarterly* **24**, 265–273.
20. Hauerwas, S.: 1975, 'The Idea of Character: A Theological and Philosophical Overview', in *Character and the Christian Life: A Study in Theological Ethics*, Trinity University Press, San Antonio, pp. 1–33.
21. Hofstadter, A.: 1949, 'Some Reflections on the Problem of Man', *Philosophical and Phenomenological Research* **10**, 25–35.
22. Jonas, H.: 1968, *The Phenomenon of Life: Toward a Philosophical Biology*, Dell Publishing Co., New York.
23. Jonas, H.: 1974, *Philosophical Essays: From Ancient Creed to Technological Man*, Prentice-Hall, New Jersey.
24. Lifton, R. J.: 1979, 'Advocacy and Corruption in the Healing Professions', in W. R. Rogers and D. Barnard (eds.), *Nourishing the Humanistic in Medicine*, University of Pittsburgh Press, Pittsburgh, pp. 53–72.
25. Mayo, B.: 1978, 'Moral Integrity', in G. Vessey (ed.), *Human Values*, Royal Institute of Philosophy Lectures, Vol. 11, Humanities Press, New Jersey, pp. 27–43.
26. Mayo, B.: 1962, 'Thomas Jefferson's Faith in Human Integrity', in J. M. Dorsey, *The Growth of Self-Insight*, Wayne State University Press, Detroit, pp. 7–29.
27. 'Morality, Courage, Common Sense – Qualities Leaders Need Most', *The United States News and World Report* **16**, p. 29.
28. Norton, D. L.: 1976, *Personal Destinies*, Princeton University Press, New Jersey.
29. Rawls, J.: 1971, *A Theory of Justice*, Harvard University Press, Cambridge.
30. Storr, A.: 1961, *The Integrity of the Personality*, Atheneum, New York.
31. Trilling, L.: 1972, *Sincerity and Authenticity*, Harvard University Press, Cambridge.
32. Walzer, M.: 1977, *Just and Unjust Wars*, Basic Books, New York.
33. Williams, B. and Smart, J. J. C.: 1973, *Utilitarianism For and Against*, Cambridge University Press, London.
34. Winch, P.: 1972, 'Moral Integrity', in *Ethics and Action*, Routledge & Kegan Paul, London, pp. 171–192.

WILLIAM B. BONDESON

CONSULTING WITH INTEGRITY: SOME REFLECTIONS ON TEAM HEALTH CARE AND PROFESSIONAL RESPONSIBILITY

The moral confusion present in health care is compounded by the number of emerging professions which are seeking their own identity and integrity as part of the health care team. The leading example of such a profession is nursing. Christine Mitchell's essay, "Integrity in Interprofessional Relationships", speaks well to the needs of a profession which is developing a strong sense of its own integrity and responsibility. There are additional, more recent examples, however, in which new groups of health care professionals are seeking recognition and responsibility. At my institution, for example, the roles of patient representative, risk-manager, and patient-educator have been created only within the past few years. On a national scale, these professionals are seeking recognition for themselves. As these groups develop their own sense of identity and integrity, the problems associated with the team delivery of health care will undoubtedly become magnified.

An interesting point has been made regarding the nature of undergraduate training for health care professionals and its relation to team decision-making.[1] Most students acquire the necessary knowledge to be scientists, humanists, social scientists, or physicians in a highly individualistic educational mode. Although a great deal of time is spent in class and in discussions, the basic mode of learning has been highly individualistic. That kind of understanding and learning is intensified by the nature and style of graduate study, although there may be some modification in the sciences, for example, when a student becomes part of a large-scale research effort. Students are given virtually no training for team decision-making and in fact the whole character of their education works against the development of such skills. If that situation is the case, then the undergraduate and professional health care educational system needs to be re-designed in such a way that team decision-making and the skills involved in it are a basic part of the curriculum.

These points have been made by way of introduction to my commentary on the essays of Mark Siegler and Christine Mitchell. Both are concerned with the nature of the physician-patient relationship and how that relationship bears upon other members of the health care team, especially consultants and nurses. Both are concerned with the hierarchy of personal, role, and social responsibilities within health care teams and with ways of reconciling conflict-

George J. Agich (ed.), Responsibility in Health Care, 185–192.
Copyright © 1982 by D. Reidel Publishing Company, Dordrecht, Holland

ing responsibilities. Both authors lament the decline of the traditional physician-patient relationship viewed as a personal and intimate relationship not unlike friendship, a relationship which is at once voluntary, cooperative, mutual, and goal-oriented. In Mitchell's terms (implicitly at least), the traditional physician-patient relationship has declined or disappeared in the modern highly technologized hospital. It has been replaced by a nurse-patient relationship which, even though more limited and episodic than the traditional physician-patient relationship, is the best available, given the complexities of high technology and specialized medical care. However, there appears to be a fundamental agreement between Siegler and Mitchell on the actual nature of the traditional physician-patient relationship and the parallels between it and the nurse-patient relationship, and both authors probably would find much to agree with in Stanley Hauerwas's comment in "Authority and the Profession of Medicine" that medicine can be viewed as an educational process for both health care professional and patient.

But to say that there are parallels between the physician-patient relationship and the nurse-patient relationship is surely not enough, especially in the context of the papers in this volume. Both Siegler and Mitchell have idealized conceptions of the relationship they discuss, and both seem to assume that each relationship is dyadic. That, of course, cannot be the case. Neither paper gives us even a hint as to how the relationship between physician and nurse ought to be characterized. It could be inferred, though perhaps without warrant, that both Siegler and Mitchell have described their respective relationships with the patient in such an exclusive, dyadic, and personal way that conflicts between nurse and physician seem almost inevitable. The concept of a team thereby goes by the board.

Siegler's paper, "Medical Consultation in the Context of the Physician-Patient Relationship", proposes a solution to the classic problem of the primary obligation of the consultant by bridging the alternatives of obligation to the primary physician on the one hand and obligation to the patient on the other in a deft move that makes the primary physician-patient relationship central to a proper understanding of the consultant's obligations. Although the consultant's loyalties are to both parties in the primary dyadic physician-patient relationship, this relationship itself is centered around the patient's own autonomy and integrity. Thus, Siegler seems to be arguing that the consultant's obligation is not to persons labelled "patient" and "primary physician" but rather to persons related in a physician-patient kind of way. It becomes the consultant's obligation to protect and enhance that relationship. The triangle has been inverted: the physician-patient relationship is at the apex and all other relations are relegated to positions at its base. And this raises the question as to how the nurse-patient relationship fits into Siegler's analysis. Is the nurse, for example, like another consultant? Or is the nurse a provider of services and thus a means of fostering the primary physician-patient relationship though not a part of Siegler's triangle? My reading of Siegler's paper leads me to believe that the latter is closer to his conception.

There are two areas in which Siegler's paper might benefit from further analysis. The first concerns the adequacy of Siegler's taxonomy of consultative relationships. Since his claim is that the nature of the consultative relationship may be affected by the service requested from the consultant, or perhaps even by the relationship (for example personal or professional) between the primary physician and the consultant, a comprehensive taxonomy is fundamental to Siegler's effort. Those who are more familiar with the empirical realities of consultative situations than I are better able to pass judgment here. I do want to raise a subsidiary point nonetheless. Siegler seems to assume that the consultative relationship is a patient-physician-physician relationship. This raises the question as to whether there are consultative relationships which are not of this kind and, if so, whether these other consultative relationships may have substantially different purposes.

If, as Siegler claims, the consultant generally is called in to provide diagnostic information and judgment by analyzing some aspect of the patient's condition or to provide therapy by performing some procedure, the terms *diagnosis* and *therapy* need not be limited to biomedical, physiological, and pathological conditions. I can think of at least four kinds of activities (all performed by non-physicians) for which the term *consultation* might be appropriate and in which the term actually is used.

First, most large medical centers routinely have social service consultations. Are these different in principle from the consultations Siegler's patients receive from the neurologist, anesthesiologist, surgeon, ophthalmologist, and endocrinologist? If there is a difference, how does it affect the primary physician-patient relationship? Second, could a consultation be obtained from one of the therapy services (occupational therapy or inhalation therapy, for example), which does not involve physician-consultants? Third, could a consultation be obtained from a non-medical professional who has a special relationship with the patient and who can provide insights, especially when the patient is not able to do so, concerning the patient's wishes (for example, the patient's clergyman)? Fourth, can the term *ethics consultation* be employed usefully? To be sure, this term requires a careful definition. Although I hesitate to acknowledge a special group of individuals as moral experts, I do acknowledge the fact that there are cases in which the moral issues in a patient's care require the skills of someone uniquely able to analyze these issues and able to present at least some kind of clarification, if not a final judgment. Although these points may involve borderline cases, they do signal the need for an extension of Siegler's taxonomy or at least a reconsideration of its extensiveness.

Even though Siegler states that his analysis is limited to consultations requested of other physicians, I do not believe it to be the case that other health professionals are called in for a consultation only on occasion. Using consultations these days seems to be the rule rather than the exception. Nor is it clear that his analysis applies equally well to these other kinds of consultations in the absence of his giving an appropriate taxonomy of the entire range of consultations. An analysis of these other kinds of consultations could shed considerable light on many of the dilemmas of health care in teams and perhaps even on the nature of consultation itself.

My second question involves a point at the end of Siegler's essay in which he discusses some of the conditions under which the consultant would be justified in stepping outside that relationship in order to take special action with regard to advising the patient. There may indeed be cases in which there are irreconcilable differences between consultant and primary physician. Siegler offers the dissenting consultant the option of directly confronting the patient or of withdrawing from the case after telling the patient that a serious difference of opinion exists. I think Siegler's analysis would be helped considerably if this choice of two morally different actions could be elaborated.

Given a difference of opinion between consultant and primary physician, directly confronting the patient seems a relatively straightforward action to take even though it could ultimately destroy the basic relationship between patient and primary physician. That action, however, is entirely different from withdrawing from the case while simply telling the patient that a serious difference of opinion exists. Given such a situation, it is easy to imagine how uneasy a patient would feel without any further information as to the nature of the difference of opinion. Siegler needs to explore these two alternatives in greater detail. It simply is not enough to rest the consultant's decision on criteria such as the degree of the difference of opinion or the closeness of the call. This example becomes an important boundary case because the relationship at stake is no longer merely that between consultant on the one hand and the patient-primary physician relationship on the other, because there are overriding obligations to the patient first of all, and perhaps to the patient-primary physician relationship only secondarily.

These boundary cases raise questions about Siegler's general approach. Not every primary physician-patient relationship these days has the ideal characteristics which Siegler would like it to have and, in fact, this kind of relationship may have substantially disappeared. Although the empirical point concerns whether such a relationship really exists, the more important and related normative point is whether such an ideal is appropriate, given the highly technologized team character of contemporary health care, especially in the hospital. The boundary cases raise questions about who should intervene when the primary physician-patient relationship is fragmented or, even worse, is itself diseased. These cases pose the question of authority when one finite professionalized body of knowledge confronts another equally finite body of knowledge or when one moral point of view confronts another. In these cases, the obligations may be to the patient qua autonomous human being apart from any other kind of relationship, professional or otherwise.

Christine Mitchell's paper, "Integrity in Interprofessional Relationships", can be read in at least three interdependent ways. First, as many non-physician members of a health care team – especially nurses – undoubtedly will recognize, she expresses very effectively the frustrations, felt conflicts, and divided loyalties which nurses experience in their personal and professional lives. As such, Mitchell's paper is an expression of the lack of authority, responsibility, and power which nurses see as characterizing their professional roles. On this view, Mitchell has provided a moving expression of a core experience of many health care professionals.

Second, Mitchell's paper can be read as an empirical analysis of the conflicts which nurses face when dealing with patients and physicians in terms of a single concept, that of integrity.

Third, Mitchell also wants to provide a normative analysis. She is attempting to articulate a concept which is often invoked or appealed to in various forms of human activity and which, given a correct analysis and account of the concept, can be used prescriptively.

Two questions emerge from these readings: Whether the empirical analysis of the dilemmas nurses face can be adequately described using the concept of integrity and whether the normative analysis of the concept adequately characterizes all the moral issues involved? I have no doubt that the kinds of conflicts which Nurse Sharon faces are real and pressing, but I am not certain that Mitchell's analysis of integrity has sufficient richness to capture either the empirical or normative complexities in the situation. The empirical analysis in Mitchell's paper would be benefited by a taxonomy of nursing relationships in the same way that a taxonomy of consultative relationships would benefit Siegler's paper. I want to concentrate instead on her use and analysis of integrity as a normative concept.

Mitchell analyzes the integrity of individuals, health care teams, institutions, and professions in terms of her analysis of the component parts of integrity: truthfulness, fairness, pureness, fittingness, and wholeness. I have two questions concerning this analysis; the first is whether the component parts she identifies in the concept are really as distinct from one another as the describes and the second is whether her list of component parts is complete.

As far as the first question is concerned, I have some doubts as to whether she has drawn too sharp a line between pureness and wholeness. Both concepts are internal to the individual or entity said to have integrity, whereas truthfulness and fairness relate the entity which has integrity to something other than itself (other individuals, for example). Pureness and wholeness accordingly could be viewed under the general heading of completeness. If an individual has integrity in the sense of pureness, it is not affected by any outside interferences or imperfections; and if an individual has integrity in the sense of wholeness, all of its parts fit together coherently. Both of these notions imply that the entity which has integrity in these senses is a complete and functioning thing of its particular kind. Thus we can speak of the integrity of an entity as being free of defects. Part of the meaning of not having any defects actually involves having all of its parts in their proper relations one to another. Accordingly, there are senses in which integrity as completeness can capture – I am almost inclined to say "integrate" – the meanings of integrity as pureness and as wholeness.

There is a second problem with her analysis which concerns the completeness of her list of the component parts of integrity. If an individual is said to have integrity, it may mean that the individual is reliable, keeps commitments and promises over sustained periods of time. Fidelity seems to be an important addition to the concept of integrity, especially as it relates to persons. But whatever the details of the analysis of integrity, the concept when applied to persons presupposes self-knowledge and therefore competency. Someone who has no understanding of himself and is without some minimum level of competency, however defined, could hardly be said to have any of the component parts of integrity analyzed above.

Mitchell contrasts two concepts of health care – a mission model and a sympathy model – and then claims that these two conceptions cannot be successfully combined in a single personality because the nurse cannot act with integrity under both systems. Mitchell thus makes integrity at the personal level the focal point for talking about integrity in general and especially for talking about other kinds or levels of integrity, such as the integrity of health care teams, institutions, and professions. Given the conflicting models of medicine as a mission system on the one hand and as a personalized system on the other, the nurse is left in a moral dilemma as far as her personal integrity is concerned because, Mitchell claims, it is not possible to have both integrity based on obedience and integrity based on sympathy. Mitchell's analysis thus seems to presuppose that the integrity of individuals is primary and that other kinds of integrity (that of teams, institutions, or professions) are secondary. In this analysis integrity is an intra-systematic notion rather than an inter-systematic notion.

This view comprises another difficulty I find with Mitchell's essay. Her analysis is extremely helpful in demonstrating how the concept of integrity can be used to talk about the concept at the levels of person, team, institution, or profession. Unfortunately, her analysis does not provide a way of using integrity to cross the boundaries between these four different kinds of integrity. As a result, her essay is not helpful in describing the ways in which personal integrity may or may not relate to the integrity of these other entities.

A more fruitful analysis of integrity seemingly would involve an analysis of that concept in terms of obligations, duties, and responsibilities. In his essay, "The Concept of Responsibility in Medicine", George Agich delineates distinguishing characteristics of task responsibilities, social role responsibilities, and personal or individual responsibilities. Task responsibilities, Agich claims, tend to be non-deliberative and can be delegated. Social role responsibilities and personal responsibilities tend to require rationality and diliberation and cannot be delegated. And both social role responsibilities and personal responsibilities are a function of the agent's competency and knowledge. If the concept of integrity in terms of responsibilities to one's self, teams, institutions, and professions could be clarified, it would be easier to understand Nurse Sharon's dilemma.

It is here that the understanding of social role responsibilities and personal responsibilities becomes crucial. The main question seems to be: Can I take upon myself the responsibility of assuming a set of social role responsibilities even though doing so may involve conflicts between my personal responsibilities and my social role responsibilities? If in fact such an action is possible, then there are ways in which one could effectively use the concept of integrity, now redefined in terms of responsibilities, to provide an analysis making integrity an inter-systematic notion instead. If I can assume responsibilities as a member of a team, an employee of an institution, or a member of a profession, and if that assumption of responsibilities is coherent with my personal responsibilities (probably because I as an agent freely take those responsibilities upon myself), then although there may be conflicts of responsibilities, I have already committed myself to some way of resolving them. Thus, it is not the existence of different models of medicine which seems to create the nurse's dilemma, but the lack of an adequate account of the relationship among different kinds of responsibilities.

University of Missouri, Columbia

NOTES

[1] I owe this point to an important observation by Stuart Spicker at the symposium from which this volume is drawn.

EDMUND L. ERDE

LOGICAL CONFUSIONS AND MORAL DILEMMAS IN HEALTH CARE TEAMS AND TEAM TALK

The call for teams of health care professionals is pervasive ([8], [12], [56]). The language of teams and teamwork – what I shall call "team talk" – in medical contexts apparently dates from the earlier decades of this century ([5], [8]). In this essay, I will offer what I believe Theodore Brown was calling for in "An Historical View of Health Care Teams", namely, a philosophical analysis of the concept of *team* with applications of that analysis to the medical context. My goal is to articulate a synthetic understanding of the salient features of the ethos, ideology, rhetoric, and ethics of teams in health care. I will discuss all four (in various degrees) since I do not believe that any could be understood properly in isolation. Beginning with some brief historical, sociological, and attitudinal observations, I will discuss some ethical issues which emerge from a consideration of medical culture and from the larger social setting of workers' rights. Finally, I will outline the rhetoric of team talk and critically discuss the ethics of this rhetoric.

I

The historical source of the use of *team* as imported into health care is not easily determined. The term has roots in agriculture (as in a team of oxen), in business (as in a managerial team), in the military (as in a team of commandoes), and in sports (as in a football team). Perhaps the central aspect of the notion of *team* which gives it applicability to agriculture, business, military, sports, and medicine is the idea of a group (of two or more members) wherein the members are bound together in some appropriate way and work toward a common end. Oxen are bound by a yoke, but teams of people would be bound by humane or human relations – by means "better" than a mere harness.

A distinctly human relation is one which binds humans by their own sense of commitment through culture and language. The complexities of contemporary health care are so great that delivering it requires group effort. But must these groups always be *teams*? What are the gains and losses, the implications and presuppositions of team talk? My contention is that team talk or team orientation is good for people if it honestly gives them a sense of

George J. Agich (ed.), Responsibility in Health Care, 193–213.
Copyright © 1982 *by D. Reidel Publishing Company, Dordrecht, Holland.*

recognition, of being non-servile, or of having a role in a significant project, if they feel recruited and accepted, and if they feel free of totalitarian authority in that they understand and endorse the project on which they are working, its plan, its leaders, and other workers, as Vance Packard implies ([47], p. 180). The rhetoric of team talk is bad for workers and those with whom they work if it coerces, misleads, or gives a distorted sense of their task as Packard also indicates it may ([47], pp. 184–5). How could this distortion take place? To answer, I will draw on a study of what one author terms "cognitive dissonance" (a kind of perplexity about things not fitting together in the expected way) involved in team membership.

II

Peter New lists six generally false "political" assumptions about team structure made by persons who are on teams:

(a) all members have equal authority and competence;
(b) each will be fully truthful with the other;
(c) specialized experts need a broad range of other experts;[1]
(d) there is equal entrenchment of professions;
(e) all work for a common good (goal?);
(f) the domain of work to be done is equally open to the efforts of all [45].

The cognitive dissonance with which New is concerned arises, he claims, from a conflict of the real structure and functioning of a team with these six idealized assumptions. His point is psychological, intended to explain why people feel confused. An analogous conceptual point is that *team work* and *teamwork* are different. *Team work* is the work the team has to do. The work the team has to do can be compromised by motives and ideas of people on the team, including those ideas involved in the six assumptions. To the degree that the work of the team is not compromised, teamwork is occurring. *Teamwork* depends upon members' insightful *understanding* of the actual structures, relationships, and limitations of the situation *together with ability to accept* them. As a step toward that understanding, a philosophical account of the concept of team is required.

Instead of trying to define "team", however, I will adopt an inventory of kinds of teams from David Londey [35]. Londey looks at the kinds or categories of action which teams seem capable of doing or undertaking and thus supplies an analytic framework for identifying and understanding three kinds of teams. The point is to distinguish the *logical* properties of the concept of teams from the ideals and *ideologies* associated with the word.

The first model can be labeled the *institutionalized assembly model*. The label derives from the fact that teams are derived to perform institutionalized actions. (Londey's appeal to institutionalized actions is very reminiscent of John Rawls's in his important essay, "Two Concepts of Rules" [49].) The idea is that certain kinds of actions are highly conventional; they require rules of enactment – rules defining a practice as opposed to just rules of thumb.

For example, that a football team can score or win logically requires rules that define the game. These rules specify what constitutes playing and scoring and define positions and roles. In any given case of scoring, an individual will usually score on behalf of the team, perhaps as a result of cooperation among the teammates. While scoring and kicking may be individual actions, many actions logically require the group. Cooperating thus seems to be a team action rather than an individual action. Nevertheless, it is not a formal action defined in the rules of the game. It may be required by peer pressure or by human nature, and it may facilitate success. In fact, cooperation is called for more by strategies of good playing than by the logic of the rules of play. In this regard, cooperating is like other team actions which are not assignable to individuals in the way kicking a ball might be. These other actions include, for example, pressuring the opponent team.

Londey likens the actions of such teams to the actions of constituted assemblies. Although this is not an entirely apt comparison, Londey implies that a logical feature of assemblies is the (moral?) interchangeability or fungibility of its members. He must be assuming that debating and voting are the only actions of its members and that an equality among members is true of all such assemblies. Of course, that may be a natural assumption in contemporary society. However, assemblies need not be constituted by equals. For example, there could be weighted ballots where greater voting power is attached to merit or to what is thought to be privileged birth. Nevertheless, the concept of equality is something Londey affirms and which most team talk also seems to presume.[2] It is a powerful ethnocentric value and it may be that when the team is democratically organized, it runs more efficiently – this, too, may be true because of the particulars of our culture or because of human nature, rather than the logic of the team.

Londey's second model of teams can be termed the *goal efficiency model*. Such teams need not be assembled in a spatio-temporal sense. Londey's example is drawn from a military context rather than from sports. He discusses a team of signallers which passes messages. Each member may have materially crucial roles depending on his technical knowledge and abilities or the physical arrangements involved, and each may perform part of the action, but only the team performs the complete action. A classic division of labor thus arises.

Such teams need have no institutionalized requirements. It is not apparent how they could break the rules or logic of the practice of transmitting the message and still function as a team of signallers, though surely they can break the rules of thumb – including some dealing with interpersonal relations. These teams mainly function to surpass individuals in efficiently carrying out complex actions such as passing messages, whereas the first kind of team performed in a way logically and structurally different from individuals. Londey's first model thus was of teams as institutional assemblies; his second is of teams as efficient mechanisms.

Londey's third model is that of a class or group of individuals who engage only in individual activities. Although these individuals are grouped as a team, the team exists for reasons other than engaging in its own formal activities. Administrative and pedagogical convenience or cost-efficient traveling would constitute reasons for constructing such a team. Londey mentions swimming teams, in which individuals compete in meets even against teammates. This third model can be appropriately termed the *heap model* of the team.

Each of these models is present in health care settings. The heap model clearly applies to teams designed solely to provide knowledge, skill, or experience to individuals. An example is found in the teaching of junior medical students, which could be accomplished on a one-to-one basis. This practice, however, is generally thought to be administratively inconvenient and costly. Accordingly, some trainees are herded together to meet as a group with the same resident and/or professor. There *need* be no real group effort in the actions of the students, although there *may* be cooperation in the form of "covering for" one another, moral support, or even the tacit agreement among the students that patient care goals be sought in a fashion reminiscent of other team models.

The second or goal efficiency model applies to a surgical team. Even if one surgeon might have been able to do all that is required in a particular operation, that surgeon could still benefit greatly from the utilization of a team of helpers. Other specialists often need assistance, too. Psychiatrists may utilize nurses, social workers, occupational therapists, pharmacists, or others. The group that the specialist utilizes could be called a "team" of the goal efficiency sort. This indeed seems to be the most common and most typical use of "team" in health care. Unfortunately, much of the aura of the first model, the institutional assembly model, is imported inappropriately (along with its fallacy about the necessity of equality) into the context of the goal efficiency model. To note this is to make a logical or conceptual complaint. But because the importation is destructive, it becomes a *moral* complaint. Because the moral complaint emerges from the conceptual, I will discuss the conceptual claim first and aspects of the moral claim second.

Londey helps clarify how the assumptions New identifies and calls into question could come to have been made. People could be adopting the ideology of equality and democracy attached to the institutional assembly model as though it applied to all teams, especially the goal efficiency model [24]. For example, sports ideologies about institution assemblies can be applied to goal efficient health care groups.

The following table maps Londey's categories onto New's assumptions:

New's Assumptions List		*Londey's Categories*
(1) equal authority and competence	←——→	institutional assembly
(2) truthfulness	←——→	institutional assembly
(3) various specializations needed	←——→	goal efficiency
(4) equally entrenched members	←——→	institutional assembly
(5) work for common good (goal?)	←——→	goal efficiency and institutional assembly
(6) domain (nonterritoriality)	←——→	institutional assembly and (to a degree) goal efficiency

If a team is of the goal efficient sort, a serious "category mistake" is made when it is identified with features which only are true of institutional assemblies. Assumptions (3), (5), and (6) may apply to both kinds of teams, but this clearly does not imply that Assumptions (1), (2), and (4) hold of both. Some actions of a medical service may be institutionalized and involve units which are considered interchangeable. Perhaps the clinical service should have a certain patient count to assure a certain level of income; perhaps it should win the race to perfect a transplant technique or cut its death rate. There actually may be a great deal of such team activity in health care delivery. Nevertheless, even if (or especially if) a team member considers his team an institutionalized assembly, a puzzle about how people in a group should conduct themselves results. For example, should they obey orders they believe are inappropriate or morally compromising, or should they "blow the whistle" on someone in the group? In effect, the varying structures of teams may have varying implications for the ethics of the health care team.

II

There is a line of argument which maintains that a person – for example, a nurse – is duty bound to refuse to obey a morally problematic order. Refusing to obey orders on moral grounds sometimes is morally desirable. Some have even called for a program which teaches disobedience [40]. To be sure, a person cannot always morally claim as justification or as an excuse that "I only work here" or "I was just following orders" [30]. Benjamin Freedman calls this non-transferability of blame for actions in compliance with orders "the opacity of moral responsibility" [17]. This doctrine denies that there is a conductive chain of moral responsibility. In other words, on this view, each person consummates his own action and as each agent acts, he consummates the particular harm and bears the particular responsibility being assessed for that particular action.

Nonetheless, Freedman acknowledges that being a subordinate can serve to exculpate in three ways. First, there are coercive and/or enticing aspects to being a subordinate within a hierarchy. Second, there is an ambience which leads subordinates to develop a sense of "justified reliance" upon superiors due to the superiors' authority, experience, or reputation. Third, there are factors in the hierarchical context which mask the moral issues to be faced, and may mask them so extensively that the subordinate may not notice any of them.

Basing his critique on Robert Veatch's pointed essay about the generalization of expertise [57], Freedman writes:

> The physician's expertise in questions of medicine does not necessarily carry over, to confer upon him an expertise in questions of medical ethics. A junior resident's, or nurse's proper attitude towards an attending physician is not one of generalized awe: and care must be taken that acceptance of an authority's judgment on matters falling within his competence does not slosh over to a general acceptance of his judgment ([17], p. 38).

Freedman argues that if the institutional superior has greater empirical understanding and if that understanding is relevant to the decisions called for, there are justified grounds for reliance on the superior. Still, Freedman insists that a subordinate's dependent adherence to a superior's judgment about a moral issue is not morally acceptable. In part, Freedman bases his argument on the nature of a profession.

That a practice is a profession implies that the practice has a significant kind of autonomy – of training, of certification, or judgment, and of action. Being a professional further implies that there is an area of duties belonging first and foremost to that profession. Freedman calls these duties "initial responsibilities" and he asserts that the current interprofessional struggles involve what profession gets which kind of initial responsibilities. Freedman makes two claims about responsibilities on the basis of this understanding of professionalism. The first is debatable: that it is *more* obligatory for a subordinate to "blow the whistle" when the superior has misappropriated the subordinate's duties rather than when the superior has mishandled one of his own jobs. The second seems clearly right: that there is a duty to be watchful for a patient's general welfare, even though "absolute surveillance" would be supererogatory.

A strong underpinning for a position such as Freedman's may be derived from Richard Flathman's analysis of *The Practice of Rights* [15]. Flathman argues that a working system of political rights requires rights holders, correlative duty-owers, a system of enforcers (such as police and judges), and a system of witnesses (such as the press and the electorate who will vote out the poor enforcers). A practice of patients' rights, then, would require that health care workers, in addition to being duty-owers, be like police, judges, the press, and the electorate.[3] So Freedman's position has powerful foundations.

However, a complex argument can be made against his general position. One premise has already been stated. It is a conceptual, non-moral premise based on Londey's team models: that certain actions can only be performed by a group. The second is a moral premise: that blame and responsibility are not distributive concepts – one cannot always distribute either blame or responsibility from a group to its separate members [19]. Indeed, it is a consequence of the truths of these two premises that certain powers and capacities are created which are of special social significance; certain organizations are created by society to allow certain actions to be done for which no one is responsible.

Jack Katz would likely grant that Freedman is right in rejecting as morally repugnant *some* appeals to claims such as "I was just following orders" ([29], p. 12). Still, he would insist that we acknowledge the moral trade-offs involved in creating groups. Rawls's position – that joining a social practice has moral-logical force – is also crucial here [49]. When someone joins a practice which has multiple goals and values, he can expect to be in situations in which important principles conflict. No matter which course of action is chosen, an important principle will be violated in an important way [39]. If the practice being joined is on its face and in its intent morally acceptable, such a "no-win" situation may well involve moral dilemmas. For example, insurance companies serve a moral purpose by enabling individuals to make reparations to those injured, but the existence of such companies may only be feasible if subscribers agree never to admit a fault or apologize until a claim is settled.

My point depends upon a recognition of the complexity of social and organizational arrangements (*pace* Christine Mitchell in "Integrity in Interprofessional Relationships"). To adopt for my own purposes a distinction of John Wisdom, one might say that if the goal or "fundamental logic" of a practice – for example, delivering fine patient care to a large population – is morally secure, then much dilution of it by its own function – its own "domestic logic" (with limitations of staff and money) – is regrettable, inevitable, and excusable ([61], p. 130). Joining a group often involves accepting this sort of moral trade-off. When it does, the appeal to following orders may be more than an excuse; it can be a moral justification. When obedience is involved, however, disobeying requires strong moral reasons.

A proper moral posture in such situations is to regret. That is, because multiple goals, values, and principles can conflict when applied to particular cases, and because a lexical ordering of these is implausible (or, at any rate, unavailable), any choice may involve injury or injustice; thus, regret may be the most one can do. It is a proper part of the fabric of moral life [39]. Morality may further require that the regret be silent, at least on the part of people who are committed to the group's existence and security. In a particular case, a reasoned, moral silence may therefore be justified as required by the trade-offs. Silence may be an ingredient to moral life as much as whistleblowing. In our world there is an ever-increasing visibility of and an accountability for work.[4] This is thought proper in some circles and no doubt is so. One of the high costs that goes with it, however, is that not only are dishonorable behaviors inhibited, but so are some honorable ones ([10], p. 353). Fear of being a whistleblower, who may also suffer from moral lapses and thereby be vulnerable, and fear of escalating the demands of morality (to a point over the brink of the reasonable and proper and into the petty and vindictive) are appropriate fears [37]. Even when one is innocent or right, throwing the first stone could be difficult – for good moral and social reasons. Thus, one might want to disobey without being a whistleblower or even obey for the sake of the practice [36]. Similarly, one may be judged to be obliged to "blow the whistle" if the infractions of the fundamental logic are severe and/or there is a serious violation of the trust involved in the *real* social contract that binds the group together – as opposed to the mythical contract implied by team rhetoric.

Whether silence or whistleblowing is appropriate depends in part upon the commitment to group work in general, the way one got into his particular group, the purpose of the group, the design of the group, the history of the group's behaviors, the context in which the group operates, and the particulars of the cases confronting the group. Some of the particulars will include the gravity of the consequences involved, but other factors are also important. Indeed, some of the particulars include whether the group fashions itself as a team and what kind of team it is, given Londey's taxonomy. It will be useful to turn to an analysis of how "team talk" fits into our culture generally, followed by a discussion of the culture of health care delivery in particular.

III

John Ladd argues that there can be a high emotional cost in doing group work as it needs to be done [31]. He argues that a degree of schizoid living, self-withdrawal, or self-alienation seems required by the logic of formal organizations. He contends that the impersonality of the organizational context, the operative (albeit tacit) distinguishing of personal responsibility from the responsibility of the office, the expectations of loyalty and obedience that emanate from the top down, and the notion that one has joined the organization (making membership seem akin to a social contract) place the employee in a complex bind. To this list should be added the general tendency to obey even immoral authority – a topic which has recently received a great deal of attention from psychologists ([42], [65]). Ladd, in effect, arrays the structure of the cultural context supporting the "cognitive dissonance" identified by New.

The result is a tension between obedience due the organization and autonomy. The tension tends to suffocate the individual who may be exempt from personal liability from outside the organization while still feeling responsible. Ladd calls the result "moral schizophrenia" because it leads to a double standard of right and wrong: what is right from a personal standpoint is wrong from an organizational orientation ([31], p. 501). More confounding to individuals in these circumstances is the fact that an officer is held to individual moral standards vis-a-vis the organization. That is, with the organization, but not with the public, the officer is supposed to be honest, forthright, and loyal.

Although I think Ladd is wrong in arguing that moral schizophrenia is a *necessary* result of formal organizations and that such organizations cannot have norms other than economic ones, Ladd's account is highly typical of *being professionalized* insofar as the professions are highly bureaucratized.

The tension involved in being a professional in a highly interdependent context of practice can produce a crisis of integrity. For at least thirty years, "team talk" has been one approach to dealing with such crises of integrity. In 1951, for example, an editorial in *Fortune* contained the following:

> The concept that appears to be emerging, as the answer of the modern individual to this challenge [to his individuality from the modern corporation], is the concept of the team. It is an old concept but it is being put to new uses. As a member of a team an individual can find full opportunity for self-expression and still retain a dynamic relationship to other individuals .... [T]he concept of the team has the power to challenge the individual to seek his self-expression, not along purely egoistic channels .... A community – big or little – is created, and through it the individual finds a higher expression of himself ([16], p. 176).

Here, in the society of a generation ago, teams are appealed to as a way of fostering individuality. However, the *Fortune* editorial is concerned primarily with managers, whereas the concern today is much more democratic. For example, David Ewing writes: "When we recall that throughout most of human history, servants have been regarded as property, as chattels of the masters, it is no wonder that legal thought has favored the employer rather than the employee" ([14], p. 54). Ewing argues that the image of the worker as merely an economic creature is *passé*. In effect, Ewing is arguing that the ideas resulting in what Ladd calls moral schizophrenia are now being rejected.

There is evidence for this in managerial practice [34]. And the courts have begun radically to reconceive workers' rights. The judiciary seems to be acting under the realization that the organization for which someone works will permeate his entire life. This idea is powerfully expressed in the following passage quoted by Ewing:

> A business corporation, like a university, or a government agency, or a large hospital – each with its hierarchy and status system – is now a lifetime experience for many of its members. Necessarily, therefore, it can no longer be an instrument satisfying a single end – in the case of the business corporation, only turning out its goods and service – but it has to be a satisfactory way of life for its members. It not only has to satisfy its customers; it has to be agreeable to its "self" ([14], p. 49).

This allusion to the hospital helps narrow the inquiry, for the hospital is full of strife and much of it is analogous to the strife in the broader culture [51].

In support of the claim that the kind of disquietude identified by Ladd is anticipated of someone who is becoming a health professional, consider a comment by Chester Burns. Burns writes: "The hallmark of being a professional person is that an individual is willing to undergo a transformation of his personal and social values, is willing to profess special personal and social values; and is willing to self-regulate his behavior in terms of these special values" ([9], p. 184). One way of construing this remaking of values is that it exemplifies the call to the forces producing moral schizophrenia.[6] The forces are ingrained in society. Ladd, for example, believe that people can forsake neither organizations nor personal integrity, and so our culture contains (or creates) a terrible dilemma [31].

The horns of the dilemma gore deeply in health care. A great deal of literature suggests that, regarding patients, many hospitals are correctly described as human rights wastelands. George Annas, in "The Hospital: A Human Rights Wasteland", compares entering the hospital with entering a prison [3]. He provocatively alludes to the depersonalizing clothing, identification number, and the loss of privacy and autonomy in each. But note how ironic it is that workers in the hospital also feel the loss of their own rights and dignity as a function of the power of physicians ([28], [60]). So Annas's title seems applicable to the situation of employees (including nurses, occupational therapists, physical therapists, technicians, and medical records administrators) as well as to patients. It seems that persons employed in a hospital would have two types of moral concerns: what they see happening to patients and the friends and families of those patients, *and* what they see happening to their own co-workers as persons and to the "lesser" professions in general. Radical writings have emerged from this second concern. For example, Jo Ann Ashley's *Hospital, Paternalism and the Role of the Nurse* is particularly outspoken about the long-lived economic and social exploitation of nurses by physicians [4]. Team talk is thus part of the general cultural response to feelings and outcries such as hers. How responsible is this team rhetoric?

IV

Plato, in the *Phaedrus*, seems to have been arraying both good and bad rhetoric and identifying good rhetoric with love. Most team talk is destructive, although some – that which comes out of team experiences – can be stimulated by some of the most fulfilling or humanizing experiences a person can have.[7] But the meaning of "team" and experiences associated with teams all too often amount to bad rhetoric, to being unloving in Plato's sense.

After quoting that *Fortune* editorial which touts teams as the answer to the conflict of individualism with interdependency, John William Ward declared:

> If one stops as one reads that the individual is to realize himself as part of a team, if one stops to wonder what happened to that reactionary proletarian danger of immersing the individual in a group, one will see the same thing happened to it that happened to that independent individual. The group has become community; interdependence has become team play; complicated relationships have become dynamic relationships. "Community", "team", "dynamic": these are all plus words. We respond to them positively and happily, perhaps even mindlessly. Unless we watch the verbal magic, we will not notice that the individualism put in the hat at the beginning is not the individualism that pops out at the end ([59], p. 40).

Ward is charging that the team talk of *Fortune* is just verbal magic. And I think he is right. It is deceptive suddenly to change labels and metaphors about work without providing the other humanizing changes that are called for. Such rhetoric might work to quiet the unrest and foster cooperation as an opiate for the masses of employees, but it may be immoral if it is deceptive. (Of course, it may be moral if it is done explicitly and frankly just to bring a cooperative attitude to persons functioning within the inequalities which everyone knows will continue.)

How could this change of label alone work with regard to health care? For one thing, the term *teams* – having a primary association with sports – has its psychological base in practices that most health care deliverers probably never experienced, since most workers are women. Part of the literature of business management written for women makes clear how distant the metaphor of team is to its intended readership. For example, *The Managerial Woman* recounts a woman's childhood memories of her older brother. The boy would play with other boys whom he disliked because the team needed eleven players ([26], pp. 31–3). The brother learned to cooperate with people he did not like but needed. As an adult, the sister claimed she had no occasion for such learning. The norm for the brother was to be a player on a team. The team experience helped him learn. The sister seemed perplexed and envious. The authors suggest that the sister's experiences are typical. This, they argue, explains why women in health care and in business have had difficulty relating to norms implied by team talk, although they could have a longing to experience what they have imagined team membership is.

In *Games Mother Never Taught You*, Betty Harragan is more sarcastic. She writes:

> It should be clear from our aerial survey of the business landscape that women who enter the working world with a continuous career in mind must be prepared to deal with the realities involved. Foremost among these are the rigidities of the military hierarchy; the team sports philosophy which management uses to coordinate work and interrelationship of employees; and the male-culture jargon which is the primary mode of communication as well as the expression of conscious and unconscious attitudes toward women ([25], p. 117).

Harragan argues that knowledge, competence, and good-will are not sufficient for a woman to be a success, "to get in the ballgame and stay on the team . . . . " She takes the team talk in the business world to be pervasive, normative, and misleading to women. She advises her readers to listen carefully for which sport is the dominant model in their particular settings.[8] She also warns that women who try to join their male co-workers by talking of teams and discussing happenings in the sports world will be looked upon as odd ([25], p. 106). Perhaps even adopting team language would be looked upon as awkward and weird.[9]

However, team metaphors and team spirit do not just lead or mislead women. They can lead or mislead men as well.[10] Saad Z. Nagi remarks that "team approaches are viewed as matters of morals" ([44], p. 75). Compromise and cooperation seem to be primary associations in team talk. Together with productivity, they can be enhanced or diminished by group structures ([21], [55]). A leader's early conforming to group norms – as a way of gaining "credits" – can later enable the leader to deviate from such norms without disapproval [27].

Such skills of leadership constitute pressures against whistleblowing or leaking information to outsiders. The skills also constitute pressures based on the apparent social contract nature of team membership. Thinking of membership as a contract makes it seem like a democratic institution, like subscribing as an equal to a set of rules or practices which will retain or even enhance equality. The professional freely joins a team for purposes of furthering his potential for serving professionally. This altruistic, though self-interested, joining seems to bind each person to the group and to its hierarchy in such a way that the in-house protocol for registering differences of opinions is considered essential to the group's ethics.

Other norms of being on teams carry over from the military. Teammates are supposed to obey orders. One source of such orders is a captain, and "captain" is a term of leadership rank in sports and in the military. Both military life and team membership can be humanizing. Jane J. Mansbridge asserts that "War, working together under stress, a common 'transcendent' experience, or self-revelation in consciousness-raising sessions and in encounter groups can quickly create mutual identification, empathy, and respect" ([38], p. 250). Mansbridge comments that a meaningful common history is built up among members of a group which has undergone intense interactions. The implication of her account is that the group will protect its individual members when the group has achieved this sense. The result is that a sense of identity arises from the members in an otherwise too large, too anonymous, too morally schizophrenic world. Sports teams and the smaller military groupings of people involve courage, practicing together, and strength. In short, they require Homeric excellence, heroic medicine, and sometimes even heroic antics [13]. Group norms of honor foster the efficacy of the group by enhancing group autonomy ([29], p. 11). The trouble is that the devices involved in doing this can be dehumanizing as well. Furthermore, teams and team talk not only can militate against members' independent choices, they can coerce patients who may have a hard enough time resisting the pressures of professionals as individuals.[11]

These points can be shown to be especially relevant when applied to health care. In it, many uses of the word *team* seem morally unproblematic, even utterly innocent – meant only as a synonym of *group* [63]. This seems true of the earliest physician-written essay I have seen which uses the term *team*. In 1922 Lewellys Barker called for each physician to have a formal, coordinated group of various medical specialists to call upon to insure comprehensive patient care because, he claimed, there is too much medical knowledge for one physician to master.[12] Aside from such innocent uses of *team*, there are other uses that are not so much descriptive as manipulative, seductive, or extravagant. For example, the American Hospital Association's efforts for National Hospital Week (May 11–17, 1980) involved sending members a packet containing suggestions for hospitals to use in preparing their participation in the week's activities [41]. The theme of the week was to be "health care teams". Suggestions made in the packet for local development and tailoring included sample news releases, editors' proclamations, employee recognition activities, community activities, hospital events, and potential community resources. The pages were decorated by stars reminiscent of the American flag, and the suggestions specifically encouraged tying the activities to the Olympics and to local teams as well as prominent athletes. Here the importing of sports norms and models into health care is glaring.

Also, in "The Physician as a Health Care Team Leader", C. E. Lewis, a confessed football buff, indicates strategies for patient management with diagrammed medical "plays" [33]. He supposes the doctor to be the quarterback. He wants to dissolve the strict military ambience that is predominant in the hospital and replace it with "team-matery". Lewis seems to think that teams are less authoritarian than military chains of command. His mistake is understandable given our customary associations, because, as we saw above in the use of Londey's "institutional assembly" model, patterns of uses of *team* and team talk are closely associated with democratic ideology.

V

I have tried to show that the concept of team is ideologically laden or normative. Expectations abound in team talk about sticking together, about practice, about supporting problem-ridden teammates, about winning, about cheating together, about losing, and about primary loyalties.[13] To understand the norms within groups in general and teams in particular, a grasp of extensive sociological and anthropological studies would be required – how group size [43] and group design ([11], [32], [52], [53]) affect behaviors. Questions of insurgency and the like within groups [64] and risk-taking of groups [54], acceptance within groups [18], socialization processes and group norms [6], as well as how group process is affected when a group is under pressure or "seige" would all be of interest.

A full account of teams as a special case of groups would include the point that sports teams sometimes represent a city, a country, a school, or a department – though sometimes they do not. Teams seem to require more than one member, but if a country sent just one athlete to the Olympics, we could say of him that he is its team. Teams seem to have to be competitive or set against some other team – some only metaphorically as when a team of mountain climbers competes against an anthropomorphized mountain. Other tasks of teams could not be put in competitive terms at all – "transition teams" of federal administrations or negotiating "diplomatic teams". Typical of these sorts of teams (but perhaps not so of health care teams) is that the former do not have *institutionalized* ingredients of a divided loyalty. All team players are supposed to be for the team. But professionals on health care teams may be committed by their code of ethics to be at odds with other professional groups. For example, until 1980 the American Medical Association Code ignored or condemned other groups [58]. The American Nursing Association Code asserts professional independence ([1], articles 3 and 10). Until what Burns considers comes to pass, health care teams will have a different domestic logic and social character than other teams. Burns writes: "It might be possible to prepare a code of medical ethics that would be suitable for the majority of health professionals, including physicians" ([9], p. 186).

Could such a code be non-platitudinous? Is it realistic to set out to accommodate the autonomy of each profession and aim to respect the integrity of each individual? Burns has called for an awareness on the part of neophytes that they redefine their values and themselves in being professionalized. Not only the patients' personhood but the personhood of the professional is at stake.

I want to sugggest that there are two ways to think of this personhood. One is modeled on the legal view – where persons are autonomous, independent, responsible atoms of agency. They are duty-bound and by and large free (as Freedman seems to cast them). The other model takes persons to be creatures of their culture – having strengths and weaknesses and being in need of protection, support, and freedom. This is the focus of Ladd's view and is the focus of the social sciences.

The tension caused by the partial truth within each model affects moral reflection about how professionals should interact both with patients and with other professionals, groups, and practices. Apart from prudential concerns, there is the commitment to groups, the desire for acceptability, the recognition of widespread frailty, and the plurality of goals which can yield conflicts. Under this tension of models what seems most needed for groups and teams to improve is their increased awareness of the values motivating them and of what – if anything – is morally problematic with their motives and their actions. In this way, both models of personhood may be enacted in the moral milieu of the workplace even though the tensions between models of person and between efficiency and institutionalized equality may continue. If the understandings are made explicit, the ties between people can be humanized. If that happens, the rhetoric of team talk will be good rhetoric and will be vindicated.

University of Medicine and Dentistry of New Jersey
New Jersey School of Osteopathic Medicine

NOTES

* This paper developed from a National Endowment for the Humanities Summer Seminar (Grant # FP–00033–79–1380) I co-directed with James B. Speer, Jr., for

teachers of health care deliverers at the University of Texas Medical Branch in Galveston. I would like to acknowledge everyone concerned with the Seminar but especially Henry Sepulveda, Jr., our research assistant.

1 New puts it thus: " ... training is so specialized and so narrow that we must have people from a wide variety of occupations and professions to tackle a problem" ([45], p. 33). His use of "to tackle" indicates how pervasive the sports influence (whether football or fishing) is.

2 The meaning of "equality" is vague here, and that vagueness has implications for criticisms made later in my essay. Still, it must be noted that equality to compete is a feature of modern sports [24] and a feature of assemblies as presumed by much contemporary political philosophy [46], [48].

3 Institutionalization of the requirement to whistle-blow includes actions by the law. Universally in American jurisdictions, one must blow the whistle on any suspected child abuser [50]. And some states are now requiring health care personnel to report incompetent practitioners [23]. Even some professional codes of ethics seem to recognize that as a duty ([1], article 3).

4 With regard to sports teams, think of team films, instant replay, etc.

5 Brill's [8] is a good attempt.

6 But we must also acknowledge with Alasdair MacIntyre: "It belongs to the concept of a practice ... that its good can only be achieved by subordinating ourselves to the best standard so far achieved, and that entails subordinating ourselves within the practice in our relationship to other practitioners" ([36], p. 32).

7 Witness Senator Bill Bradley's autobiography, *Life on the Run*. This book concerns Bradley's life with the New York Knickerbockers. It is replete with powerful descriptions, of which the following embodies the entire perspective: "I believe that basketball, when a certain level of unselfish team play is realized, can serve as a kind of metaphor for ultimate cooperation" ([7], p. 60). The camaraderie of a lasting team, the thrill of victory, company in agonizing defeat, the joy of meshing and of being led are given great testimony by Bradley.

8 Although Harragan does not help us understand what the variations from sport to sport are or how they can apply, Guttmann's masterful book can [24]. He shows how baseball fills the need in America for a pastoral occasion combined with a pervasive fascination with quantification while football's violence and unpredictability fits as an antidote to the tedium of life (largely among college graduates).

9 Although I must confess that after studying the concept of *team*, I find all "team talk" in medicine alien, I also find Harragan's prediction powerfully fulfilled by my reaction to the article "You Can't Be a Team by Yourself" [22]. The word "team" in the title actually was printed in such a way that each of its letters was composed of several capital letters of its own kind. Thus, the "T" was composed of nine regular capital "Ts", the "E" by thirteen "Es", the "A" by nine "As", the "M" by seventeen "Ms". The echo of letters within letters is uncomfortably reminiscent of cheerleading.

10 This is true outside of health care, too. See ([2], pp. 51; 60–1).

11 At the symposium where aspects of this essay were presented, Arthur F. Kohrman reported to me that his experience with handicapped patients confirmed that once a patient is informed of a team position on a "management" problem, the patient has greater difficulty exercising choice.

12 [5]. Barker seems never to have considered the possibility that persons besides

physicians would be on the team. Sometimes, even recently, nurses have taken analogous positions. For example, in "You Can't Be a Team By Yourself", the authors are concerned about good nurse-nurse communication and consider their team to be composed solely of nurses [22].

[13] One of the reasons whistleblowing on teammates may often be unthinkable is that "game films" make the whistleblowing unnecessary and provide a forum for group critique. Whistleblowing is, after all, an act of the referees. I own to Christine Mitchell my awareness of the near pun relating "whistle-blowing" to whistles used in sports. I intended to show why whistleblowing is prohibited by the social norms implicit in the team metaphor. No football player would tell the referee, "My teammate was illegally holding the opponent on that play." But if, in the huddle, a plan to injure an opponent severely were proposed, informing the appropriate parties would seem morally required.

Empirically, this may seem utterly naive or worse. See William Furlong on how even physicians who are team physicians may be compromised by the sports model ([20], p. 126). Even the practice of injuring in games could be defended by a position like Robert Paul Wolff's, where it is suggested that the tacit social contract of a constituency can vary and include such things [62], pp. 223–224). This expectation of hurting may be part of the allusions to sports found so offensive to people socialized as women were "supposed to be" socialized. In other words, this presumption about acceptable injuring may make team membership undersirable and alien to many persons. But, if we agree with Annas that the hospital is a human rights wasteland, we cannot suggest that the social contract among teammates in the hospital is of sufficient moral force to permit teams to fail to respect patients' rights [3].

BIBLIOGRAPHY

1. American Nurses' Association: 1973, 'Code for Nurses With Interpretive Statements', in *Perspectives on the Code for Nurses*, pp. 44–60.
2. Anderson, R. M., Terrucci, R., Schendel, D. E., and Trachtman, L. E.: 1980, *Divided Loyalties*, Purdue University, West Lafayette, Indiana.
3. Annas, G.: 1974, 'Hospital as a Human Rights Wasteland', *The Civil Liberties Review* **1**, 15–35.
4. Ashley, J. A.: 1976, *Hospitals, Paternalism, and the Role of the Nurse*, Teachers College Press, New York.
5. Barker, L. F.: 1922, 'The Specialist and the General Practitioner', *JAMA* **78**, 773–79.
6. Bosk, C.: 1979, *Forgive and Remember*, University of Chicago Press, Chicago.
7. Bradley, B.: 1976, *Life on the Run*, Quadrangle/The New York Times Book Co., New York.
8. Brill, N. I.: 1976, *Teamwork: Working in the Human Services*, J. B. Lippincott Co., New York.
9. Burns, C. R.: 1974, 'Comparative Ethics of the Medical Profession Outside the United States', in *The Humanities and Medicine*, Special Issue, *Texas Reports on Biology and Medicine* **32**, 181–190.
10. Collier, A. T.: 1964, 'Conflicts of Interest in the Glass Age', *Federal Bar Journal* **24**, 351–357.

11. Coleman, A. D. and Bexton, W. H. (eds.): 1975, *Group Relations Reader*, GREX, Sausalito, California.
12. Ducanis, A. J. and Golin, A. K.: 1979, *The Interdisciplinary Health Care Team*, Aspen Systems Corporation, Germantown, Maryland and London.
13. Erde, E.: 1981, 'Pathos and Pathology: Physicians in *The Last Angry Man, M*A*S*H*, and *The Magician', Studies in Science and Culture* 1(in press).
14. Ewing, D.: 1977, *Freedom Inside the Organization*, D. P. Dutton, New York.
15. Flathman, R.: 1976, *The Practice of Rights*, Cambridge University Press, Cambridge.
16. *Fortune* editorial, February 1951. (This issue was under the general editorship of Russell Davenport.)
17. Freedman, B.: 1980, 'A Prolegomenon to the Allocation of Responsibility and Hierarchical Organizations: The Hospital Context', *Legal Medical Quarterly* **4**, 35–43.
18. Freidson, E.: 1970, *Profession of Medicine*, Harper and Row, New York.
19. French, P.: 1975, 'Types of Collectivities and Blame', *The Personalist* **56**, 160–169.
20. Furlong, W. B.: 1980, 'Football Violence', *The New York Times Magazine* **130**, 38–41; 122–134.
21. Gibb, J. R.: 1976, 'Dynamics of Leadership and Communication', in W. R. Lassey (ed.), *Leadership and Social Change* (2nd rev. ed.), University Associates, La Jolla, California, pp. 85–99.
22. Gordon, E. and Adams, P.: 1971, 'You Can't Be a Team By Yourself', *International Nursing Review* **1**, 76–79.
23. Graham, S.: 1981, 'States Move to Catch Incompetent Doctors, But Progress is Uneven', *The Wall Street Journal* **104** (May 1, 1981), 1.
24. Guttmann, A.: 1978, *From Ritual to Record*, Columbia University Press, New York.
25. Harragan, B. L.: 1977, *Games Mother Never Taught You*, Warner Books, New York.
26. Henning, M. and Jardim, A.: 1977, *The Managerial Woman*, Doubleday, New York.
27. Hollander, E. P.: 1964, *Leaders, Groups, and Influence*, Oxford University Press, New York.
28. Kane, R. L. and Kane, R. A.: 1969, 'Physicians' Attitudes of Omnipotence in a University Hospital', *Journal of Medical Education* **44**, 684–690.
29. Katz, J: 1977–78, 'Cover-up and Collective Integrity: On the Natural Antagonisms of Authority Internal and External to Organizations', *Social Problems* **25**, 3–17.
30. Lachs, J.: 1978, '"I Only Work Here": Mediation and Irresponsibility', in R. T. DeGeorge and J. A. Pichler (eds.), *Ethics, Free Enterprise and Public Policy*, Oxford University Press, New York, pp. 201–13.
31. Ladd, J.: 1970, 'Morality and the Ideal of Rationality in Formal Organizations', *The Monist* **54**, 488–516.
32. Lassey, W. R. (ed.): 1976, *Leadership and Social Change* (2nd rev. ed.), University Associates, La Jolla, California.
33. Lewis, C. E.: 1968, 'The Physician as a Health Care Team Leader', *Group Practice* **17**, 20–24.

34. Lohr, S.: 1981, 'Overhauling America's Business Management', *The New York Times Magazine* **130**, 14–27; 42–43.
35. Londey, D.: 1978, 'On the Action of Teams', *Inquiry* **21**, 213–218.
36. MacIntyre, A.: 1981, 'The Nature of the Virtues', *The Hastings Center Report* **11**, 27–34.
37. Manning, B.: 1964, 'The Purity Potlash: An Essay on Conflicts of Interest, American Government, and Moral Escalation', *Federal Bar Journal* **24**, 239–256.
38. Mansbridge, J. J.: 1975, 'The Limits of Friendship', in J. R. Pennock and J. Chapman (eds.), *Participation in Politics, Nomos* **XVI**, Leiber-Atherton, New York, pp. 246–275.
39. Marcus, R. B.: 1980, 'Moral Dilemmas and Consistency', *The Journal of Philosophy* **77**, 121–136.
40. McCarthy, S. J.: 1979, 'Why Johnny Can't Disobey', *The Humanist* **39**, 30–34.
41. McMahon, J. A.: 1980, Letter about National Hospital Week.
42. Milgram, S.: 1968, 'Obedience and Disobedience to Authority', *The International Journal of Psychiatry* **6**, 259–276.
43. Miller, E. J. and Rice, A. K.: 1975, 'Selections From Systems of Organizations', in A. D. Colman and W. H. Bexton (eds.), *Group Relations Reader*, GREX, Sausalito, California, pp. 43–68.
44. Nagi, S. Z.: 1975, 'Teamwork in Health Care in the U. S.: A Sociological Perspective', *Milbank Memorial Fund Quarterly* **53**, 75–91.
45. New, P. K.: 1968, 'An Analysis of the Concept of Teamwork', *Community Mental Health Journal* **4**, 326–333.
46. Nozick, R.: 1974, *Anarchy, State, and Utopia*, Basic Books, New York.
47. Packard, V.: 1957, *The Hidden Persuaders*, Pocket Books, New York.
48. Rawls, J.: 1971, *A Theory of Justice*, Harvard University Press, Cambridge.
49. Rawls, J.: 1955, 'Two Concepts of Rules', *The Philosophical Review* **64**, 3–32.
50. Robertson, J. A.: 1977, 'Involuntary Euthanasia of Defective Newborns: A Legal Analysis', in D. J. Horan and D. Mall (eds.), *Death, Dying and Euthanasia*, University Publications of America, Inc., pp. 139–195.
51. Rogers, D. W. and Blendon, R. J.: 1978, 'The Academic Medical Center: A Stressed American Institution', *New England Journal of Medicine* **298**, 940–950.
52. Sherif, M. and Sherif, C.: 1964, *Reference Groups*, Harper and Row, New York.
53. Sherif, M. and Sherif, C.: 1969, *Social Psychology*, Harper and Row, New York.
54. Siegel, S. and Zajonc, R. B.: 1967, 'Group Risk Taking in Professional Decisions', *Sociometry* **30**, 339–349.
55. Spotts, J. V.: 1976, 'The Problem of Leadership', in W. R. Lassey (ed.), *Leadership and Social Change* (2nd rev. ed.), University Associates, La Jolla, California, pp. 254–74.
56. Tichy, M.: 1974, *Health Care Teams: An Annotated Bibliography*, Praeger Publishers, New York.
57. Veatch, R.: 1973, 'Generalization of Expertise', *Hastings Center Studies* **1**, 29–40.
58. Veatch, R.: 1980, 'New Principles for Physicians?', *The Hastings Center Report* **10**, 16–19.
59. Ward, J. W.: 1964, 'The Ideal of Individualism and the Reality of Organization', in E. F. Cheit (ed.), *The Business Establishment*, John Wiley and Sons, Inc., New York, pp. 37–76.

60. Whitehouse, F. A.: 1951, 'Teamwork – A Democracy of Professions', *Exceptional Children* 18, 45–52.
61. Wisdom, J.: 1965, *Paradox and Discovery*, Basil Blackwell, Oxford.
62. Wolff, R. P.: 1973, *The Autonomy of Reason*, Harper and Row, New York.
63. Yanda. R. L.: 1971, *Doctors as Managers of Health Teams*, AMACOM, New York.
64. Zald, M. N. and Berger, M. A.: 1978, 'Social Movements in Organizations: Coup d'Etat, Insurgency, and Mass Movement', *American Journal of Sociology* **83**, 823–861.
65. Zimbardo, P. G.: 1972, 'Pathology of Imprisonment', *Trans-Action* 9, 4–8.

RUTH B. PURTILO

RESPONSIBILITY AND HEALTH CARE TEAMS: A HEALTH PROFESSIONAL'S PERSPECTIVE

In his essay, "Logical Confusions and Moral Dilemmas in Health Care Teams and Team Talk", Ed Erde helped set the direction for this commentary by noting that "team talk comes out of team experience." The comments expressed here are rooted in experience – the experience of team talk and team work from the perspective of a seasoned health professional.[1] In this commentary *health professionals* includes allied health professionals, social workers, and nurses, since these health care providers, and not the physician, will serve as the focal point for discussion. When the term *team* is used, however, physicians and administrators are included.

In all probability, many readers have had first-hand experience with health care teams and are familiar with variations on the following scenes:

(1) I am sitting at a long table in my white coat, eating a sandwich and wiping crumbs from my notes about Mr. Carlson's condition, while listening to another professional present an evaluation of whether the patient is ready for discharge;

(2) I am standing near the nurses' station with one eye on the clock, a pair of crutches dangling from my left arm, talking with the physician and nurse about Mr. K's recent setback;

(3) I am talking on the telephone with the occupational therapist;

(4) I am in a cafeteria line or on a crowded elevator with Dr. C., whispering in hurried and hushed tones about Miss H., who threw her oatmeal at the medical technologist this morning, confirming my suspicion that she seems angry about something these days;

(5) But most of the time I am going about my job, subtly aware that "out there somewhere" my team mates are taking their turns in the management of their patients' day and treatment. The team is a great cloud of witnesses whose presence is felt but with whom I may have little or no contact during a day's (or several days') work.

Although the team concept takes several forms, its essential feature is *patient management*.

Erde notes correctly that there are also other goals of team activity. He surely would agree that when discussing teams with the majority of health

George J. Agich (ed.), Responsibility in Health Care, 215–223.
Copyright © 1982 *by D. Reidel Publishing Company, Dordrecht, Holland.*

professionals, the goal of *patient management* is the phrase most associated with the team concept. For these professionals, the verbalized object of their responsibility becomes *good patient care*. From a psychological perspective, however, the work of patient management highlighted in the examples above is more consistent with Erde's notion of *team work* (doing the work of a team) than of genuine *teamwork* (activity based on insightful understanding of the authority relationship involved, in addition to the knowledge and acceptance of limits of what a team can accomplish).

Most health professionals do not seem to acknowledge that such a difference exists, and regularly substitute the first for the second type of activity. Far from having benign results, the price exacted for this substitution is a shift in effort from trying to achieve effective patient management to trying to foster effective interaction among members of the team. Often, neither is achieved. Erde's paper lends insight into how the notion of *equality*, as it is misused, misunderstood, and misinterpreted, is at the root of this hapless state of affairs. A brief review of Erde's discussion of equality as it pertains to the goal efficiency model will be followed by personal observations as to how the illusion of equality develops in the first place. The essay will conclude with a description of how responsible action by health professionals is affected by this state of affairs. Throughout the preparation of this essay, Erde's careful assessments provided insight and direction.[2]

I. EQUALITY AND TEAMWORK

Drawing on the models developed by Londey, Erde describes three categories of action which teams are capable of taking. The models are:

(a) Institutionalized assembly model;
(b) Goal efficiency model; and
(c) Heap model.

Erde explains that the notion of equality is appropriate for the institutionalized assembly model but not for the others. I agree with him that if equality is smuggled into the goal efficiency model as a device for continuing unequal modes of decision-making, then the result is moral damage to health professionals. Erde maintains that this is precisely what happens, and spends considerable time showing how the problem affects team talk and teamwork. While there is much substance to these arguments, I think too much of this diagnosis rests on at least the implication that the physician (the authority figure in patient management) assumes his place on the team with the stated intent of equality, but actually uses talk of equality to gain or maintain power. I believe that it is not physicians, but other team members, who actually bring the notion of equality to the patient-management context of the goal efficiency model. While most health professionals do not like the ambiguity associated with not knowing how much their contribution is going to count in patient management decisions, they probably do not think about it very much on a day-to-day basis. This, however, does not signal that all is well. Under the stress of managing a critically-ill patient, the unequal-but-efficient mode of patient management decisions often is put to a test. At this juncture, the notion of equality is raised as a battle banner by health professionals themselves. Discussion in the following pages will revolve around the origin of this societal ideal within health care and why health professionals reckon that it belongs to team activity.

Before proceeding, however, the reader should be reminded that Erde does not argue for the necessity of equality in order for good teamwork to be realized. Citing Packard, he proposes that a good team either exercises equality (i.e., does not smuggle in the rhetoric only) *or* exercises explicitly understood and agreed upon inequality. For instance, a good team could be one that gives health professionals only a small role in a significant project, but with the agreement that they understand and endorse the plan, leaders and workers.

Since inequality exists, and can be justified in some contexts, is it important to discuss the point further? Erde provides direction in his observations that equality (in the form of equal respect) is among the most cherished of societal ideals. Equal respect supposedly is the moral right of all persons in virtue of their being rational and free agents. It is therefore not surprising that I propose that all types of team members wish to be treated with equal respect and to treat other team members with equal respect. This *societal ideal* is perceived as a right which ought to be honored within any context – including the team context. Though the *institutional ideal* of efficiency is applied to patient management decisions, the ideal of equal respect creates an active tension with the obvious inequalities present in efficient decision-making. To relieve this tension, the societal ideal of equality becomes expressed within the team, albeit within the context of the team model that Erde all too facilely dismisses – the heap model.

Recall that in the heap model no real *group* effort exists, although there is cooperation, "covering for", and moral support. Examples Erde provides are of teams which get together for convenience of administration or to travel cheaply (and I might add, as in some marriages). While he convincingly points to difficulties which arise when the moral notion of equal respect fallaciously is superimposed on the goal efficiency model of the team, he also should realize that serious difficulties arise when equality is imported into the heap model.

The heap model is indeed familiar to many health professionals in that it characterizes a substantive part of the loosely coordinated and ill-defined activity that they engage in as *team* members. What emerges, then, are two models of the team operating simultaneously – the goal efficiency model and the heap model. Within the context of the heap model equality *does* exist. There is equal ability and opportunity to cooperate, cover for, and support. The *esprit de corps* that develops in such a team is heartening to observe and delightful to experience. The problem is that in order to work, the focus of attention and effort must shift, usually subtly, from the institutional ideal of efficiency (allowing unequal decision-making related to patient management) to the societal ideal of equal respect (experienced among teammates). Members can quite independently perform tasks in which they are clinically competent, while continuing to disregard equality-related problems pursuant to team-oriented patient management decisions.

In short, heap model *team work* supports a more fragmented patient treatment approach by each team member and places less emphasis on *teamwork* (which has coordinated patient management as its goal). With regard to the patient, the situation seems more like the *team work* Erde described and less like genuine *teamwork*. This looser approach to patient management enables each person to experience the gratification that comes from receiving and giving as equals.

None of these considerations is surprising. Most people want as much equal respect as they think they deserve and can get. Health professionals are no exception. One result of this circumstance would be two models operating compatibly – one with activity fostering team rapport, the other dealing with patient management. Such an arrangement is not realistic, however, in that health professionals are mainly patient-oriented. Therefore, both physicians and health professionals justify the equal support, cooperation, and "covering for" of the heap model activity by appealing not to team rapport, but rather to good patient management. (N. B. The patient's well-being is usually the justification used for everything in health care.)

It should not be surprising, then, that health professionals who enjoy equal status imagine that the equal give-and-take also applies to the patient management arena in critical situations. This illusion is not put to the test until a physician and a health professional disagree about the proper course of action when a patient experiences acute distress. The following exchange between Mr. Anderson and Kim Segard provides one illustration of when such a team problem arises:

Mr. Clayton Anderson, a 43-year-old contractor, fell from a scaffold, fracturing his right tibia. A month earlier he had consulted his physician of 20 years, complaining of unusual fatigue. Tests revealed no abnormal findings, and Mr. Anderson returned to work. He believes he "blacked out" prior to the fall, but this is fuzzy to him.

Since the fracture is healing very slowly, Mr. Anderson has been hospitalized for three weeks. The social worker, Kim Segard, has been visiting him often, at Mr. Anderson's request. Mr. Anderson is discouraged about his slow recovery and worried about his wife and three children because he is self-employed, and every day away from work is a financial loss. Kim has been working to help Mr. Anderson arrange financial matters and provide support for the whole family. In the fourth week of hospitalization, Mr. Anderson develops a fever during the night. The symptoms persist the next day, so that all treatments must be cancelled. Another series of tests is run, this time revealing a lymphosarcoma involving the bone (a type of cancer that is likely to be fatal within a year).

The physician telphones Kim to report the diagnosis and its implications for treatment. He says he is quite certain that Mr. Anderson would not want to know that he has cancer. Kim asks the physician why he has come to this conclusion, and he explains that Mr. Anderson once said of a friend who had died of cancer, "He stopped living as soon as he found out." The physician also tells Kim that he has spoken to Mrs. Anderson, who concurs with his judgment. He asks if Kim has had any discussion with Mr. or Mrs. Anderson that would provide insight into whether Mr. Anderson would want to know. Kim tries to think of something he may have said, but is unable to recall any discussions that would clarify this difficult decision. Kim believes that both the Andersons have always confronted problems directly and honestly, and says so. There is a pause. The physician says, "Well, I've pretty much decided not to tell him. I think all in all it's better for him not to know."

Kim Segard goes on seeing Clayton Anderson. About ten days later Clayton says to Kim, "You know, we have talked often, and I have come to trust your judgment. I'm grateful for the help you've given me and my family. You know I've tried to cooperate with the doctors and everyone, but I have a feeling that something funny is going on that I can't get at. My wife and the doctor are acting strange and that is scaring me. I couldn't sleep all last night and so I decided to ask you. I know you will level with me . . . . Do I have cancer or some fatal illness?" ([2], p. 87).

This situation can be intensified by assuming that, based on his experience with Mr. Anderson and the physician, Kim fully is persuaded that Mr. Anderson is asking him for a diagnosis, fully is persuaded that the physician will *not* provide the information, and believes he is the only one who will tell Mr. Anderson the diagnosis. Kim either can tell or not tell Mr. Anderson he has cancer.

This is not a comfortable moment for any member of the health care team. But the thoughts going through Kim's mind at this moment are quite different than they would be if he were an "equal" with the physician or were in fact a physician. Kim probably is worrying about what his course of action will mean in terms of his relationship to other team members, coupled with what effect it will have on Mr. Anderson. He wants to act responsibly, and also to keep his status, not be mention his job. In order to describe Kim's present dilemma, it is necessary (at last!) to turn to the notion of responsibility.

II. RESPONSIBILITY, EQUALITY, AND HEALTH CARE TEAMS

Erde did not attempt a definition of responsibility and neither will I. It seems more appropriate to use the term in two of its most commonly understood connotations – *accountability* and *response*. A responsible person charts a course between "an ethics of conformity to a law or an order – and an ethics that reacts in utter open endedness to whatever is happening" ([1], p. 13). People who are at the extreme accountability end of the continuum are excessively scrupulous and duty-bound. They "keep promises" or "refrain from harming" but in the process lose all sight of the complexity of the circumstances calling for the responsible action. In contrast, people at the extreme open-ended response end of the continuum act in what appears to be a chaotic fashion characterized by excessive diffusiveness of response. These people transform creative action into a whirlwind which finally destroys the very structures supporting their freedom of response ([1], p. 14).

In the thinking of health professionals, the notion of responsibility correctly is associated with having authority to make decisions for which each professional must be accountable *and* which demonstrates the creative ability of each. Such a notion has appeared with increasing frequency as various Codes of Ethics are updated.[3] Clearly, as health professionals judge themselves to be approaching equal status *qua professionals* with physicians, their sense of responsbility also increases. Within the heap model they act responsibly in their cooperative, supportive, and even "covering for" activities, and are treated as equals. Only when the test case of patient distress arises and a decision about patient management must be made do their attempts at continuing to act responsibly lead to action which fails to steer the middle course embracing both accountability and creative response.

Consider the situation of Mr. Anderson and Kim Segard. Kim, wanting to act responsibly, has decided to risk erring on the side of over-scrupulous accountability.The team members are likely to respond angrily to the fact that this lone professional has tried to exercise equality by assuming authority which "belongs" only to the physician. Both the equal respect of the heap model and the efficient (though ambiguous) decision-making of the goal efficiency model are perceived by team members as breaking down. In the ensuing battle attention usually is diverted increasingly from the patient and focused on the interaction among team members. When confronted with the possibility that assuming a disproportionate responsibility was not necessary, health professionals often proclaim that what was done needed to be done to rescue the patient from distress. Health professionals with this attitude usually hope that other team members will support them and thereby affirm the status of equal respect. Often, however, the opposite happens.

A second course of action Kim could take is to hedge and dodge. Under no circumstances is Mr. Anderson going to be told that he has cancer. Since Kim believes that Mr. Anderson is asking for that information, however, Kim is faced with the perplexity of how to act responsibly. He executes daring verbal gymnastics and dizzying psychological spins, an equal to anyone in his display of creative alternatives. He is willing to continue to err on the side of creative response, knowing that it may dissipate into chaos. At no point, however, does he edge close enough to accountability to justify his being termed "responsible".

The repercussions of this mode of behavior sometimes go unnoticed to all but the health professionals involved. The equal respect of teammates may continue with the result being that Mr. Anderson's management may proceed "efficiently" until he dies.[4] (No good teammate makes waves!) But Kim, as *one member of the team*, has lost self-respect (and experiences a loss of respect for the physician) by knowingly acting in a manner that he judges is not in the best interests of the patient.

III. TOWARDS RESPONSIBLE TEAMWORK

Given the complexity of the present health care system, it would be impossible to pretend that the plan for assuring responsible teamwork has been delineated in this essay. The following suggestions, however, should serve to point health professionals in the right direction:

(A) *Affirm existing strengths*. The extent to which equal respect is operative within team activity and teamwork and the shared sense of responsibility for good patient care should be fostered.

(B) *Look more rigorously at the trade-offs between efficiency and more equal modes of decision-making in patient management*. Clearly not every health professional needs to be involved in every health care decision. Under what conditions should efficiency be sacrificed for more democratic procedures?

(C) *Try to reduce ambiguity*. The criteria suggested in (B) can help determine how much equality is desirable at various junctures in decision-making and what constitutes the limits of the goal efficiency model.

These practical suggestions seem consistent and complementary to the underlying philosophical and logical issues that Erde suggests health professionals must confront. I agree with his contention that the tensions between equality and efficiency will continue for a long time to come. By moving in the directions suggested in both our essays, I hope that health professionals will make their undertakings more humanized.

Massachusetts General Hospital
Institute of Health Professions

NOTES

[1] Since Erde's and my papers are only two of many in this volume addressing responsibility and health care, I spent considerable time deliberating about what responsible course I might take to add to the richness and breadth of discussion as it has already developed.

I decided my own experiences in the health field could provide more than adequate background for such a discussion. Prior to creeping up to and peeking into the crystal cave of philosophic thought and reflection, I spent six years as a physical therapy clinician working with patients. For four more years I was the clinical coordinator for health professions students at Boston University. Having found that there is life after the dissertation, I am presently teaching humanities courses to graduate students in nursing, physical therapy, dietetics, social work, and other health-related professions.

[2] The reader who has digested Erde's highly provocative and thorough paper will understand my dilemma in having to pick and choose a few aspects of the paper to develop in this response.

[3] A prime example is the Code of Ethics of the American Social Worker's Association adopted in 1980. The entire code is designed around the language of responsibility.

[4] Many readers know the situation often is worse than I describe here. The patient who has risked such a frightening question expects an honest answer. The eventual realization that he has cancer likely will lead to an outraged sense of having been betrayed by Kim, whom Mr. Anderson thought he could trust.

BIBLIOGRAPHY

1. Gustafson, J. and Laney, J.: 1968, *On Being Responsible*, Harper and Row, New York.
2. Purtilo, R. B. and Cassel, C. K.: 1981, *Ethical Dimensions of the Health Professions*, W. B. Saunders Company, Philadelphia. The excerpt quoted here is reproduced with permission.

SECTION IV

LEGAL AND POLITICAL RESPONSIBILITY IN HEALTH CARE MATTERS

PETER C. WILLIAMS

LEGAL RESPONSIBILITY IN HEALTH CARE: WHOSE FAULT IS IT ANYWAY?

Dr. Eddingfield was a general practitioner. He had been the family physician for the Hurley family for some time and was the only physician in the area available to the Hurleys. One evening Mr. Hurley became critically ill and sent a messenger to Dr. Eddingfield's house seeking help. The messenger arrived at Dr. Eddingfield's house, informed him of Hurley's dangerous condition, offered to pay the fee before services were rendered and asked Dr. Eddingfield to come visit the patient. Without any reason whatever, Dr. Eddingfield refused to go to Hurley's aid. No other patients were requiring the doctor's services, and he could have gone to Hurley's aid had he been willing to do so. No other care was available for Mr. Hurley. Because of lack of attention Hurley died of his illness. Mr. Hurley's estate sued the doctor for failure to render services and lost the suit. The court said then in 1901, as it would now, that in the absence of some special contract or other commitment, physicians have no obligation, *no legal responsibility*, to treat people [12]. The law does not require health care providers to be even minimally good samaritans.

The point of this story is not criticism of Dr. Eddingfield's behavior – though criticism could certainly be adduced; rather it is to highlight in a dramatic way the separation between notions of legal responsibility and moral responsibility.

I. LEGAL VS MORAL RESPONSIBILITY

In Anglo-American law what individuals are bound to do and what they legally can be held accountable for diverge significantly from what even the most callous moralist says they ought to do or are obligated to do. Only a cursory look at tort law is sufficient to manifest the separation of morality – that is, moral responsibilities – from the requirements of law. This separation runs both ways, with the dictates of morality sometimes being more and sometimes less onerous than those of the law.

In many instances in which we would hold someone morally responsible the law does not. Good samaritan cases such as *Hurley v. Eddingfield* substantiate this point. While individuals may be morally required to aid others

George J. Agich (ed.), Responsibility in Health Care, 227–243.
Copyright © 1982 *by D. Reidel Publishing Company, Dordrecht, Holland.*

in distress, the law does not hold them blameworthy for failure to do so. In his famous treatise on tort law, William Prosser remarks that the "law has persistently refused to recognize the moral obligation of common decency and common humanity, to come to the aid of another human being who is in danger . . . " ([20] , p. 336). Statutes of limitation provide another example of the lesser stringency of legal than of moral responsibility. The law's interest in efficient administration of courts often precludes people from effectively holding others legally accountable, even though their moral culpability is clear.

A third example of the law holding someone to a lesser standard of responsibility than morality is found in the defense of contributory negligence. This doctrine states that an injured party cannot recover damages from a blatant wrongdoer if the victim himself was negligent "in any degree, however slight" ([20] , p. 431). No account is taken of the degree of the fault involved. Finally, in negligence cases the standard of care required of people has been determined by reference to customary practice, i.e., what others in the community or enterprise usually did. The now largely discredited locality rule in tort law allowed individuals to adopt a low standard of care if their local colleagues used the same low standard. While morality might require that individuals act morally, the locality rule requires only that they do what others do. All four of these examples – good samaritanism, statutes of limitation, defenses like that of contributory negligence, and the standard of customary practice – are examples of the law allowing people to escape legal responsibility for behavior most would think morally questionable or wrong.

At the same time, the law has held people accountable for behavior that most would concede was morally blameless. Two common examples illustrate this point. First, sometimes responsibility is assigned to one person who himself had done no wrong but who is held liable because of the negligence of another. *Vicarious liability* would hold a master responsible for the wrongdoing of a servant, in spite of the former's proper oversight of the latter; employers are responsible for the misfeasance of employees; physicians are responsible for the negligence of people who work under them. In these cases of vicarious liability a person is held legally liable though having done nothing morally wrong. The second example of the law affixing greater responsibility than do moral codes is *strict liability*. Throughout the history of tort law certain classes of people – keepers of dangerous animals, for example – have been held liable for injuries that occur even though nothing reasonable could have been done to prevent those injuries. It is generally conceded that impossibility is a bar against holding individuals morally responsible or accountable for what they have done. Society cannot morally blame people for something they could not help doing. And yet, in both civil and criminal law this excuse is occasionally unavailable. Individuals are sometimes legally "blamed" for unavoidable accidents.

Given these numerous examples of the differences between law and morals, any discussion of the notion of legal responsibility in health care must begin with the realization that concepts of moral responsibility are only marginally helpful. As this essay will demonstrate, the notion of moral culpability is becoming less and less important in many areas of the law – a change which may in fact be salutary.

II. LIMITING THE INQUIRY

This paper will outline possible topics in legal responsibility and focus on a few of the more relevant ones. First, the concept of responsibility will be discussed only as it relates to civil law – criminal justice system relationships will be omitted. Because of the need to limit topics, there will be no discussion of the obligations and liabilities that grow out of contracts and little attention devoted to changes in statutory law or regulations promulgated and enforced by administrative agencies. Rather, the focus will be on tort law and more particularly on accidents – what can be termed *medical maloccurrences* – and their treatment in the court system.

Second, there are various categories of health care that could be analyzed with regard to legal responsibility. Discussion here will be limited to a few pertinent categories, least justifiable of which is the almost exclusive attention to accidents arising from actions (or inactions) on the part of physicians. This limitation is somewhat unfortunate since it perpetuates a bias in most discussions of health care. Professionals in the areas of nursing, allied health, and public health receive far too little attention. This bias is particularly egregious in view of the fact that a great preponderance of health care is delivered by non-physicians. Nevertheless, there are two reasons for examining physician practice in particular. Most of the legal doctrines that affect health care workers have been developed in case law arising out of physician behavior. Additionally, as other health professionals – in particular nurse practitioners and physician's assistants – gain independent status, the legal doctrines that will apply to them are assuredly those that have been developed in regulating the conduct of physicians. Consequently, a discussion of the law relating to physicians will by implication be a discussion of the law that has or will relate to other health care professionals.

To say that this essay will focus on the responsibility of physicians would still be too broad a declaration. Of primary importance is the relationship between physicians and patients in the clinical setting. Issues of responsibility in research or in more general areas of public or environmental health will be excluded. Since the most salient issue of responsibility in clinical medicine concerns accidents that occur in physician/patient interactions intended to benefit the patient directly, the focus will be on iatrogenic disease or injury.

There is a third general limitation accompanying these remarks. A number of distinctions dealing with the notion of responsibility could be analyzed. Although concepts of moral responsibility do not always parallel legal responsibility, there are some common elements. In neither morality nor law is there one single and clear idea of what responsibility is, but both legal and moral scholars note the difference between descriptive responsibility and prescriptive or normative responsibility [17]. As George Agich points out in "The Concept of Responsibility in Medicine," the former is a retrospective view of responsibility, focusing on notions of cause and control; the latter is a prospective view, dealing with what people ought to do. The law usually combines – one might even say confuses – these two notions. To use distinctions drawn by J. Roland Pennock, the two major ideas that comprise the literature of responsibility in the legal system are capacity responsibility and accountability [17].

Capacity responsibility perhaps can best be explained through an example. Usually when a court holds someone responsible, it presupposes a claim about that person's capacities. Here a legal scholar could discuss notions of intentionality, deliberation, purpose, and other characteristics of people who use free will, who deliberate and choose alternatives, and who exercise discretion. Attention of legal scholars would be drawn to the insanity defense, the grounds for civil commitment, excuses such as ignorance, immaturity, and the like. From Aristotle to Austin, philosophers have noted the important connection between individuals' capacity as agents and the degree to which they would be held accountable for their behavior [6].

The second major focus in legal discussions involving responsibility has to do with accountability – that is, liability for the consequences of one's act. When and for what may individuals be held accountable? As noted above, this is not a question about moral blame, though during some periods in legal history the two were more closely tied than they are today [11]. Rather, it is a question about compensation and requital. The concern here will be with this second sense of responsibility, that of accountability or liability. The question is: *How has legal responsibility, that is, liability, been affixed*? Prior to any examination of this historical question, the general goals of tort liability will be delineated. The essay will conclude with suggestions as to the direction legal responsibility in health care will and should go.

III. THE GOALS OF TORT LIABILITY

Civil liability in general and tort liability in particular are designed to accomplish four oftentimes competing goals: prevention, compensation, retribution, and administrative efficiency. An understanding of and evaluation of any system of assigning legal responsibility must be cast in terms of these four goals.

Prevention of accidents is sought through deterrence, the effort at keeping people from causing injuries to others by censuring, admonishing, or punishing those who do. The goal is a reduction in the number and severity of accidents, thereby reducing the costs arising therefrom. When most people think about medical maloccurrences, they tend to categorize them in terms of such costs as the loss of productive time or capacities. The question to be addressed here is: What kind of fault assignment would be best at keeping iatrogenic accidents from happening?

Compensation is an effort at returning an injured person to the state that person would have been in had the injury not occurred. This effort can be satisfied through a number of devices – for example, through compensatory damages or schemes of social or injury insurance. Two complementary notions rationalize the compensatory role of tort liability: the formal ideal of reparation and the utilitarian goal of minimizing the costs consequent to accidents. The former seems intuitively clear. Individuals are bound to remedy prior wrongs. The questions to be addressed regarding the utilitarian goal are the following: Is it less expensive to let victims of medical accidents pay for their own injuries; or to make parties causing the injury bear those costs; or to pick another mode of payment, such as social insurance, to spread the burdens over time or across groups of people?

Retribution for wrongdoing usually is considered central to criminal law, although on occasion it is appropriate to civil law as well. The question in terms of retribution becomes: Is tort law used to exact a penalty from wrongdoers so as to deter future injury and at the same time satisfy a desire to retaliate for past wrongs? Even though this function was central to the creation of tort law in medieval England, it has come to play an ever decreasing role. Nonetheless, there still is an element of retribution when courts allow punitive damages for especially serious injuries or intentional malfeasance ([20], pp. 9–11). A full evaluation of methods of legal responsibility must include some attention to this feature.

Administrative efficiency pertains to the cost of administering any system of liability. The question in this case is: How expensive is it to identify and punish a wrongdoer? An important point needs to be made here. Moral judgments are made by individuals or groups of individuals in the absence of bureaucratic structures. Thus in applying moral principles, the costs of administration are seldom considered. If they are addressed, it is normally in terms of the emotional distress that often accompanies decision-making, or in terms of the fallibility of decision-makers. A strictly economic analysis is seldom deemed appropriate. In the legal system this is not the case. The economic burden of a system of allocation is of extreme importance, and, as will be evident, discussions of assigning responsibility in the legal system have tended more and more to focus on administrative expenses.

As was pointed out earlier, these four goals of a system of assigning liability – prevention, compensation, retribution, and administrative efficiency – are often inconsistent. The disadvantages of one of these goals will have an impact on the other three. For example, one of the arguments against the current malpractice system is that the administrative costs of trials are inordinately high. Professionals such as trial lawyers, who earn their living from these administrative costs, often argue against any changes in the system of assigning responsibility which lessen the need for litigation. When, for example, no-fault automobile insurance schemes – which require fewer negligence trials – were proposed in many states, groups who earned their living from these procedures fought the changes vigorously. The rationale for their opposition was that such change would have a negative impact on deterrence, compensation, and retribution, whereas few doubted that the system actually would lower adminstrative expenses.

IV. THE HISTORY OF TORTS

With these considerations in mind, the history of assigning legal responsibility – that is, legal accountability or legal liability – in Anglo-American law can be examined. The earliest response to injury caused by other people's action was self-help. Alone or with a family, an individual would exact reparation from an alleged wrongdoer. Retribution was a major goal, and family or clan warfare sometimes ensued. In English law the state, in order to assure domestic tranquillity, took over the functions of securing redress for injuries one person caused another ([21], p. 1). Prior to the nineteenth century, under common law individuals acted at their own peril. If someone behaved in a way directly causing injury to another, he was liable for that injury; the resulting harm was his responsibility irrespective of any wrongdoing. To quote the classic *Case of Thorns* from 1466:

> Though a man doth a lawful thing, yet if any damage do thereby befall another, he shall answer for it, if he could have avoided [the activity causing the damage] [5].

Modern notions of wrongdoing would have been considered irrelevant in those times. In explaining the law of 1466, the court stated:

> If a man assault me, and I lift up my staff to defend myself and in lifting it up hit another, an action lies by that person and yet I did a lawful thing. And the reason of all these cases is, because he that is damaged ought to be recompensed [5].

By the middle of the nineteenth century, notions of legal responsibility for injury began to change. Though there are a number of explanations given for this change, the standard view is that growing urbanization and industrialization caused a drastic increase in the number of injuries. The growing complexity of society and the increase in the number of total strangers who came into contact with one another gave rise to many more law suits. Coupled with a strong impetus to encourage industrialization and economic activity at this time, these forces prompted the development of a new standard for assigning legal responsibility for injuries.

A characteristic case illustrating this change arose with facts and events almost identical to the hypothetical example mentioned in the *Case of Thorns*. In an effort to break up a dog fight, George Kendall raised a stick to hit the fighting dogs. He accidentally struck George Brown, who was standing behind him. Brown sued Kendall for the consequent damages and lost. In announcing the new standard of liability the court stated:

> Plaintiff must come prepared with evidence to show either that the intention was unlawful or that the defendant was in fault; for if the injury was unavoidable, and the conduct of the defendant was free from blame, he will not be liable. [Citations omitted] If, in the prosecution of a lawful act, a casualty purely accidental arises, no action can be supported for an injury arising therefrom [1].

This court was one of the first to enunciate the standard of ordinary care, namely "that kind and degree of care which prudent and cautious men use ... " [1]. This decision was an important turnabout from the standard view of earlier centuries as expressed in the *Case of Thorns*. The notion of wrongdoing was now self-consciously introduced; merely causing an injury was no longer sufficient to cause liability to be assigned. The newly-enunciated general principle of law was that a loss from an accident must normally lie where it falls [11]. The starting point for assigning liability, for affixing responsibility, had shifted from the actor to the victim. In most areas of accident law, individuals would not be held accountable for everything they did; rather, negligence had to be established. A victim had to demonstrate that the person causing the injury had not lived up to the standard of care that an ordinary and prudent person would exercise. Applied to professionals (and this is where the issue of malpractice enters), the standard of care is the behavior of a reasonable practitioner. That standard grew rapidly in popularity until a court in 1873 stated " . . . the rule is, at least in this country, a universal one, which, as far as I can discern, has no exceptions or limitations, that no one can be made liable for injury to the person or property of another without some fault or negligence on his part" ([14], p. 491).

Though direct, this statement was simply incorrect. There were then as there are now numerous exceptions to the negligence standard. Strict liability – legal responsibility without showing of fault – had existed before the industrial age and in major areas continued. Liability for dangerous things or animals is one example [22]. *Respondeat superior* is another; non-negligent masters were still responsible for the negligence of their servants. Nonetheless, the trend after 1850 was clear and consistent for fifty years or more. The standard of reasonableness as determined by customary practice was predominant. It has been estimated that between 1875 and 1905 no case occurred in which an enterprise was ruled negligent for not introducing a new safety measure not required by customary practice [19].

In a sense, two standards of assigning legal responsibility ran concurrently. In the latter part of the nineteenth century, negligence played a progressively larger role, while strict liability saw a continuation and then a slow expansion. If the development of negligence rather than the persistence of liability without fault is examined, other elements in assigning legal responsibility become important.

Injured parties sometimes were simply barred from recovering the costs of injuries they received at the hands of negligent others. The strong social policy which favored expansion of industry and business led to extensive protection of business from suits by employees. A rule called the Fellow Servant Rule precluded suits by one employee against a company for the negligence of another ([20],pp. 551–553). This rule marked out an enormous exception in the principles of vicarious liability and left a large class of workers unprotected. Discussing the trend toward letting the cost of injuries fall upon victims, Oliver Wendell Holmes, Jr., wrote in *The Common Law* in 1881:

> The state might conceivably make itself a mutual insurance company against accidents, and distribute the burden of its citizens' mishaps among all its members . . . . As between individuals it might adopt the mutual insurance principle . . . and divide damages when both are at fault . . . or it might throw all loss upon the actor irrespective of fault. The state does none of these things, however, and a prevailing view is that its cumbrous and expensive machinery ought not to be set in motion unless some clear benefit is to be derived from disturbing the status quo ([11], sec. 14).

In this famous passage, Holmes was rationalizing the refusal of the state to assign legal responsibility to those who had not committed fault. He also noted that the state was not likely to adopt policies in court or in the legislature to compensate the victims of mere accidents. Nonetheless, it was not long before the ambit of strict liability began to grow and compensation for injuries in the form of workers' compensation statutes began to appear.

The development of insurance schemes had and continues to have a significant impact on the legal system's response to injuries. It became apparent at the turn of the century that there were a number of enterprises creating hazards for which there was no indemnification within the tort system. Not only did the negligence standard rule out recovery for mere accidents, but the Fellow Servant Rule or the Doctrine of Contributory Negligence, which barred recovery for plantiffs who had been at fault to any degree, limited the class of successful plaintiffs even further. Concern for the welfare of workers in the now more mature industries prompted the passage in many states of workers' compensation statutes. The kind of social insurance scheme that Holmes had ridiculed three decades before became a reality:

> Workman's compensation statues eliminated (or tried to) the process of fixing civil liability for industrial accidents through litigation in the common law courts. Under the statutes compensation was based on set schedules and the responsibility for initial determination of employee's claims was taken from the courts and given to an administrative agency ([7], p. 70).

This marked a drastic change in the view society began to take toward injury. The goal of compensating people for injuries rapidly grew in importance. Concomitantly, in the late nineteenth century, the view that victims should bear the costs of injuries unless the injuring party were blameworthy waned.

Declining in popularity also was the assumption that a major purpose of tort law was retribution. Compensation became a major focus. In addition to the development of compensation statutes for industrial and railroad accidents, liability insurance was developed as a way for employers to protect themselves against suits resulting from the negligence of their employees. By the 1930s liability insurance had become very popular. The growth of insurance was central to a dispute that began after the end of the Second World War – namely, whether tort law would be viewed primarily as an instrument for deterring unwanted conduct or primarily as a means for compensating those who had been injured. The goal of retribution had all but disappeared:

> If "blameworthiness," as reflected in the "fault" requirement of much of tort law, was the standard of conduct that triggered compensation, injurers could expect, since the compensation of injured persons was deemed a desirable social goal, that they would more regularly be found "blameworthy," or liable in tort. Accordingly they could be expected to protect themselves against the risks of having to compensate others. Liability insurance secured them this protection ([26], p. 149).

Assignment of legal responsibility thus began to reflect an interest in social efficiency and compensation much more than in deterrence or retaliation. The application of the concept of strict liability grew rapidly, for example. Legal responsibility without wrongdoing for defective products and foodstuffs became an established doctrine by the middle of the twentieth century. In the 1960s, recovery for automobile accidents was moved largely out of the negligence system as no-fault automobile insurance became more common.

But what of health care? For what were health care providers legally responsible? Until quite recently, the negligence standard has been consistently applied to health care providers. Liability would not be found unless the provider had done something that fell below the standard of other providers. Nonetheless, the negligence standards for health care providers have come under heavy attack.

V. CHALLENGES TO THE NEGLIGENCE STANDARD

The major arguments against the negligence theory in health care have referred to all four goals of tort law: prevention, compensation, retribution, and administrative efficiency. *Prevention* should deter unwanted behavior and minimize the incidence of accidents. It is an effort to make physicians more careful, to prompt retaining when necessary, to abandon procedures that are apparently too risky, and to implement safer practices. A great deal of evidence suggests that the negligence standard does not meet these ends.

There have been a number of attacks on the application of this standard and its effectiveness as a deterrent for unwanted conduct.

The negligence standard traditionally has relied on custom. The question becomes: What would a comparably-situated, reasonable practitioner do in these circumstances? To answer this question requires expert testimony. Because of this requirement two problems arise: a situation which has been called the conspiracy of silence and the resultant fact that the customary standard may be too low. A patient who has been injured in contact with a physician will have difficulty establishing negligence if no other physician is willing to testify that the customary procedure is more exacting than the one used by the defendant physician in the situation. It should be conceded that there has been little systematic research on the conspiracy of silence issue. Whatever its merits in the past, the sheer number of successful malpractice suits being brought today seems to demonstrate that plaintiffs have some access to expert witnesses willing to break the "conspiracy".

The second difficulty with the customary standard of negligence, however, is more substantive. It is possible that the customary practice of the profession is simply too low. In this event the standard applied by the courts would protect neither social interests nor plaintiffs' interests. The court does have the power to set a standard higher than the community's standard and occasionally (though very seldom) does so [10].

A second argument that the negligence standard does not deter injurious conduct turns on the availability of liability insurance for physicians. The notion of liability insurance contains two difficulties, both of which shield wrongdoers from their wrongs. First, the wrongdoer gets compensated by an insurance company for any costs that are incurred. Any incentive to avoid costs is thereby diminished. Second, even extremely careful physicians do not have very strong incentive to be careful since their insurance rates are set by members of the group in which they practice. The persons who set insurance rates do so in the aggregate, and thus are not very sensitive to the particular carefulness or carelessness of individual practitioners. This insensitivity is obvious to all safe drivers when they pay auto insurance sufficient to cover the accident costs incurred by less careful drivers in their class. It should be recognized that notoriety and inconvenience can accompany being named a defendant in a malpractice suit. The availability of malpractice insurance, nonetheless, largely shields practitioners from deterrent effects of those suits.

A third argument against the effectiveness of the negligence standard as a deterrent focuses on the characteristics of possible plaintiffs. Many people are either too ignorant of the fact that they have received insufficient care or are too poor to bring suit. Others are unwilling to sue, whether for financial reasons (the amount of recovery may be too small to justify the expense) or because they are not litigious. If the negligence standard is to work as a deterrent to inadequate practice, those injured by that practice must bring suit. Research indicates that only a small percentage of the people who might successfully bring negligence suits actually does so ([4], p. 250; [23], p. 1286; [8]; [13]).

A fourth potentially most damaging argument against the negligence standard involves criticism of the general level of care given in the United States. If the purpose of negligence as a system is to optimize care, there is little evidence that it has been successful. Critics who rely on international comparisons of health status – for example, infant mortality – often argue that American care is good for some, but certainly less than optimal in the aggregate. This conclusion, however, may be as much a result of maldistribution of health care as it is low quality care delivered. Nonetheless, some studies conclude that quality itself is low ([15], [18]).

A final argument against the negligence system arises from what is called defensive medicine. Fear of law suits seems to encourage practitioners to protect themselves through excessive diagnostic or other testing. The introduction of third party payment for many of the additional tests and procedures thereby ordered removes what used to be an economic disincentive for such behavior. In addition to its economic costs, the additional risks borne by patients attendant to many diagnostic procedures must be also considered. Defensive medicine simply increases the bill that the negligence system imposes.

If any one of these five contentions is correct, then the power of the negligence standard to deter iatrogenic harm is severely diminished. But what of its worth as a system of compensation? Here we encounter some of the most cogent criticisms of the negligence standard. The first criticism concerns the question of fairness or justice. If legal responsibility is assigned only when there is fault, a number of injuries go uncompensated. Two patients could be injured equally in their contact with physicians and yet only one compensated under the negligence system. The reason for this is that the availability of compensation depends on the behavior of the provider. When an injury was caused through negligence, the injured party can recover; if negligence does not exist, recovery is not possible. The claim of justice implicit in this critique is that equal injuries deserve equal compensation. Need, not characteristics of the causal agent, should be the criterion for recompense. But even if everyone did not share this particular standard of justice, a principle of beneficence would argue in favor of compensating all iatrogenic injuries. This principle, too, is certainly precluded by the negligence standard.

It is important to recognize that the likelihood of compensation is not simply limited by the existence or absence of malfeasance. Remember that a significant number of victims who are unaware that negligence has occurred or who are unwilling or unable to bring suits are also denied compensation. Anyone familiar with the actual operations of hospitals is well aware of the large number of incidences which could create legal liability but which either are not discovered or not pursued by potential plaintiffs.

The third criterion used to evaluate the method of affixing legal responsibility for iatrogenic injuries is: How well does the system serve the end of retribution? This criterion is not consequentialist (i.e., does not refer to future costs or benefits of punishment); rather, it focuses solely on the past actions of people, inflicting harm only on those who have done wrong. First, *lex talionis* – the legal version of the doctrine of an eye for an eye – plays an ever decreasing role in tort law. Punishment of wrongdoers has been of steadily diminishing concern. Second, as liability insurance, corporate medicine, and group practice shield wrongdoers from most court-determined punishment, the goal of retribution is frustrated.

The fourth and final goal of a tort system is administrative efficiency. Consonant with the other goals, legal responsibility should be assigned in the way that most reduces costs. The enormous administrative costs of the negligence system are a prime target for those who argue in favor of strict liability in health care. It is estimated that between seventeen and thirty-four cents of every dollar in malpractice insurance premiums is paid to successful claimants. Fifty cents of that same dollar is donated to the legal system ([4], p. 246; [23], p. 1287). This figure is more meaningful when compared to the eight-eight cents of every premium dollar reaching patients who have health insurance. If the goal of the negligence system is to line the pockets of those responsible for its inception and maintenance, then it has been highly successful. That does not, however, seem to be a goal normally espoused by advocates of the negligence system. As a system of transferring funds from injurers to victims, it is very inefficient.

VI. SUGGESTIONS

In summary, it is apparent that the negligence method of assigning legal responsibility does not well serve any of the ends of the liability system. What alternatives have been suggested? The most promising seems to be an analogy to strict liability and workers' compensation. Under this system patients who have been injured in the course of treatment of a disease would be compensated by an insurance scheme funded by users of that system. Perhaps an apt name would be "medical maloccurrence insurance". Money for the program would be exacted from health care providers, with an understanding that they will continue to pass on these costs to consumers.

This suggestion is not original. A form of this system has been employed in Sweden [3] and suggested by others [9], [16]. As stated at the outset, medical maloccurrence insurance could not be expected to satisfy equally well the four goals in assigning legal responsibility. The strongest case in its favor is that it compensates people for injuries occurring in health care. Medical maloccurrence insurance achieves this regardless of fault. Of course, the number of compensable events would be greater, increasing costs concomitantly.

The argument that this insurance would be an administratively efficient system is also strong. As with workers' compensation, it would avoid the costs of deciding whether a physician, nurse, physician's assistant, or anyone else was negligent. Medical maloccurrence insurance admittedly would give rise to difficult law suits as to whether a condition were a "maloccurrence" and, if so, whether it was the result of medical treatment or the manifestation of prior or subsequent illness. Just how great the real administrative savings under a medical maloccurrence insurance program would be is uncertain. It could hardly eliminate disputes and litigation. If the program were patterned after the workers' compensation plan, an administrative agency might well lessen the costs of determining whether a particular outcome – hepatitis, for example – was an antecedent condition, was iatrogenic, or was contracted after a patient's contact with the health care delivery system.

The major problem with this proposal is the way in which it would affect deterrence and retribution. Some argument could be made that care would worsen with the removal of the deterrent effects of negligence suits which the malpractice method of assigning legal responsibility carries. There are three responses to this argument, though none of them is wholly adequate. First is a reiteration of the fact that deterrence under malpractice is itself none too effective. Second is the hope that deterrence and retribution can be achieved through other mechanisms that to date have not been impressively effective (such as licensing and P. S. R. O.'s). There is also some hope that the development of prepaid health plans will provide internal policing within the profession, as groups of physicians and other health care providers become economically interested in improving the performance of their colleagues. Third is the argument that even with strict liability, deterrence can be achieved

[25]. The fact that a health care provider is financially responsible for *any* maloccurrence may well prompt good care. Admittedly, though, defensive medicine is the opposite side of this coin. Deterrence may also be a contributing factor in the sort of strict liability recommended in this essay in that the less competent might be kept out of the field of health care or out of specialties within health care that are particularly subject to compensable events. Unfortunately, the competent yet timid professional might be discouraged as well.

By far the most serious problem in assigning responsibility in health care arises from the fact that patients have more to do with their health status than the input of physicians and other health care providers. Assigning responsibility for compensation of iatrogenic problems to health care providers might well be economically beneficial in that any risk is spread out. Such a decision, however, ignores the major role that patients have in instigating physician/patient contact (the risky encounter) and in the success of therapy. The incentive on the part of citizens to maintain their own health consequently may be lessened.

Two responses seem appropriate to this powerful objection. The first would be to tax whenever possible behavior that contributes to illness. As Robert Veatch notes, "additional health fees on health-risk behavior calculated to reimburse the health care system would redistribute the burden of the cost of such care to those who have chosen to engage in it" ([24], p. 51). For an activity like smoking, this incremental tax would be easy. How stress or failure to exercise could be taxed is less clear. The real answer seems to be the second mitigating factor to this objection – namely, that those who take health risks have more contact with the health system and, through the bills they pay, thereby would contribute an appropriate share.

It seems that the strongest argument in favor of medical maloccurrence insurance is its value as a compensatory system and its high potential as an efficient means of allocating costs of injuries. This insurance would remove the stigma often attached to practitioners for unfortunate outcomes of medical procedures. It would also act as a stimulus for health care providers to put greater emphasis on preventive medicine. This suggested program admittedly is no panacea. Society will still bear the costs and the responsibility for the collective health of its members.

Any choice among methods of assigning responsibility unavoidably places much of the burden of that loss on consumers. But it is time to admit frankly that responsibility is collective and to argue for cessation of the excessively expensive and traumatic task of having courts attempt to assign blame to individuals. The ends of punishment – deterrence and retaliation – can be served better if separated from the goal of compensation to injured patients.

State University of New York
at Stony Brook

BIBLIOGRAPHY

1. *Brown v. Kendall*, 60 Mass. (6 Cush.) 292 (1850).
2. Calabresi, G.: 1970, *The Cost of Accidents*, Yale University Press, New Haven.
3. Cooper, J.: 1976, 'Sweden's No-Fault Patient Injury Insurance', *New England Journal of Medicine* **294**, 1268–70.
4. Cooper, J. K. and Stephens, S. K.: 1977, 'The Malpractice Crisis: What Was It All About?', *Inquiry* **XIV**, 240–253.
5. *Case of Thorns*, Y. B. 6 Ed. 4, 7a, pl. 18. (1466).
6. Fearey, R. A.: 1954, 'Concept of Responsibility', *Journal of Criminal Law, Criminology and Political Science* **45**, 21–28.
7. Friedman, L. M. and Ladinsky, J.: 1967, 'Social Change and the Law of Industrial Accidents', *Columbia Law Review* **67**, 50–82.
8. Gunther, J.: 1977, *The Malpractitioners*, Doubleday, New York.
9. Havighurst, C. and Tancredi, L. R.: 1973, 'Medical Adversity Insurance – A No-Fault Approach to Medical Malpractice and Quality Assurance', *Milbank Memorial Fund Quarterly* **51**, 125–16.
10. *Helling v. Carey*, 83 Wash. 2d 514, 519 P. 2d 981 (Superior Court of Washington; 1974).
11. Holmes, O. W., Jr.: 1881, *The Common Law*, Lec. III, Little, Brown and Co., Boston.
12. *Hurley v. Eddingfield*, 156 Ind. 416, 59 N. E. 1058 (1901).
13. Lander, L.: July, 1978, 'Why Some People Seek Revenge Against Doctors', *Psychology Today* **12**, 88–104.
14. *Losse v. Buchanan*, 51 N. Y. 487 (1873).
15. McCleery, R. S., *et al.*: 1971, *One Life – One Physician: An Inquiry into the Medical Profession's Performance in Self-Regulation*, Public Affairs Press, Washington, D. C.
16. Note: 1975, 'Comparative Approaches to Liability for Medical Maloccurrences', *Yale Law Journal* **84**, 1141–1163.
17. Pennock, J. R.: 1960, 'The Problem of Responsibility', in C. F. Friedrich (ed.), *Responsibility*, Liberal Arts Press, New York, pp. 3–27.
18. Peterson, O. L., *et al.*: 1956, "An Analytical Study of North Carolina General Practice, 1953–4', *Journal of Medical Education* **31**, Special Supplement Part 2, 1–165.
19. Posner, Richard A.: 1972, 'A Theory of Negligence', *Journal of Legal Studies* **1**, 29–83.
20. Prosser, W.: 1964, *The Law of Torts*, 3rd ed., West Publishing Company, St. Paul, Minnesota.

21. Rabin, Robert L.: 1976, *Perspectives on Tort Law*, Little, Brown and Co., Boston.
22. *Rylands v. Fletcher*, L. R., 3 H. L. 330 (House of Lords, 1868).
23. Schwartz, W. B. and Komesar, N. K.: 1978, 'Doctors, Damages and Deterrence', *New England Journal of Medicine* **298**, 1282–1289.
24. Veatch, R. M.: 1980, 'Voluntary Risks to Health', *JAMA* **243**, 50–55.
25. Wasserstrom, R.: 1960, 'Strict Liability in the Criminal Law', *Stanford Law Review* **12**, 731–745.
26. White, G. E.: 1980, *Tort Law in America*, Oxford University Press, New York.

ROBERT F. RICH

REACHING CLOSURE ON HEALTH-RELATED CONTROVERSIES

> . . . Science cannot tell us how many potential human cancers swim in a can of diet soda, though it has made some guesses. What can be shown is that a weak cancer can be induced by saccharin in rats, but only under unusual conditions whose relevance to human risk is obscure. From epidemiology we learned that the number of human bladder cancer cases that might currently be caused by past patterns of saccharin use is certainly small, and perhaps zero. We know, on the other hand, that it is at least plausible that saccharin offers substantial health benefits to certain groups of people, that these benefits need not be large in order to offset saccharin's slight risk, and that, unless we know for sure that the benefits are imaginary, it would be reckless to gamble with the public's health to compel a ban on diet food products. We know that a simple program of informing the public would accomplish by itself most or all af the aims of wise policy. And we know that the impetus for a ban does not issue from a proven public injury but from a well-intentioned legalism whose full consequences probably were not foreseen. Finally, we know that the public has spoken against a ban not just patiently and politely, but with a mass roar ([3], p. 24).

With this statement, William Havender put himself on public record as questioning the validity of banning saccharin from the market. A biochemist researching environmental carcinogens at Berkeley, Havender has taken his colleagues to task and called the scientific evidence into question. He argues for the public's "right" to choose freely and to procure its desires through the majority rule common to a democratic system. He also cites growing distrust of professionals – whether in medicine or government – and resentment of paternalistic attitudes, coupled with mounting public support for deregulation as justification for this popular majority rule notion.

Havender inadvertently raises the question of what the responsibility of medical practitioners and bio-scientists really is. One might simply argue that responsibility in medicine – especially for physicians – involves providing the best possible care to individual patients on a case-by-case basis. The physician has taken an oath to provide high-quality care. In the ideal case, decisions concerning the patient are made solely on the basis of medical needs, available technology, and preferences of the patient and his family. Within this context, physicians are held accountable primarily on the basis of self-adherence to the highest professional standards and review by peers through professional organizations. Medical practitioners are of course also accountable to patients

George J. Agich (ed.), Responsibility in Health Care, 245–259.
Copyright © 1982 by D. Reidel Publishing Company, Dordrecht, Holland.

and their families. This "ideal type" represents the model which hitherto has been accepted in defining physician responsibility, both on the part of the practitioners themselves and the society as a whole.

More recently it has been asserted – by consumer groups and "public interest lobbies" in particular – that responsibility in health care extends beyond the sacred physician-patient relationship. Moreover, its standards for accountability need to be expanded to include consumer preference in addition to strict professional standards. The physician's responsibility to his patients on a case-by-case basis thus is seen as only one dimension in a broader "corporate" sense of accountability. Since medicine is a publicly regulated activity and profession, physicians are seen as having social duties relating to the "public interest" as well as more narrowly defined medical ethical duties.

In responding to this corporate sense of responsibility, physicians and other medical scientists are placing health care at the center of political controversy. Havender's statement clearly defines responsibility in terms of political criteria. When a scientist such as Havender, *qua* scientist, takes a position of this kind, the public's health may be jeopardized. It seems clear that Havender has employed primarily non-scientific criteria as the basis for his position, rather than trying to balance the corporate responsibility with the professional responsibility which dominated medicine in the past.

This essay will examine the trade-offs involved in defining health responsibility issues strictly in terms of political and social accountability (that is, in the corporate sense) as opposed to balancing scientific and political criteria. It is interesting to note that the corporate sense of responsibility is being equated with policies that are "in the public interest". Politically, the public interest is seen as responding to consumer demands and the "will of the majority". Alternatively, it is clear that the public interest could be defined in terms of what is *objectively* correct – defined in terms of the best professional practices.

Over the last twenty-five years, there has been extraordinary pressure put on politicians, consumer advocates, and scientists in government to formulate policies which are consistent with the corporate sense of the public interest. The arguments for the public's right to define its own preferences threads it way through the speeches of officials such as Senator Stephen Symms of Idaho. Symms is among the most vocal representatives of issues alluded to in Havender's statements:

> Freedom is the issue. The American people should be allowed to make their own decisions. They shouldn't have the bureaucrats in Washington, D.C., trying to decide for them about what is good and what is bad, as long as it is safe . . . .

> The FDA is typical of what you get in regulatory agencies – a very protective mentality by bureaucrats who want to protect their own jobs and own positions. It's easier for them to say "no" to a product – Laetrile or anything else – than it is to say "yes" . . . .
>
> Stringent drug regulation for society as a whole limits therapeutic choice by the individual physician, who is better able to judge the risk and benefits for the individual patients.[1]

It is obvious that the standards for public policy-making should be guided by the public interest. The confusion comes, however, in the determination of just what constitutes the public interest. In the health field, disagreements arise over such matters as the sale of products containing saccharin, for example, in which consumer concerns must be balanced with concerns of safety and efficacy. The subsequent controversy illustrates differences between criteria for formulating health policy as opposed to criteria for other social welfare policies. Consumer groups lobby successfully for positions with public agencies, state legislatures, and Congress. The issues which public debate and the media focus on usually involve broad political concerns such as government interference and freedom of choice, as opposed to scientific concerns. In some cases it seems as if decisions on technical or scientific issues are being made independently of the available scientific evidence.

It is possible to argue that decisions *should not* be made exclusively on the basis of the available scientific evidence. On the other hand, it seems important to question the extent to which consumer public interest groups should be concerned with the safety and efficacy of potentially dangerous or harmful substances. How are issues of cost savings, fraud, and abuse to be balanced against safety and efficacy concerns?

Generally, public policy is made on the principle of achieving the greatest good for the greatest number. In the area of health policy, however, it seems appropriate to raise an additional set of concerns: How "safe" is "safe"? What "dangers" or risks are acceptable? How can scientific evidence be balanced with the articulated preferences and demands of the public? On what basis should scientists make their recommendations to legislators and political executives? Should they rely on the tested, empirical results published in scholarly journals or should they take equity, social welfare, and cost considerations into account? Which criteria should be foremost in the medical practitioner's mind?

This essay will explore the *scientific* and *political* foundations employed in reaching closure on health-related controversies. Discussion will include an analysis of what constitutes "responsible behavior" on the part of public policymakers. In exploring these issues, controversies in the pharmaceutical industry will be used to exemplify the kinds of problems and questions being posed. It should become apparent that the best scientific evidence is not necessarily consistent with "legitimate" public policy adopted by elected representatives.

I. WORKING TOWARD THE PUBLIC INTEREST

Governmental bodies supposedly operate under mandates generated from public interest. Presumably, a great deal of conflict and controversy in democratic politics focuses on alternative means for achieving the public interest.

In the United States, society has developed mechanisms designed to transfer the private interests of groups and individuals into something with the adjective "public" before it: elections, referendums, executive orders, the legislative process (including hearings), Supreme Court decisions, and the judgment of experts. These mechanisms for translating private interests into public interests are obviously not mutually exclusive alternatives. In most of these cases procedures are designed to settle controversies or competing claims among competing interests. Settlement or closure simply reflects the fact that the majority of stakeholders are willing to allow the decision-making process to move forward. No substantive decision may actually be taken; alternatively, there may even be a conscious decision "not to decide" (not to formulate a policy). The important point is that procedures for *negotiating a settlement* among competing interests have been put into place.[2]

Within this context, the question arises as to whether there is something special about scientific controversies (or rather, political controversies with a scientific content). As Jean-Jacques Salomon points out, there is no reason to believe that policy with a scientific content necessarily is handled differently from other forms of politics and policy ([9], p. 197). In any society it is important to understand how political controversies are resolved. It is also essential to examine whether the established mechanisms and "ground rules" are successful in working with competing interests, competing claims for scarce resources, and other forms of conflict.

Attempting to resolve controversies in a political environment characterized by distrust and demands for autonomy is complex and difficult. In recent years, controversies that involve "scientific issues" (or simply have a "scientific content") *have not* been resolved in any sense of the word. Public officials who have the formal responsibility for reaching decisions find it difficult to integrate their own individual and ethical social values with "facts" from scientific experts.[3]

C. P. Snow once observed that there is a gap between the culture of science and the culture of politics [10]. Scientists have well-developed procedures for working on scientific controversies. There are rules for "settlement"; there are rules for what types of evidence are acceptable; there are rules for how to present challenges to "state-of-the-art" findings; and there are institutional procedures for deciding disputes. In the field of science, decisions are not necessarily made through a process of negotiation and bargaining among competing political constituencies. Instead, by using well-developed canons of research and evidence, a procedure is legitimately developed for settlement of disputes without having to rely on negotiation.

Disputes are settled through procedures which are accepted by practicing scientists. Scientists develop hypotheses based on past research or ideas. These hypotheses are then tested and submitted for publication and subsequent examination by peers. "Validity" of new findings is based strictly on the judgment of experts working in the same field as the scientist presenting the "new research". Judgments are binary: an article is accepted or it is not; findings are valid or they are not. To the extent that there are questions, they are not settled through a process of negotiation; instead, new evidence is sought to clarify any ambiguity. Scientists characterize this process as a "rational one".

In a polity, the process employed for reaching a decision is different, and can be accurately characterized as one which maximizes the interests of each group with a stake in the ultimate outcome. Thus, when science enters the political arena, it is not necessarily a unique or unusual event from the perspective of policy or the political process. It is, however, a unique and often "shaking" experience for scientists who are accustomed to different rules and procedures for reaching rational decisions which are thought of as having withstood the tests of judging evidence and feasibility. Most of the time scientists must play by political rules. For example, in the controversy over recombinant DNA research, scientists had to appear before community-planning groups and city councils to justify their views. Similarly, laetrile proponents argued their respective cases in public debates, often to full legislative sessions and television cameras. The issue of public accessibility to generic drugs has been argued by numerous consumer groups intent on getting their complaints across to the largest constituencies possible. All this activity has been performed in the name of the "public interest".

Although scientific bodies have also taken up these disputes, their decisions have not governed the procedures for deciding upon these questions in the political arena. It would be unfair, however, to say that science has not had a major role in helping to define how political problems are addressed.[4] Critical issues in the realm of science usually are not resolved by elected officials; rather, they are assigned to regulatory or judicial bodies for resolution. The courts are then put in the position of having to balance strongly-held convictions and competing sets of values. In cases like the one involving he laetrile controversy, the circuit courts have often acted in contradictory ways, even to the point of passing the buck to the Supreme Court. In turn the Supreme Court has tried to select a narrow issue or technical area of law on which to base its decision, utilizing none of the official channels to set a consistent policy.

The courts are clearly uncomfortable in being the final arbitrators in these kinds of cases. This prompts a question: Should the courts be in the business of formulating science policy? ([7], p. 95–96) There is the alternative view that one policy is not more scientific than another policy merely because it deals with issues of science. Some policies have scientific and technical subject matter, but the policies are merely one among others of a country's general policy [9].

II. MODELS OF RESPONSIBLE BEHAVIOR

In settling any public policy controversy, a number of questions must be considered. It is essential to determine first just who the stakeholders are and to whom they are accountable. Next in importance is the question of the appropriate and proper function for a political executive. What actually is the function of a bureaucracy? Should it have a direct role in the policymaking process through implementation or should it simply be the administrative apparatus for the executive? What is the appropriate and proper role for scientists?

These questions are at the heart of a debate between two famous political scientists, Herman Finer and Carl Friedrich ([1], [2]). The debate is over the "political" versus "technical responsibility" of public officials. These same concepts can be appealed to when making judgments about scientists acting in the public arena. Both scholars have defined their own ultimate standard or ideal type of responsibility.

Finer argues that the ultimate standard of what administrative actions are acceptable in a democratic soceity is quite simple: those that are consistent with the legislative intent or mandate of elected representatives [1]. Political executives (governors, presidents, and legislators) are elected by the people; they are expected to be "protectors of the public interest". The actions of these executives can be challenged in court; this is a sufficient "check and balance" on their priorities.

Friedrich, on the other hand, contends that these principles are necessary, but not sufficient conditions for responsibility [2]. He believes that the responsible official is one who emphasizes two dominant factors: technical knowledge and popular sentiment.[5]

According to Friedrich, when modern society is faced with decisions that require increasingly sophisticated knowledge and expertise, it needs to be able to rely on experts to specify the right solution. Clearly, this reliance on expertise is limited to decisions where it can be appropriately applied. Experts should be responsible and have the authority to set policy for issues that require professional and technical decisions. Friedrich labels this *technical responsibility* and contends that it protects the public good

> . . . whether we call it "objective" or "functional" or "technical", the fact remains that throughout the length and breadth of our technical civilization there is arising a type of responsibility on the part of the permanent administrator, the man who is called upon to seek and find the creative solutions for our crying technical needs, which cannot be effectively enforced except by fellow-technicians who are capable of judging his policy in terms of the scientific knowledge bearing upon it. Nature's laws are always enforced, and a public policy which neglects them is bound to come to grief, no matter how eloquently it may be advocated by popular orators, eager partisans, or smart careerists ([2], pp. 13–14).

It is often the case in health-related controversies that neither of these pure types really operates. Instead, a kind of "hybrid" model emerges in which proponents argue that decisions are made to protect the public, when in fact elected officials take one set of actions in the policymaking process through passing legislation, but then ultimately take another set of actions through the implementation process. Bureaucrats and scientists are often relied upon to *modify* or *contradict* the legislative intent through the writing of regulations that will be consistent with the available scientific evidence.

In Finer's terms, a weaker form of "political responsibility" could manifest itself if elected officials *consciously decided* to allow the technicians/bureaucrats to set official policy through regulations. If the will of the scientists and technicians is *consciously acquiesced to*, it can be argued that elected officials give active approval to this form and style of policymaking. Alternatively, legislators may demur to the will of the technicians by default or without articulating any contrary position.

Hence, it is appropriate to think of "political responsibility" as being based on the formal and informal actions of elected officials in the name of the public. Technical responsibility is based on scientific standards. Bureaucrats with expertise in a particular substantive area are balancing the best available scientific knowledge with the public's wishes as articulated through their elected officials. In health-related controversies, the two different kinds of responsibilities are mixed.

The Generic Drug Controversy

A number of years ago, consumer advocates and public interest groups became concerned about the staggering costs of pharmaceutical products. The major drug companies were accused of monopolizing the market, thus forcing consumers to pay higher prices than necessary. (This controversy actually has proven to be part of a more general controversy over the rising costs of medical care.) Some groups felt that American consumers would save hundreds of millions of dollars if physicians and pharmacists were encouraged, or even forced, to engage in the practice of generic substitution of brand-name drugs.

Consumer groups tried to examine and hypothesize about the prescribing behavior of physicians. The general consensus was that physicians were greatly influenced by the promotional activities of drug manufacturers. Many people subscribed to the "iron triangle" view of the relationship among physicians, drug companies, and pharmacists, all concerned with promoting each others' profits. Physicians were accused of not using their professional judgment in their prescribing behavior.

The Scientific Evidence

The original debate over generic substitution focused primarily on consumer-related issues: cost savings, informing patients as to the interchangeability of products, and breaking up the iron triangle [7]. Consumer groups seemed almost as a matter of faith to believe that generic substitution was the answer to problems in medical care.

In an attempt to resolve the issue of generic substitution of drug products in the midst of a lively controversy, the Congressional Office of Technology Assessment (OTA) assembled a study panel in 1974 to examine the relationships between the chemical and therapeutic equivalence of drug products and their generic substitutes. This panel was asked to assess the capability of the current technology (short of actual therapeutic testing on humans) to determine whether drug products with the same chemical and physical composition could produce comparable therapeutic effects [7].

In concluding their investigation, the OTA panel noted some serious scientific concerns about *bio-equivalency, bio-availability*, and *therapeutic equivalency.*[6] The final report submitted to Congress recommended that methods be developed to insure uniform and quality bio-availability and bio-equivalency. Quality control and good manufacturing procedures were seen as essential in meeting these goals and the report called for a distinction to be made between drugs for which there are no bio-equivalency problems and those for which there may be. Finally, the panel urged that when the technology was in place, both federal and state governments should begin to develop a listing of interchangeable products.[7]

The OTA report represents the scientific state of the art at the time, and it is significant that it raised serious scientific questions concerning the interchangeability of drug products. Since that report was made public, about forty-six states have enacted drug product selection laws, which have effectively cancelled out earlier anti-substitution legislation. The new selection activities permitted by law vary greatly among states and are restricted to the use of specific drugs to be administered under conditions dictated by physicians. (In some states, however, consumers could demand generic substitution even if the physician thought it unwise. Thus in some states, the ability to substitute is quite broad.) Many states have prepared "formularies" as guides to the pharmacists regarding product selection. Given the fact that in testimony before the Senate, OTA panel members suggested that it may take ten to twenty years to develop appropriate technologies and formularies, one wonders about the basis for proceeding so quickly with current policies in this area. In this context, scientists would want to assess one critical question: Are substitutes for brand-name products indeed the same? ("Sameness" breaks down into two important components: therapeutic equivalency/bio-equivalency on the one hand and bio-availability on the other.)

The Food and Drug Administration has been called upon to provide a perspective. In an official publication entitled "Generic Drugs: How Good Are They?", Annabel Hecht starts off by asking:

> Are generic drugs as good as brand-name products?
>
> The answer to that frequently asked question is, for the most part, "yes" according to the Food and Drug Administration. As FDA Commissioner Donald Kennedy has said, "There simply is no evidence to support the notion of serious quality differences between generic and brand name drugs."

> The differences are largely semantic. All drugs have a generic name, also called the "official" or "nonproprietary" name . . . .
>
> Certain drugs have shown inconsistencies in their absorption rate or in how long they remain in the bloodstream. For example, tests may have shown that different batches of the same durg made by the same manufacturer have differed in their absorption rate. In other instances, a drug made by one manufacturer may have shown a different absorption rate than the same drug made by another manufacturer. When this occurs, the drug is said to have "bioequivalence" problems, which means that there has been difficulty in assuring that different batches of the drug will always behave in the body in the same way . . . .
>
> As the public and the medical, pharmacy, and other health professions gain more understanding of the quality assurance programs enforced by FDA, generic prescribing and purchasing is likely to increase. The result should be lower cost, but equal quality health care ([4], pp. 17–20).

The FDA notes that some drugs pose bio-equivalency problems and that this is a cause for concern. The FDA policy statement is interesting especially because the official position is that there is no evidence to support the notion of serious quality differences. However, the FDA notes that for the most part there are no bio-equivalency problems.

Current State of the Scientific Evidence

In an interview Kenneth Melmon, one of the leading pharmacists on the OTA panel, suggested:

> The science or the information related to drugs has not changed at all [since the 1974 OTA study], so you are still in the same situation you were when you knew that a few drugs are very important in terms of the bio-availability that related to non-generic products and you know that most drugs probably could be given the generic substitution, but the problem is that you don't know which ones those most are and the data that relate to the bio-availability of those drugs is not good data to make the decisions on, and the politics of the circumstance was to make the decision without the data . . . [8].

A review of the current literature and a series of intensive follow-up interviews with OTA panel members show that there are serious and significant problems with the practice of interchanging drug products:

(a) viable testing procedures to determine bio-availability and bio-equivalency have not been significantly improved;

(b) testing procedures have been particularly poor for those drugs involving potential or real problems;

(c) inadequate information has been submitted to the FDA for drug clearance;

(d) bio-equivalency and bio-availability data testing standards are established on "normal, healthy males", a procedure that does not account for significant differences among women, children and elderly.[8]

What is most striking in reviewing this case is an apparent difference between the judgment of scientists in their role as scientists and the judgment of policy-makers on the one hand, and the judgment of scientists when acting as policymaking advisors on the other. It seems that scientists and non-scientists believe in the concept of substitution based on a non-scientific, normative judgment: for the vast majority of drugs "there appears to be no problem." Reading scientific journals and conducting a series of intensive interviews nevertheless reveals that scientists are quite concerned with a variety of serious and critical problems still facing researchers and the public with respect to formulating a list of interchangeable drug products.

Based on the evidence collected in studying this case, it seems that political pressure has had a major effect in influencing the policy decisions concerning generic substitution. It is striking that political considerations seemed to be foremost in the minds of all interested parties, including the scientists who were asked to give advice based on their scientific expertise. Scientists may inadvertently have based their judgment on normative considerations such as strong ideological beliefs, while still maintaining that they were providing unbiased, technical judgment. (In this case, the line dividing science from politics is very thin.)

With regard to generic substitution of drug products, it seems that although some scientists readily accept substitution, their numerous scientific reservations have become obscured by their enthusiasm for the concept of substitution. Clearly, political and ideological considerations have taken precedence over scientific evidence. This kind of decision-making represents what might be expected from politicians and consumer-advocates, but not from scientists. It is not that political and economic considerations are inappropriate in making policy concerning health care. Rather, it is unfortunate that medical and technical considerations are given low priority in the formulation of some types of health care policy. In the case of generic substitution, it seems wise that the public should be informed of the medical costs and benefits of their choice. It is clear that from the consumer-advocate's point of view and from the FDA's point of view that the public interest is being served. From a medical practitioner's point of view, however, one might ask whether the public's health and safety is being adequately protected.

The case for and against generic substitution is thus an excellent one for contrasting professional and consumer perspectives on responsibility in medical care. In examining the facts of this case, one is tempted to reflect on the fact that physicians are also medical practitioners who have (and should have) as their primary responsibility concern for the therapeutic effectiveness of the treatment provided to their patients – including generic drugs. The effectiveness of pharmaceutical products is part of the responsibility and accountability of practitioners; the preferences of consumers and advocate groups cannot be the criteria that are relied upon exclusively.

The Laetrile Case

The laetrile controversy actually is a debate about several different issues:

(a) whether laetrile should be publicly available;
(b) whether it should be available to terminally ill patients;
(c) whether the government (in the form of the FDA has the right to ban laetrile from the market;
(d) whether the government has a right to intervene in the process of free choice.

There has been little debate, however, over the efficacy and safety of laetrile itself. Not even the proponents of laetrile make any claims for its efficacy. Some claim that it is safe. In this case, *all of the scientific evidence* points to the fact that laetrile is in no way effective in treating cancer, but some significant scientific evidence suggests that it is unsafe in that it causes cyanide poisoning.

The laetrile controversy can only be understood as part of an overall political process. This political process is one that has been dramatized in attempts to legalize laetrile in forty-six states, to repeal the 1962 amendments to the Food, Drug, and Cosmetic Act, and to amend drug testing procedures so that laetrile can be tested.

The proponents of laetrile have used the political process to its best advantage and consequently have been largely successful in their drive for nationwide legalization. Twenty-five states have legalized the drug for sale in intra-state commerce. Laetrile is currently being tested on humans – an unprecedented step that breaks all FDA traditions in terms of clinical trials. The FDA has been pushed into the position of feeling that it must attempt to "resolve" the laetrile issue, *even though there is not a shred of scientific evidence that points to its effectiveness.*[9] This is evidently a case in which the scientific evidence has not played a significant role in the overall political process. It is interesting to point out that the FDA has tested what has been called "laetrile" over thirty times and found thirty different chemical formulations. The FDA is particularly concerned because cancer patients forego what is known to be effective treatment in place of what they feel is a "quack cure".

III. CONCLUSION

This essay has contrasted different conceptions of responsibility and accountability in health care. In particular, the traditional model of physician accountability has been differentiated from a "corporate" perspective on accountability. Conceptions of responsibility and accountability are particularly appropriate in examining how controversies are resolved. In this essay I have attempted to illustrate the effects of allowing social and political considerations to provide the primary (if not the sole) basis for resolving controversies and making decisions in health-related matters. There appears to be a growing number of cases in which public policies and decisions reflect deliberate non-utilization of the available scientific evidence. This fact raises great concern as to whether the public health and safety is being protected adequately and whether the public interest actually is being served.

Princeton University

NOTES

[1] This quotation is from an interview Senator Symms granted to *United States News and World Report* in the issue dated June 13, 1977, pp. 51–52.

[2] [7]. In this context, it is also noteworthy to realize that controversies can be settled at either a *micro-level* or *macro-level*. Controversy in *micro-level* disputes may be centered on particular procedures or rules. They may also be over a specific case of a more general principle (for example, should laetrile be given to a specific terminal patient?). The mechanisms outlined above are well-suited to settling these *micro-level* types of disputes.

Macro-level disputes involve much broader questions concerning many competing interests. In order to negotiate a settlement for this type of dispute (for example, a policy for dispensing or not dispensing laetrile to the public as a whole), an agreement would have to be reached which could leave several significant questions unanswered. For example, when the Carter Administration formulated its health insurance program, it realized that in order to negotiate a settlement within Congress, certain questions would have to be excluded from the formal legislation.

[3] As matters now stand, public officials are left to rely largely upon intuition and *ad*

hoc procedures. Politicians, especially legislators, have been reluctant to choose between the consequences of the "Faustian" bargains facing them: between gaining a competitive edge in international trade and limiting the mobility of citizens who do not believe that there is a "true energy crisis"; between producing a potentially valuable source of energy (nuclear) and unknown but potentially serious risks to the environment; between increasing the speed with which American manufacturers produce a highly efficient engine and easing the pressure on meeting environmental standards; between increasing the speed with which the oil pipeline between California and Texas is completed and meeting local safety and environmental standards.

4 Jerome Weisner, for example, points out that the "state-of-the-art" within a scientific discipline can and does affect policy making. If the Secretary of Defense knows that a weapon system is being developed, it will potentially affect arms control negotiations ([6], p. 31). U. S. interests and future investments in hard technology are affected by knowledge which can be assumed at the time a decision is made.

5 Norton Long underscores this perspective when he writes:

The doctrine of the political supremacy of the elected over the non-elected branch of government has inspired the delusion that to be politically supreme the legislature must not only make final decisions on policy but also must have primacy in the whole process of policy formulation. The bureaucracy should be an instrument and not a brain. The necessities of the case have forced the abandonment of this view save as folklore and political metaphysics. In practice it must be recognized that the bureaucracy is a part, and a highly important part, of the collective brain that somehow thinks or emotes a government policy ([5], p. 29).

6 These are the technical terms used to describe official testing procedures. *Bio-availability* simply refers to the fact that the same ingredients are being used in a drug; *bio-equivalency* refers to the fact that drugs have the same chemical content and that the ingredients interact with each other in the same way; *therapeutic equivalency* refers to the fact that different drugs have the same effect on a given patient.

7 The OTA panel was very concerned with the state of current technology and the scientific basis on which to develop lists of interchangeable drug products. One panel member summarized the views of his colleagues in a recent interview by saying: "I think they were very good recommendations because they really studied the subject and the meanings were very pointed in frank outright discussions. I think we did what we could in the time that we had and, in retrospect, I don't see anything we said, even with the critiques that were made on my report, that invalidates any point we made." This study was a follow-up on the findings of the OTA panel. The results of this study are soon to be published [6].

8 One of the former OTA panel members who felt that the scientific problems were so serious pointed out that the only thing that was really protecting the public was biology itself: "Oh, I think biology protects them [the public] from any kind of political move; we're just basically meant to survive and it is very hard to insult biology with drugs and so that is what is protecting the public; the public is protecting itself" [8].

9 This position is made clear in testimony by the FDA before state legislatures and in the official publications of the FDA. It is also interesting to note that proponents do not base their arguments on scientific evidence.

BIBLIOGRAPHY

1. Finer, H.: 1941, 'Administrative Responsibility in Democratic Government', *Public Administration Review* **1**, 335–350.
2. Friedrich, C. J.: 1940, 'Public Policy and the Nature of Administrative Responsibility', in C. J. Friedrich and E. S. Mason (eds.), *Public Policy*, Harvard University Press, Cambridge, pp. 3–24.
3. Havender, W. R.: 1979, 'Rumination on a Rat: Saccharin and Human Risk', *Regulation* **3**, 17–24.
4. Hecht, A.: 1978, 'Generic Drugs: How Good Are They?', *FDA Consumer* **12**, 17–20.
5. Long, N. E.: 1954, 'Public Policy and Administration', *Public Administration Review* **15**, 22–31.
6. Rich, R. F.: 1981, 'Knowledge in Society', in R. F. Rich (ed.), *The Knowledge Cycle*, Sage Publications, Beverly Hills, California, pp. 11–39.
7. Rich, R. F.: 1981, 'The Political Implications of Laetrile: Who Gets What, When and How', in G. E. Markel and J. C. Peterson (eds.), *Politics, Science, and Cancer: The Laetrile Phenomenon*, AAAS Selected Symposium Series, Westview Press, Boulder, Colorado, pp. 73–97.
8. Rich, R. F. and Schwartz, L.: 'Resolving Political Controversies: Are All Drug Products the Same?' (unpublished manuscript).
9. Saloman, J. J.: 1974, *Science and Politics*, MIT Press, Cambridge.
10. Snow, C. P.: 1962, *Science and Government* (Harvard University Godkin Lectures), New American Library, New York.

BRUCE L. MILLER

RESPONSIBILITY AND PUBLIC POLICY IN HEALTH CARE: COMMENTARY ON ESSAYS BY WILLIAMS AND RICH

The many nuances of the idea of responsibility in health care are evident in the essays in this volume. When issues of public policy are added to responsibility and health care, the problems engendered by their inclusion become staggeringly complex. To eliminate some of this complexity, a few preliminary definitions and distinctions seem in order.

I. RESPONSIBILITY

The term *responsibility* does not have one central usage upon which all other usages can rest; rather, there are four senses of *responsibility* ([3], pp. 211–230). *Role responsibility* is the idea of a set of specific responsibilities (obligations or duties) which are attached to a distinctive position, role, or office within a social organization. The idea of a role in this case is more vague than the sociological notion of role, because it includes temporary tasks assigned to a person as well as the more enduring role of fatherhood, etc. Role responsibilities are provided in answer to the question: What are the responsibilities of an "X" where X can have as substitution instances such things as lawyer, teacher, parent, patient, nurse, and physician? Role responsibility is used in a commendatory sense with the statement that "Jones is a responsible person" (in the sense of teacher, neighbor, etc.) – the implication being that Jones takes his role responsibilities seriously and nearly always fulfills them.

Liability responsibility is the sense of responsibility used in legal and moral contexts to assert that someone is, or should be, held responsible for some harm to another. In the standard cases of liability responsibility, two conditions must be met: first, the actor must have some causal connection with the harm of another; and second, the actor must have acted in some faulty manner. There are two ways, then, to escape liability responsibility: to argue that one was not causally involved (or only in an incidental manner) and to claim that though one was causally involved, the conduct which caused the harm was not a failure to meet the standard appropriate to the situation (for instance, that it was unavoidable, an honest mistake, or not negligent). The standards for fault are often set by role responsibilities. For example, whether a physician can be held responsible for the harm suffered by a patient – harm

George J. Agich (ed.), Responsibility in Health Care, 261–275.
Copyright © 1982 *by D. Reidel Publishing Company, Dordrecht, Holland.*

caused by medical treatment – depends on whether the physician fulfilled his role responsibilities, that is, the specific responsibilities of a competent physician.

Causal responsibility is often confused with liability responsibility. When it is said that some human act or omission, or some event or condition, is responsible for some harm, sometimes we only mean that the act, omission, event, or condition caused the harm. These two senses of responsibility are run together because "responsible for" may be used in place of "caused" when the result is harmful or in some way unfortunate and the causation is an element of liability responsibility. These are distinct uses in common parlance. One can say that the administration's monetary policies are responsible for (caused) the increased inflation without at all meaning that the administration should be blamed or held responsible (liable) for the unhappy result.

Capacity responsibility is that sense of responsibility used to assert or deny that a person has the appropriate level of understanding, reasoning, or control over some area of conduct. A statement such as "Smith is not responsible for what he does" implies that Smith lacks the capacity to act otherwise, and indicates that he should not be assigned (role) responsibilities or be held responsible (liability) for what he does. "Responsible" and "not responsible" in this sense are roughly equivalent to "competent" and "not competent". Capacity responsibility is an important notion, but it is not central to the discussion of responsibility and public policy which follows. Rather, it is the role responsibility of policy-makers which is of most importance to Robert Rich's essay, "Reaching Closure on Health-Related Controversies," and the liability responsibility and causal responsibility of physicians which is the focus of Peter Williams's essay, "Legal Responsibility in Health Care."

There are several additional distinctions of importance. The first distinction is between a concept of responsibility and the objects of responsibility. The rough account given earlier of liability responsibility as requiring the faulty performance of an action that is causally connected with a harm explains the concept of liability responsibility but does not relate the things for which an individual should be held responsible. The criminal law employs a concept of liability responsibility similar to the one explained here, but the criminal law also includes a set of rules which specifies the things for which a person will be held liable. Specifying the objects of liability responsibility requires specifying kinds of harms, kinds of casual connections, and ways of acting faultily.

The second distinction is between the descriptive and normative use of concepts of responsibility. There is a difference between what the responsibilities of a given role are and what they ought to be. The laws and customs of our society do not place much responsibility upon one citizen to benefit another, absent the existence of some special relationship. It can be argued that social norms ought to recognize a higher degree of responsibility to benefit others. Similarly, what law and custom in fact hold an individual responsible for and what they ought to hold an individual responsible for in the sense of liability responsibility are different. Under current law, physicians are held responsible only for those harms which they negligently cause patients in the course of treatment. Williams argues that physicians ought to be held strictly liable, independent of negligence or any other sort of fault.

Discussion of role and liability responsibility in the descriptive and normative senses must appeal to rules or other sorts of standards. Rules and standards comprise a practice if there is general observance of them. That is to say, they are complied with and regarded as reasons for acting. A practice is possible if there is a set of values shared by nearly everyone, and if nearly everyone believes that complying with the rules will realize or promote these shared values. A descriptive analysis of role or liability responsibility must state the existing rules and other standards and determine what values they serve. A normative position about role or liability responsibility must state what the rules and standards should be and defend them by showing which values they serve. Often, the argument which emerges is that some set of rules better serves a shared set of values than the existing rules.

II. PUBLIC POLICY

Public policy is the set of rules established by legislatures, executives, administrative agencies, and courts which establishes patterns of rights, liberties, privileges, and benefits on the one hand and responsibilities, obligations, and burdens on the other. For example, the Medicare and Medicaid programs are two of the most significant pieces of public policy regarding health care. These programs established the legal right to government-financed health care for certain classes of citizens. In so doing, they imposed a tax burden on all citizens and created responsibilities for various government agencies and private institutions. In the past, destitute citizens could only seek medical care and hope that someone or some institution would provide needed care in recognition of an obligation to be charitable. Now these same citizens can demand medical care as a right. Medicare and Medicaid are thus dramatic examples of public policy creating new patterns of rights and responsibilities. On most occasions public policy does not work in such a large-scale manner to alter rights and responsibilities. Often, public policy expands or limits an existing pattern of rights and obligations. Another way that public policy affects rights and responsibilities is to provide mechanisms for seeking redress of existing rights.

The public policy issue in Rich's essay about generic substitution involves the scope of the existing right of patient autonomy. A person has the right to seek or not seek medical treatment, the right to accept or refuse medical treatment, and the right to comply or not comply with a physician's orders. Prior to the enactment of many state laws permitting generic substitution, a person did not have the specific right to determine whether he would use a trade name drug or a generic substitute. For this right to be brought within a person's general right to autonomy in medical care, existing laws which required that prescriptions be filled as a physician wrote them had to be changed. As a result, when patients gained a right to substitute, physicians lost some authority.

A second issue of public policy in Rich's paper is what the responsibility of lawmakers should be in regard to policy in health-related matters. Must public policy be consistent with scientific evidence? Who has the responsibility for policy in health-related areas and what are the standards for carrying out the responsibility? Should scientists decide questions of policy on scientific grounds? Or should politicians decide on political grounds? What is the relationship between political grounds and scientific grounds? These are questions about role responsibility.

The issue of public policy which concerns Williams involves mechanisms for compensation of persons who are injured in the course of medical treatment. A patient has the right to competent medical treatment and a physician has the correlative obligation to provide it. What mechanisms for redress should be available to a patient when incompetent treatment results in the patient's injury? For what injuries to patients should physicians be held liable? What are the general grounds for a claim of liability? By what values or objectives should the standards of liability be judged?

These are questions about liability responsibility which clearly have implications for the role responsibility of physicians. New standards of liability can have a direct effect on role responsibility. When the doctrine of informed consent replaced the doctrine of consent, physicians gained a new responsibility to inform their patients of the risks of, and alternatives to, proposed treatments, in addition to informing them of what treatment was proposed and obtaining their voluntary permission. An alteration of rules concerning liability may have an indirect effect on physicians' role responsibility. If rules of procedure for malpractice suits were made more favorable to the patient/plaintiff (thereby increasing the likelihood of successful suits against physicians), no new role responsibilities would be imposed on physicians, but the change might affect the way in which physicians carry out responsibilities (that is, more carefully or defensively). Williams's proposal that the liability of physicians for "medical maloccurrences" should be strict liability rather than liability based on fault will not establish new responsibilities for physicians, but could have significant impact on how they carry out their responsibilities.

III. ROLE RESPONSIBILITY AND PUBLIC POLICY

There are two issues concerning role responsibility in Rich's essay. One of them is whether generic substitution should be allowed. This is a question about rights and responsibilities in the physician/patient relationship. It is not, however, the issue about which Rich is most concerned – his main concern is with another and more general issue: How should issues of public policy on subjects with a scientific, health-related content be resolved? The specific questions here are: Who should be responsible for making public policy on scientific and health-related matters and how should that responsibility be carried out? Rich sketches two alternative positions.

One of them is the position Rich attributes to Carl Friedrich and calls "technical responsibility". The main tenets of this position are that experts should set policy on matters involving significant scientific content and that a responsible official should defer to the superior knowledge of the expert. The other view is that of Herman Finer and is characterized as "political responsibility". On this view, elected officials should set policy through the political process and experts should be the instruments of the political process – that is, they should carry out the policy set by elected officials. Rich's account of how closure is reached on scientific disputes is appropriate to "technical responsibility" and his account of reaching closure on political disputes is appropriate to "political responsibility".

Rich's own position in this controversy is not easy to discern. On the one hand, he puts forward the descriptive claim that the way in which disputes in health-related matters in fact are resolved is through a mixture of technical and political responsibility. On the other hand, he seems to put forward the normative thesis that policy makers should enact policy on health-related matters consistent with scientific evidence. A specific instance is his view that the policy which permits generic substitution by a patient is inconsistent with the scientific evidence and should not have been enacted.

There are several problems with this position, and they are of such magnitude that they can only be discussed briefly. First, a policy allowing a person to substitute generic drug A for a prescribed trade name drug B cannot be inconsistent with scientific evidence. Suppose the evidence shows that A and B are not bio-equivalent. That is simply a matter of fact; the policy, however, asserts a right. A statement of scientific fact cannot by itself contradict a statement of what rights a person has. It would be inconsistent if it were assumed that a necessary ground for the right is that A and B are bio-equivalent. This brings up a second problem in Rich's position. There are two distinct situations with regard to evidence relating to the bio-equivalence of two drugs that must be considered. It may be the case that there is no evidence from adequate testing procedures to determine that a trade name drug and its generic counterpart are bio-equivalent. Another situation is that there is no evidence that two drugs are not bio-equivalent.

The crucial issue Rich ignores is which sort of evidence is required to justify the patient's right to substitute. Must it be conclusively shown that two drugs are bio-equivalent, or is it enough that for two drugs with the same chemical composition there is no evidence that they are not bio-equivalent? Rich seems to demand that the first alternative be operative, and thus a policy which allows substitution without evidence of their bio-equivalence is irresponsible. He would regard the second alternative as the political resolution of the issue, and to be rejected in favor of the first, and scientific, resolution. The problem with this view is that neither is more scientific than the other and both embody scientific statements of what the available evidence does or does not show. Thus, some argument is needed as to why one should be preferred over the other, independent of scientific evidence.

This brings up a third problem Rich ignores: What ought to be the grounds for the State to prevent a citizen from making choices regarding his health care? It can be argued that not allowing generic substitution protects the profits of the drug companies who invest millions in research on new drugs. Generic substitution may cut profits and thus be a disincentive to drug research. However, this is not an approach Rich pursues. His position seems one of paternalism – protection of citizens from their own ignorant or ill-considered decisions. Paternalistic interferences run counter to the libertarian traditions in our society, to be sure, but they are not always unjustified. A plausible approach to justification is to argue that there are certain things which every reasonable person wants no matter what else he might want; a policy which would prevent a person from pursuing courses of action which would remove or interfere with these things is a justified interference.

Specifically, every reasonable person wishes to maintain and restore health and therefore wishes to do those things which will realize that objective. In some areas of life, the ordinary reasonable person is not able to judge whether a given option will in fact realize the objective of restoring health; it requires expert knowledge to know the effects of alternatives offered in the marketplace. This justifies both the licensing of physicians and the regulations of the FDA. They limit the treatments available in the marketplace to those which experts have judged not to run counter to the public's interest in health. When a consumer makes choices in the medical marketplace, he thus can be reasonably assured that his choices will not thwart his objective. Can this approach justify Rich's view on generic substitution and his general position that policy on health-related matters ought to be consistent with scientific evidence? Neither question is easy to answer. The question of generic substitution would require returning to the problem of what kind of evidence is required to justify not allowing generic substitution. On the more general point, however, Rich would have to provide a much more detailed account of how scientific evidence can have implications for public policy on health-related matters. Until these analyses are provided, Rich's position is an interesting, but unsupported, possibility.

IV. PHYSICIAN LIABILITY AND PUBLIC POLICY

I am sympathetic to Williams's preference for a system of strict liability over the current system of fault liability for medical maloccurrences. There are, however, matters of importance in which I disagree with Williams – in particular, with some of his arguments concerning the goals of a liability system. In addition, there are important issues which he does not consider but which are central to his main concern.

Under the current system of assigning liability for medical maloccurrences, the patient/plaintiff must be ready to bring a case of negligence against the physician/defendant. The tort of negligence has four elements. The plaintiff must show that (a) a standard of care (b) was breeched by the defendant (c) which caused (d) damages to the plaintiff. The first and second elements are what make this a system of *fault* liability; to breech a standard of care is to be at fault, and so the tort of negligence is in conformity with the principle that there shall be no liability without fault. This system of fault liability is backed up by two insurance systems. Physicians carry liability insurance which will pay damages to patients. The costs of this insurance are passed on to the consumers of medical care through the fees physicians charge for their services. The second insurance system is the insurance which patients have. For medical services covered by the patient's insurance, the costs of the physician's liability insurance are passed to the patient's medical insurance. The net effect is a distribution of the costs of medical maloccurrences to the users of medical services. When medical services are covered by Medicare and Medicaid, the costs are distributed to the taxpayers.

Williams's proposal of a system of strict or no-fault liability eliminates the first two elements of fault liability. A patient would only have to show that the physician caused damages to the patient. There would be no inquiry into whether a standard of care had been breeched, either by the patient to plead for recovery or by the physician to plead against recovery. Williams compares the system to a workmen's compensation system, so I presume that physicians would pay into a central fund and awards to patients would be made by an administrative procedure or a hearing board. Whatever the method, the costs would be passed on to the users of medical services through the fees charged for the services; the distribution of costs would not be any different from the system of fault liability.

Williams says that the goals of tort liability in general and medical maloccurrence in particular are prevention, compensation, retribution, and administrative efficiency. The only quarrel I have with this contention is that he runs together two distinct ideas under the heading of compensation. On the one hand, there is the notion of giving something to the victim because of the injury or wrong done. In some cases the transfer can restore the victim to the state he would be in if the wrong had not been done – for example, by returning an object rightfully belonging to the victim or by paying monies of which the victim was wrongfully deprived. In a situation involving physical injury, it may not be possible to restore the victim, in which case the victim can be compensated only by money for the injury. Whatever the situation, the injured party is owed something because of losses incurred. In medical maloccurrences the idea of reparation, return to the *status quo ante*, is not usually possible; instead, the patient can only be compensated for the injury. Reparation and compensation are part of the idea of justice. A person who is an innocent victim has a claim on others such that he should not be made to suffer the loss.

The second aspect of compensation discussed by Williams is very different. He asks the following question:

Is it less expensive to let victims of medical accidents pay for their own injuries; or to make the parties causing the injury bear those costs; or to pick another mode of payment, such as social insurance, to spread the burdens over time or across groups of people? (p. 231)

This is a question about the costs of accidents. As such, it is distinct from the question about compensatory justice. Conceivably, the least costly way of paying for accidents would be to let victims pay for their own injuries, but this alternative runs counter to the idea of compensatory justice. Compensatory justice and considerations of cost efficiency are compatible only when the overriding concern is compensating victims in the least costly way. This is the issue with which Williams is concerned; he does not entertain the approach of letting the costs of accidents fall on the victims of accidents.

Williams's reasons for preferring a system of strict liability can be stated briefly. In terms of prevention: strict liability will be no worse than fault liability in reducing the incidence and severity of medical maloccurrences. In terms of administrative efficiency: strict liability will be much less expensive to administer than fault liability. In terms of compensation: more victims will be compensated under strict liability than under a fault liability system. I agree with Williams on all three of these claims, but it is important to note that they are empirical claims, and that there is little direct evidence to support them. There is, however, a good deal of indirect evidence from those areas of law wherein strict liability has replaced negligence law (for example, in workmen's compensation and no-fault automobile accident insurance). Arguments can also be based on general knowledge about different institutional arrangements. Williams, however, says nothing about the costs of compensation for a system of strict liability compared with a system of fault liability.

If more victims will be compensated, the total costs of compensation will be increased, though the average costs could be lessened. If less money is spent on administrative costs, more might be used for compensation. A reduction in very large awards might come about under a no-fault system, but they are probably so few that it would not have a significant effect on total costs. A great deal of analysis and evidence from other areas of law where strict liability has replaced negligence law would be required to address these concerns. The only comment Williams make about retribution is that it is playing a decreasing role in tort liability. It thus seems appropriate to consider more fully than Williams does the questions about retributive and compensatory justice regarding strict liability.

Consider the following simple situation: physician X negligently performs a surgical procedure on patient Y, and as a result, Y is seriously injured. X is a wrongdoer and Y is an innocent victim. Retributive justice requires that X be penalized for his wrongful conduct. Compensatory justice requires that Y be compensated for his injury; Y should not have to bear the costs himself.

A system of *fault liability* can realize both objectives. If a court determined that X breeched a standard of care, thereby causing damages to Y, it could order that X compensate Y for his damages; as a result X would be penalized (retributive justice) and Y would be compensated (compensatory justice). If X has liability insurance, X is not *directly* penalized, and though Y is compensated, he is not compensated by X.

If there is a system of *strict liability* and X has liability insurance (that is, he pays an amount into the compensation fund which is determined by his patient volume or some other factors not related to the number and severity of medical maloccurrences which befall his patients), X again is not penalized directly. Though Y is compensated, he is not compensated by X. Two questions arise from these observations: "Does retributive justice require that X compensate Y as X's penalty?" and "Does compensatory justice require that Y's compensation come from X?" In the context of medical maloccurrences, I believe the answer to both these questions is no [1].

Compensatory justice requires that innocent victims be compensated for their loss. The additional requirement that the compensation come from the wrongdoers who inflicted the loss is part of compensatory justice only in cases in which the wrongdoers benefit from causing loss to the victims. If Z cheats W in a business deal and Z thereby gains and W suffers a loss, compensatory justice requires that Z provide the compensation to W. Suppose Z promises to sell his car to W and accepts a down payment of $500 with delivery upon payment in full. Suppose that Z sells the car to S before W makes payment in full. W should be compensated – his $500 should be returned and any additional losses he sustained as a result of counting on his contract with Z. It is Z who should compensate W, not someone else. The idea of compensatory justice in a situation like this is to restore the parties to the *status quo ante* – to take away Z's wrongful gain and return W's losses. In a situation of medical maloccurrence, however, the wrongful physician does not benefit by causing damages to the patient, at least not directly – that is to say, the patient's loss is not the physician's gain. There *may* be some indirect gain to the physician such as time and money from a negligent shortcut, but that is not necessarily the case. Compensatory justice accordingly does not require that the wrongful physician compensate the wronged patient, only that *someone* compensate the wronged patient.

Whether retributive justice requires that the penalty for the wrongful physician be the compensation of the injured patient is a more difficult question. It depends on how the concept of retributive justice in a system of liability is understood. In both a fault system and a strict liability system, if there is an insurance scheme, the wrongful party is not penalized by compensating the victim, but there is an important difference between these systems. In a fault system, the physician is determined by a court to be wrongful – that is, the physician is shown to have breeched a standard of care. Even though the monetary penalty will be paid by a liability carrier, the physician still bears the "stain" of the court determination of wrongful conduct. In a strict liability system, however, this would not occur as the result of a determination that a patient should be compensated; all that is determined in this case is that the patient was injured as a result of the medical services of the physician. This situation can occur even when the physician was not at fault, where the best possible care was given to the patient.

Patient injuries, of course, can also be the result of physician negligence. Under a fault system, the latter would be compensated while the former would not; both would be compensated in a strict liability system. Williams argues that for this reason the strict liability system is more just than the fault system. It is more just in the sense of compensatory justice, but is it just from the point of view of retributive justice? If a physician who was at fault was not treated any differently than a physician who was not at fault in cases in which both caused injuries to patients, then retributive justice might not have been realized. There would not be any "stain" associated with the determination that a patient should be compensated.

What rationale can be given for "staining" wrongdoers in one system and not "staining" those who are wrongdoers in the other? Here the conception of retributive justice becomes important. On one view, wrongdoers should be stained in order to deter future wrongdoing by those individuals or by others. Blaming someone, over and above compensating victims, thus has deterrence as its prime justification. If medical maloccurrences would not be deterred by blaming any more effectively than through a system of strict liability, then the idea of retributive justice would not entail the fault system and so the system of strict liability would be acceptable. There is, however, another view of blaming (and thus of retributive justice) which has different implications.

Retributivists from Immanuel Kant [5] to Herbert Morris [6] have maintained that there is a moral value in blaming which is independent of its deterrent effect. One simplified version of this line of argument is as follows:

If we treat in the same way two persons, one of whom is a wrongdoer and the other not and both of whom cause injury to another, we are saying, in effect, to the person who was not wrongful, "Your adherence to the appropriate standards of care does not distinguish you from those who do not so adhere." The wrongful person thus can infer that his violation of the standard of care does not distinguish him from those who adhere to the standard. This inference betrays the standards which are supposedly applicable to everyone. For these reasons, this conception of retributive justice would require the fault system of assigning liability for medical maloccurrences.

There is a way around this dilemma. (It is tempting to find a way because the system of strict liability is preferable to fault liability on grounds of economic efficiency and an increase in the number of innocent victims who would be compensated.) If there were another system besides the system of strict liability, then retributive justice could be separated from compensatory justice. If the current system of professional review were strengthened so that every case of medical maloccurrence were reviewed to ascertain whether the physician's conduct was wrongful and if a penalty were attached on the basis of these findings, then the requirements of retributive justice could be met, whatever one's view of retribution. There is no reason in principle why this could not be accomplished if a strict liability system were adopted. Some practical considerations, however, raise doubts as to whether it would be effectively implemented. An alternative is an informal mechanism of retributive justice. Briefly, wrongful conduct would be found out by other physicians; physicians who have a bad record would be known by physicians in their community. The lack of collegial esteem, not to mention the lack of referrals, might be regarded as sufficient retribution, both as blame and deterrence.

There is a problem of theoretical and practical importance which must be resolved before a system of strict liability for medical maloccurrences is defensible. It is the problem of specifying the kinds of outcomes of medical treatment for which a patient will be compensated. Under the current negligence system, patients are compensated if they suffer an injury which is caused by their physicians' breech of a standard of care. Under the strict liability system, patients will be compensated if they suffer an injury which is caused by the medical treatment administered by their physicians. There will be no inquiry into fault, that is, into a breech of a standard of care. In these situations, though, how will proponents of the strict liability system distinguish between the side-effects of a medical treatment and medical maloccurrences or iatrogenic injury? Both are caused by the medical treatment; the latter results from a breech of a standard of care, the former does not. If no distinction is made, any undesirable consequence of a treatment could be compensable.

There are two reasons why it will be very difficult to drop the fault component from medical liability law. First, the concept of medical maloccurrence or iatrogenic injury contains an element of fault. The idea of injury or maloccurrence does not mean simply that the patient suffered as a result of medical treatment, but that the suffering involved a wrong done to the patient. For example, the pain of an intramuscular injection of penicillin is not an iatrogenic injury or medical maloccurrence, yet it is pain caused by medical treatment. An allergic reaction to penicillin is an iatrogenic injury if the physician failed to determine that the patient had previously received penicillin and had an allergic reaction. When the fault element of the concept of injury is revealed, the plausibility of a strict liability system that would preclude the costly inquiry into fault diminishes.

A second and related problem concerns that fault element in causation. The simple formula for negligence separates fault and causation – it appears as if the questions of whether a physician's action caused damages to a patient and whether the physician's action was negligent are two distinguishable inquiries. In any situation a number of factors make up the causal sequence determining what actually happened. Each factor is necessary for the final result, but no one of them is sufficient ([2], pp. 187–221). How is *the* cause determined? Or, to put it in the legal framework, which is the proximate cause?

When the purpose of the inquiry is to fix responsibility for the undesirable result, the inquiry is directed toward those factors which may have been due to a faulty human action. For example, a physician's failure to inquire whether a patient ever had an allergic reaction to penicillin is a more plausible candidate for the *cause* of an allergic reaction than the fact that the patient is allergic to penicillin, though administering penicillin and the biological condition of the patient are both *causal factors* for an allergic reaction. This interdependence of fault and cause shows that their separation in a strict liability system is not an easy task. How this problem should be approached depends on what the intended scope of the strict liability system is compared to the actual scope of the negligence system. Will the number and kind of maloccurrences for which patients are compensated be greater or roughly the same? Williams says that there will be more compensations under the system of strict liability. One of his arguments is that it is unjust for victims of medical maloccurrences not to be compensated where there is no fault.

In order to distinguish maloccurrences from side-effects, however, Williams will have to propose criteria which make no appeal to fault considerations. There is no indication in his essay how this could be accomplished.

Clark Havighurst and Laurence Tancredi have shown a different intention in their consideration of this problem [4]. They seem to expect that the combined strict liability and fault liability system they propose will have roughly the same scope as the current fault liability system. They propose that a list of "compensable events" be developed by physicians and others with expertise on medical maloccurrences. For items on the list, physicians would be held strictly liable. For items not on the list, patients may bring negligence actions. They discuss several examples of maloccurrences which would be on the list and propose three criteria for inclusion: avoidability, effect on quality of care, and administrative efficiency. Their discussion clearly implies that the list would be composed of those outcomes of medical treatment which are obvious instances of medical negligence (for example, a blood transfusion reaction due to an error in matching donor and recipient blood-type).

The criterion of avoidability is clearly a fault-related notion. An unavoidable outcome is not something for which a person is blamed; more importantly, avoidability is relative to the degree of care taken. The incidence of post-operative infections will vary with how careful physicians and other staff are to detect and prevent them. Suppose that a regimen of drugs would prevent all post-operative infections; such infections would therefore be avoidable and hence compensable. But suppose also that such a drug treatment would have unavoidable and serious side-effects which makes for an unfavorable risk/benefit ratio to accept the side-effects in order to prevent the infection.

"Avoidability" cannot be understood in the simple sense of "could-have-been-prevented"; it must also be taken in the broader sense of avoidability within some standard of what constitutes good medical practice. The concept of fault thus has not been eliminated. The only possible advantage of Havighurst and Tancredi's system is that administrative efficiency *may* be served by having an established list of compensable events on which the claims of patients can be readily adjudicated rather than doing so on a case-by-case method. Whether there would be a savings is a matter of speculation. It would depend on the ratio of cases resolved by the strict liability component to those resolved by the fault liability component and on whether the strict liability system would become bogged down in extensive fact-finding procedures.

Williams instead proposes that public policy on determining physician liability be changed from a system of fault liability to a system of strict liability. His arguments concerning compensatory justice, quality of care, and administrative efficiency are in this regard persuasive. However, from the foregoing discussion it should be clear that more analysis and research is needed to solve the problem of defining which medical maloccurrences the strict liability system will compensate. Until this problem is resolved, the strict liability system simply is not feasible.

Michigan State University

BIBLIOGRAPHY

1. Coleman, J.: 1975, 'Justice and the Argument for No-Fault', *Social Theory and Practice* **5**, 161–180.
2. Feinberg, J.: 1970, *Doing and Deserving*, Princeton University Press, Princeton, New Jersey.
3. Hart, H. L. A.: 1968, *Punishment and Responsibility*, Oxford University Press, New York and Oxford.
4. Havighurst, C. and Tancredi, L. R.: 1973, 'Medical Adversity Insurance – A Fault Approach to Medical Malpractice and Quality Assurance', *Milbank Memorial Fund Quarterly* **51**, 125–168.
5. Kant, I.: 1973, 'The Right to Punish', in J. G. Murphy (ed.), *Punishment and Rehabilitation*, Wadsworth, Belmont, California, pp. 35–39.
6. Morris, H.: 1973, 'Persons and Punishment', in J. G. Murphy (ed.), *Punishment and Rehabilitation*, Wadsworth, Belmont, California, pp. 40–63.

NOTES ON CONTRIBUTORS

George J. Agich, Ph.D., is Associate Professor in the Departments of Medical Humanities, Philosophy, and Psychiatry and Director of the Ethics and Philosophy of Medicine Program at Southern Illinois University School of Medicine, Springfield, Illinois.

William B. Bondeson, Ph.D., is Professor of Philosophy and Co-Director, Program in Health Care and Human Values at the University of Missouri School of Medicine, Columbia, Missouri.

Theodore M. Brown, Ph.D., is Mercer Brugler Distinguished Teaching Professor in the Departments of History and Preventive, Family and Rehabilitation Medicine at the University of Rochester, Rochester, New York.

Edmund L. Erde, Ph.D., is Associate Professor in the University of Medicine and Dentistry of New Jersey, New Jersey School of Osteopathic Medicine, Camden, New Jersey.

Richard E. Flathman, Ph.D., is Professor and Chairman of the Department of Political Science at the Johns Hopkins University, Baltimore, Maryland.

Stanley M. Hauerwas, Ph.D., is Associate Professor in the Department of Theology at Notre Dame University, Notre Dame, Indiana.

Arthur F. Kohrman, M.D., is Director of LaRabida Children's Hospital and Research Center, University of Chicago, Chicago, Illinois.

Christine Mitchell, M.S.N., is a Fellow in the Kennedy Program in Bioethics at Harvard University, Cambridge, Massachusetts.

Bruce L. Miller, Ph.D., is Professor of Philosophy and Assistant Coordinator of the Medical Humanities Program at Michigan State University, East Lansing, Michigan.

Ruth B. Purtilo, Ph.D., is Associate Professor of Health Care Ethics and Humanistic Studies at the Massachusetts General Hospital Institute of Health Professions, Boston, Massachusetts.

Robert F. Rich, Ph.D., is Assistant Professor of Politics and Public Affairs at the Woodrow Wilson School of Public and International Affairs, Princeton University, Princeton, New Jersey.

Guenter B. Risse, M.D., Ph.D., is Professor in the Department of the History of Medicine at the University of Wisconsin Center for Health Sciences, Madison, Wisconsin.

George J. Agich (ed.), Responsibility in Health Care, 277–278.
Copyright © 1982 *by D. Reidel Publishing Company, Dordrecht, Holland.*

Mark Siegler, M.D., is Associate Professor in the Department of Medicine at the University of Chicago, Chicago, Illinois.

Robert M. Veatch, Ph.D., is Professor of Medical Ethics in the Kennedy Institute of Ethics, Georgetown University, Washington, D.C.

Peter C. Williams, J.D., Ph.D., is Assistant Professor in the Departments of Philosophy and Preventive Medicine at the State University of New York at Stony Brook, Stony Brook, New York.

INDEX

The Philosophy and Medicine Book Series

Editors

H. Tristram Engelhardt, Jr. and Stuart F. Spicker

1. **Evaluation and Explanation in the Biomedical Sciences**
   1975, vi + 240 pp. ISBN 90-277-0553-4
2. **Philosophical Dimensions of the Neuro-Medical Sciences**
   1976, vi + 274 pp. ISBN 90-277-0672-7
3. **Philosophical Medical Ethics: Its Nature and Significance**
   1977, vi + 252 pp. ISBN 90-277-0772-3
4. **Mental Health: Philosophical Perspectives**
   1978, xxii + 302 pp. ISBN 90-277-0828-2
5. **Mental Illness: Law and Public Policy**
   1980, xvii + 254 pp. ISBN 90-277-1057-0
6. **Clinical Judgment. A Critical Appraisal**
   1979, xxvi + 278 pp. ISBN 90-277-0952-1
7. **Organism, Medicine, and Metaphysics**
   Essays in Honor of Hans Jonas on his 75th Birthday, May 10, 1978
   1978, xxvii + 330 pp. ISBN 90-277-0823-1
8. **Justice and Health Care**
   1981, xiv + 238 pp. ISBN 90-277-1207-7
9. **The Law-Medicine Relation: A Philosophical Exploration**
   1981, xxx + 292 pp. ISBN 90-277-1217-4
10. **New Knowledge in the Biomedical Sciences**
    1982, xviii + 244 pp. ISBN 90-277-1319-7
11. **Beneficence and Health Care**
    1982, xvi + 264 pp. ISBN 90-277-1377-4